PUBLIC HEALTH SYSTEM
Vision, Mission and Action

This Study is an Outcome of
the Research and Development Programme
supported by NRDMS
Department of Science & Technology
Government of India, New Delhi

About the Author

Hridai R. Yadav obtained degree of M.Phil. and Ph.D. from Jawaharlal Nehru University, New Delhi, worked with CSIR, Government of India as Research Associate and Pool Scientist Officer for eight years. He had authored 15 Books and 73 Research Papers. Dr. Yadav successfully implemented 110 Action Research and Development Projects supported by the Government. He has been the Member of National Wastelands Development Board, Government of India and nominated as UGC observer to oversee the selection process from Reader to Professor in the Universities and UGC Nominated Member in the Board of Management of Autonomous Institute of Engineering and Technology (UPTU), Lucknow. Dr. Yadav is has been former Member of Board of Management, Bhoj (Open) University, Bhopal, Madhya Pradesh.

Dr. H.R. Yadav is presently working as the Visiting Professor & former OSD at Uttar Pradesh Technical University, Lucknow. Dr. Yadav has also been the Member of various Government and Autonomous Institutions/Universities besides being Founder Member-Secretary-Director of the Institute of Wastelands Reclamation and Rural Development (1990), Institute of Science and Technology for Rural Development (1994) and University Grants Commission Accredited and Grants-in-Aid supported RIWARD Post Graduate College, Hanumanganj, Sultanpur, U.P. (2004).

Presently, Dr. Yadav is engaged in the implementation of the Bachelor of Vocation (B.Voc.) in Food Processing and Public Health System and Rural Management-Entrepreneurship & Skill Development programmes as per the guidelines of the National Skill Qualification Framework.

PUBLIC HEALTH SYSTEM
Vision, Mission and Action

Volume III
Programmes, Progress and Management

Prof. (Dr.) Hridai R. Yadav

CONCEPT PUBLISHING COMPANY PVT. LTD.
NEW DELHI-110059

ISBN-13 : 978-93-5125-212-2 (Set)
ISBN-13 : 978-93-5125-213-9 (Vol. I)
ISBN-13 : 978-93-5125-214-6 (Vol. II)
ISBN-13 : 978-93-5125-215-3 (Vol. III)

First Published 2018

Published and Printed by

Concept
Since 1974

Concept Publishing Company Pvt. Ltd.
Regd. Office :
A/15-16, Commercial Block, Mohan Garden
New Delhi-110 059 (INDIA)
Phones : 011-25351460, 011-25351794
E-mail : publishing@conceptpub.com
Website : www.conceptpub.com

Cataloging in Publication Data—*Courtesy:* D.K. Agencies (P) Ltd. <docinfo@dkagencies.com>

Yadav, Hridai Ram, 1957- author.
Public health system : vision, mission and action / Prof. (Dr.) Hridai R. Yadav.
volumes cm
Includes bibliographical references and index.
Contents: volume I. Water contamination, water-borne diseases and public health status -- volume II. Policy, planning and implementation -- volume III. Programmes, progress and management.
ISBN 9789351252122 (set)
ISBN 9789351252139 (vol. I)
ISBN 9789351252146 (vol. II)
ISBN 9789351252153 (vol. III)

1. Drinking water--Contamination--India. 2. Water-borne infection--India. 3. Public health--India. 4. Medical policy--India. I. Title.

LCC RA529.Y33 2018 | DDC 362.10954 23

PREFACE

Water Pollution denotes the contamination of water or such alteration of the physical or biological properties of water which is harmful or injurious to the public health. The domestic sewage, poor sanitation, industrial effluents and surface run-off are the primary sources, that result in several water and sanitation related problems. Water pollution is a threat to bio-diversity self, thereby adversely impacting sustainable development. Polluted water transmits bacteria and parasites which causes various diseases including diarrhoea and typhoid.

Water-borne diseases are caused by pathogenic micro-organisms that most commonly are transmitted in the contaminated fresh water. The infection commonly results during bathing, washing, drinking, in the preparation of food, or the consumption of food thus infected. Various forms of water-borne diarrhoeal diseases probably are the most prominent example and affect mainly children. According to the World Health Organization such diseases account for an estimated 4.1 per cent of the total DALY global burden of disease and cause about 1.8 million human deaths per annum. It has been estimated by the World Health Organization that 88 per cent of that burden is attributable to unsafe water supply, hygiene and sanitation.

The water-borne diseases can have a significant impact on the economy, locally as well as internationally. The infected people by the water-borne diseases are usually confronted with related costs and not seldom with a huge financial burden. This is especially the case in the remote rural areas.

The financial losses are mostly caused by, e.g. costs for medical treatment and medication costs for transport, special food and by the loss of the human beings. Many families must even sell their land and property to pay for the treatment in a proper hospital. It has been noted that on average a family spends about 10 per cent of the monthly household's income per infected person.

Significant progress has been registered in improving life expectancy at birth reducing mortality due to malaria, as well as reducing infant and maternal mortality over the last few years. In spite of the progress made, a high proportion of the population especially surviving in the remote rural areas, continues to suffer and die from the preventive diseases, pregnancy and child birth related complications as well as malnutrition.

In addition to the old unresolved problems, the health system is facing emerging threats and challenges.

The rural public health care system in the many backward regions is in an unsatisfactory state leading to pauperization of poor households due to expensive private sector health care. We are in the midst of an epidemiological and demographic transition with the attendant problems of increased chronic disease burden and a decline in mortality and fertility rates leading to an ageing of the population.

Non-communicable diseases such as Cardio-vascular diseases, cancer, blindness, mental illness and tobacco use related illness have imposed the chronic diseases burden on the already overstretched health care system.

Premature morbidity and mortality from chronic diseases can be a major loss of economic and human resources. The large disparity across the rural areas, the burden of these conditions mostly on the poor and on women, scheduled castes especially those who live in the remote villages. The equity is also related in the skewed availability of public resources between the developed and less developed areas.

The public spending on the preventive health care services has a low priority over curative health. Indian Public spending on health is amongst the lowest in the world whereas the proportion of private spending on health is one of the highest.

The private sector health care is unregulated pushing the cost of health care up and making it unaffordable for the rural poor.

Thus, it is evident that maintaining the health system in its present form will become untenable. Persistant malnutrition, high levels of anaemia amongst children and low age of women marriage and at first child birth, inadequate safe drinking water round the year in many villages, overcrowding of dwelling units, unsatisfactory state of sanitation and disposal of wastes constitute major challenges for the public health system.

Most of these public determinants are correlated to high levels of poverty and to degradation of the environment in the villages. Thus, our government has to deal with multiple health crisis, rising costs of the health care and mounting expectations of the people. The challenge of the quality health services in the remote rural areas has to be met with a sense of urgency. Under the National Resources Data Management System Programmes of the Department of Science and Technology,

Government of India, a research project has been financially supported on "Planning of Potable Water using Geo-spatial Technology, in Sultanpur District." The outcome of the implemented Research and Development Project has been appropriately documented and published in the book form in three volumes —

Vol. I	Public Health System	(Water Contamination, Water-Borne Diseases and Public Health Status)
Vol. II	Public Health System	(Policy, Planning and Implementation)
Vol. III	Public Health System	(Programmes, Progress and Management)

Given the scope and magnitude of the problems, it is no longer enough to focus on narrowly defined programmes. The urgent need is to transform the public health system into an accountable, accessible and affordable system of the quality health services at the village level for the downtrodden deprived sections of the society.

Thus, an attempt has been made to analyse the Water Pollution, Water Contamination and Water-Borne Diseases and the Public Health Status.

The health policy, public health action planning, implementation framework, strengthening the health system and quality assurance of the delivery of the public health services at the facility level has been analysed at village panchayat level in Bhadainya Block of the District Sultanpur.

Effort has been made to analyse the Public Health Programme and the progress of the public health programme and public health management as per guidelines of the Indian Public Health Standards to ensure an appropriate delivery of the public health services at the facility level to fulfil the ever increasing requirements of the downtrodden deprived resourceless, vulnerable sections of the society surviving in the remote villages.

Prof. (Dr.) Hridai R. Yadav

ACKNOWLEDGEMENTS

Water Pollution/Water Contamination causes various Water-Borne Diseases especially the children, women and downtrodden section of the society which causes financial losses and loss of the human beings.

We are highly obliged and grateful to Dr. Bhoop Singh, Adviser and Head — NRDMS, Department of Science & Technology, Government of India, New Delhi for providing Techno-Scientific-Financial support for successful implementation of the project and publication of the book.

Sincere gratitudes are recorded to Dr. A.B. Singh, G.M., N.R.H.M., U.P., Lucknow and District Programme Manager, N.R.H.M., Sultanpur for providing needful data, information and reports related to the National Rural Health Mission at National and State Level and also for the District Sultanpur because this study is based on the available information/data from the National Rural Health Mission at National Level, State Level and District Level.

We are also grateful to the official of the District Water Testing Laboratory, Jal Nigam, Sultanpur and Incharge, Primary Health Centre, Bhadainya, Sultanpur for their needful support for providing the requisite information at village level.

Kamlesh Chandra Verma deserves special thanks for typing of the data manuscript.

Master of Social Work Students, Staff and Research Team of the RIWARD Post Graduate College, Hanumanganj, Sultanpur & Mr. D.K. Tewari and Mr. R.K. Mishra deserve sincere thanks.

Sincere gratitudes are acknowledged to Sri Ashok Kumar Mittal, Managing Director, Concept Publishing Company Pvt. Ltd., New Delhi for tne publication of this study.

Last, but not the least, I am grateful and indebted to **Baba Sultan Shah, Sharmad Shah Ji** and **Late Nafees Baba Ji** and my wife Reeta and lovely son Sahit Hridai, without whose support writing and completion of this study would not have been possible.

Prof. (Dr.) Hridai R. Yadav

CONTENTS

LIST OF TABLES

LIST OF FIGURES

LIST OF MAPS

ACRONYMS

AEFI Kits	Adverse Event Following Immunization
ART	Anti Retroviral Therapy
EMTS	Emergency Medical Transport System
FIMNCI	Family Integrated Management of Neo-Natal Child Illness
FLW	Field Level Worker
FWC Training	Family Welfare Centre
GNM	General Nurse Midwife
HBNC	Home Based New Borne Care
ICTC	Integrated Counseling and Testing Centre
IFA	Iron Folic Acid
IRS	Indoor Residual Spray
LT/RTI/STI Drugs	Lab Technician/Reproductive Tract Infection/ Sexual Transmitted Infections
MDA	Mass Drug Administration
MTP Act	Medical Termination of Pregnancy Act
MPW	Multi Purpose Workers
PPTCT	Prevention of Percent to Child Transmission
PC PNDT	Pre-Conception Pre-Natal Diagnostic Techniques
PPIUCD	Post-Partum Intra Uterine Conceptive Device
RMNCHA	Reproductive Maternal Neo-Natal Child Health and Adolescent
RPR Kits	Rapid Plasma Region Kits
IUD	Intra Uterine Device
UNFA	United Nations Funding Agency
USAID	United States Agency for International Development
SIFPSA	State Innovations in Family Planning Service
VDRL	Venereal Disease Research Laboratory Test

ABBREVIATIONS

AMC	Annual Maintenance Contract
ANM	Auxiliary Nurse Midwife
ANC	Ante-natal Care
APH	Ante-partum Hemorrhage
ASHA	Accredited Social Health Activist
AWW	Anganwadi Worker
Be/MOC	Basic Emergency Obstetric Care
BA	Birth Asphyxia
BCC	Behaviour Change Communication
BCG	Bacillus Calmette-Guerin
BP	Blood Pressure
CEmOBC	Comprehensive Emergency Obstetrics and New Born Care
CFL	Compact Fluorescent Light
CHC	Community Health Centre
CME	Continual Medical Education
CSF	Cerebrospinal Fluid
DL	Deciliter
ECG	Electrocardiography
EBM	Expressed Breast Milk
EDD	Expected Date of Delivery
ELBW	Extremely Low Birth Weight
EmOC	Emergency Obstetric Care
F-IMNCI	Facility based Integrated Management of Neonatal and Childhood Illnesses
FRU	First Referral Unit
GIR	Glucose Infusion Rate
GoI	Government of India
HBNC	Home-Based New Corner Care
HEPB	Hepatitis B
HIE	Hypoxic-Ischeic Encephalopathy
HIV	Human Immunodeficiency Virus
HR	Heart Rate

IAP	Indian Academy of Paediatric
IMNCI	Integrated Management of Neonatal and Childhood Illness
IMR	Infant Mortality Rate
IANN	Indian Association of Neonatal Nursing
IV	Intravenous
IVF	Intravenous Feeding
IUCD	Intrauterine Contraceptive Device
IDU	Intrauterine Device
LHV	Lady Health Visitor
JSY	Janani Suraksha Yojana
KCL	Potassium Chloride
KG	Kilogram
LBW	Low Birth Weight
LMP	Last Menstrual Period
MAS	Meconium Aspiration Syndrome
MCH	Maternal and Child Health
MDG	Millennium Development Goals
ML	Millilitre
MoHFW	Ministry of Health and Family Welfare
MO	Medical Officer
MTP	Medical Termination of Pregnancy
MVA	Manual Vacuum Aspiration
NBCC	New Born Care Corner
NBSU	New Born Stabilization Unit
NGO	Non-Governmental Organization
NHSRC	National Health System Resource Centre
NIBP	Non-Invasive Blood Pressure
NMR	National Mortality Rate
NNF	National Neonatology Forum
NRHM	National Rural Health Mission
NS	Normal Saline
NSV	Non-Scalpel Vasectomy
NSSK	Navjaat Shishu Suraksha Karyakram
OPV	Oral Polio Vaccine
OT	Operation Theatre
PHC	Primary Health Centre
PIH	Pregnancy Induced Hypertension
PIP	Project Implementation Plan
PPH	Post-Partum Haemorrhage

PRI	Panchayati Raj Institution
PROM	Premature Rupture of Membrane
RCH II	Reproductive Child Health Programme-II
RDS	Respiratory Distress Syndrome
RL	Ringer's Lactate
RR	Respiratory Rate
RTI	Reproductive Tract Infection
SC	Scheduled Caste
SHG	Self-Help Group
SHRC	State Health System Resource Centre
SIHFW	State Institute of Health and Family Welfare
SNCU	Special New Born Care Unit
SPO2	Spot Oxygen Saturation
SRS	Sample Registration System
STI	Sexually Transmitted Infection
TSB	Total Serum Bilirubin
U5MR	Under-5 Mortality Rate
UNICEF	United Nations Children's Fund
USAID	United States Assistance to International Development
VHND	Village Health and Nutrition Day
VHSC	Village Health and Sanitation Committee
VLBW	Very Low Birth Weight
WHO	World Health Organization

1

INTRODUCTION

1. Introduction

A significant progress has been registered in improving the life expectancy birth, reducing the mortality due to Malaria, as well as reducing infant and maternal mortality over the last few decades in India. In spite of the progress made, a high proportion of the population especially the remote villages continues to suffer and die from preventable disease, pregnancy and child birth related complications as well as malnutrition.

In addition to old unresolved problems, the health systems in our country is facing emerging threats and challenges. The rural public health care system in many states and regions is in an unsatisfactory state leading to pauperization of poor households due to excessive extensive private sector health care.

Our country is in the midst of an epidemiological and demographic transition with the attendant problems of increased chronic disease burden and a decline in the mortality and fertility rates leading to an ageing of the population.

An estimated 5 million people in our country are surviving with HIV/AIDS, a threat which has the potential to undermine the health and development gains, India has made since its independence.

Non-communicable diseases such as Cardio-Vascular disease, cancer, blindness, mental, tobacco use related illness and Japanese Encephalitis and Swine Flue and Dengue Fever have imposed the Chronic Disease burden on already overstretched health care system in Uttar Pradesh.

Pre-mature morbidity and mortality from chronic diseases have been a major loss of economic and human resources. The large disparity across different places the burden of these situations affects mostly on the poor and women, scheduled caste and scheduled tribes especially those who are living in the remote villages. The equity has also been reflected in the skewed availability of public resources between the advanced and less developed villages.

It has been noticed that the public spending on preventive public health services has a low priority over the curative health as a whole. The Indian Public spending on health is amongst the lowest in the world, whereas its proportion of private spending on the health is on the highest.

It has been estimated that more than ₹ 1,00,000 crore are being spent annually as household expenditure on health care has been more than three times of the Public expenditure on health. The private sector health care is unrequalated pushing the cost of health care up and making it unaffordable for the deprived rural poor multitudes.

Thus, it is evident from the fact that maintaining the health system in its present form will become untenable. The persistent malnutrition, high levels of anaemia amongst children and women, low age of marriage and first child birth, inadequate safe drinking water round the year in many villages, overcrowding of dwelling units, unsatisfactory state of sanitation and disposal of waste constitute major challenges for the public health system in Uttar Pradesh.

Thus, most of the public health determinants are correlated to high levels of poverty and to degradation of the environment of the villages. It has been noted that State of Uttar Pradesh has to deal with multiple health crises, rising costs of health care and mounting expectations of the people.

The challenges of quality health services in the remote backward villages has to be met with a sense of urgency. In view of the given scope and magnitude of the problem, it is no longer enough to focus on narrowly defined programmes. Thus, urgent need is to transform the public health system into an accountable, accessible and affordable system of quality health services at the facility level.

It has been visioned to provide effective health care to the people living in the remote villages which have weak public health indicators and weak health infrastructure. It has also been visioned to raise public spending on health from 0.9 per cent of GDP to 2.3 per cent of GDP with the improved arrangements for community financing.

It has been visioned to undertake the architectural corrections of the public health system to enable it to effectively handle increased allocation and promote health policies that strengthen the public health management and proper delivery of public health services and to revitalize local health traditions and mainstream AYUSH into the Public Health System.

It has also been visioned to ensure effective integration of health concerns through decentralized management of District, Block and Village level with the *determinants of health like sanitation, hygiene, nutrition, safe drinking water, gender and social concerns.*

Lastly, it has been visioned to ensure an improved access to village people especially poor women and children to *equitable, affordable, accountable and effective* care of primary health services at the facility level.

2. Public Health Views

It has been strategically viewed to bringing about a dramatic improvement in the health system and health status of the people especially those who are surviving in the remote backward villages. It has also been viewed to provide universal access to equitable, affordable and quality health care which is accountable, at the same time responsive to the requirements of the village people, reduction of child and maternal deaths as well as stabilization of population, gender and demographic balance.

It has also been viewed strategically to facilitate increased access and utilization of quality health services to the needy and interested patients and forge a partnership between the Central, State and Local Governments including Panchayati Raj Institutions.

It has been viewed to set-up a platform for involving Panchayati Raj Institutions and Community in the management of Primary Health Programme and infrastructures at the facilities level.

It has been planned to provide an opportunity for promoting equity and social justice and to establish a mechanism to provide flexibility to the states and the community to promote local initiatives. Lastly, it has been viewed strategically to develop a framework for promoting inter-sectoral convergence for ensuring *promotive, preventive and curative Primary Health care* at the facility level.

3. Objectives of the Public Health Programme

Important objectives of the Public Health Programme are as follows:

- To ensure reduction in child and maternal mortality.
- To provide universal access of public health services for food and nutrition, sanitation and hygiene and universal access to public health care services with the emphasis on services addressing women's and children's health and universal immunization.

- To ensure prevention and control of communicable and non-communicable diseases including locally endemic diseases.
- To ensure access to integrated comprehensive care of Primary Health services at facility level.
- To ensure population stabilization, gender and demographic balance at the village level.
- To ensure revitalization of local health traditions and mainstream AYUSH health system.
- To ensure promotion of healthy lifestyles of the village people.

4. Expectations from Public Health System

It is being expected that the outcomes from the Primary Health System will be helpful in reducing the Infant Mortality Rate to 30/1,000 live births by 2012 and Maternal Mortality reduction to 100/1,00,000 live births by 2012 and reduction in Total Fertility Rate 50 per cent up to 2010 additional 10 per cent by 2012.

It has also been expected that the outcomes of the public health system will be helpful in reducing Kala-Azar Mortality Rate — 100 per cent by 2012 and substantial elimination until 2012 and Filaria/Micro Filaria Reduction Rate — 70 per cent by 2010, 80 per cent by 2012 and elimination by 2015. Dengue Mortality Reduction Rate — 50 per cent by 2010 and sustaining at that level until 2012.

The cataract operations increasing to 46 lakh until 2012 and Leprosy Prevalence Rate reduction from 1.8 per 10,000 in 2005 to less that 1 per 10,000 thereafter. The tuberculosis DOTS series — maintain 85 per cent cure rate through entire period and also sustain planned cases detection rate.

It has also been expected that the outcomes of the Public Health System will be helpful in upgrading all Community Health Centres to the norms of the Indian Public Health Standards and to increase an appropriate utilization of First Referral Units from bed occupancy by referred cases of less than 20 per cent to over 75 per cent and to ensure deployment of 4,00,000 female Accredited Social Health Activists (ASHAs) at the facility level.

The expected outcomes of the Public Health System at the Community level is to ensure availability of trained community level workers at village level with a drug kit for generic ailments and organize Health Day at Anganwadi level at a fixed day/month for provision of immunization, Ante/Post Natal check-ups and services related to mother and child health care including nutritional care.

To ensure availability of generic drugs for common ailments at sub-centre and at the hospital level and to provide access to good hospital care through assured availability of Doctors, drugs and quality services at Primary Health Centres/Community Health Centres level and assured referral transport communication to reach these facilities in time.

To ensure improved access to universal immunization services under the programme.

To provide improved facilities for institutional deliveries through provisions of referral transport, escort and improved hospital care subsidized under the Janani Suraksha Yojana for the Below Poverty Line families.

To provide availability of assured health care at reduced financial risk through pilots of Community Health Insurance and also ensure availability of safe drinking water and provision of household toilets.

To provide improved outreach services to the medically underserved remote areas through Mobile Medical Units and increase awareness about preventive health including nutrition, etc.

5. Strategies of Public Health System

The core strategies of the Public Health System includes training and enhance capacity of Panchayati Raj Institutions to own, control and manage Public Health Services at the facility level and also to promote an access to improved health care at household level through the female Health activities, i.e. Accredited Social Health Activists.

To ensure health plan for each village through the village health Committee of the Village Panchayat and to strengthen sub-health centres through better human resource development, clear quality standards, better communication support and untied funds to enable local planning and action and more multi-purpose workers at village level.

The core strategies also include the strengthening of the existing Primary Health Centres through better staffing and human resource development policy, clear quality standards, better community support and untied funds to enable the local management committee to achieve the norms of the Indian Public Health Standards.

It has been strategically planned to ensure the provision of 30-50 bedded Community Health Centres per lakh population for improved curative care to a normative standards of Indian Public Health Standards defining personnel equipments and management standards, its decentralized administration by a hospital management committee and the provision of adequate funds and powers to enable these committees to reach desired levels of the Public Health System at the facilities level.

The core strategies of the Public Health System has been to ensure formulation and implementation of an inter-sectoral District Health Action Plan, Block Health Action Plan and Village Health Action Plan formulated by the District Health Society, Block Health Society and Village Panchayats Health Society respectively including drinking water, sanitation, hygiene and nutrition.

To ensure vertical integration of health and family welfare programme and technical support to the Public Health Management at the facility level and strengthening capacities for data collection, assessment and review for evidence based planning, monitoring and supervision.

The strategies of the Public Health System has been to strengthen capacities for data collection, assessment and review for evidence based planning, monitoring and supervision and to formulate the transparent policies for deployment and career development at the facility level.

It has also been strategically planned to develop capacities for preventive health care at all levels for promoting healthy lifestyles, reducing in consumption of tobacco, alcohol, etc. and also promoting non-profit sector particularly underserved or unserved backward remote villages.

An additional strategy of the Public Health System has been to ensure regulation for Private Sector including the informal Rural Medical Practitioners to ensure availability of quality services to the people at the reasonable cost and to ensure promotion of Public-Private-Partnership for achieving the goals of the Public Health System.

The supplementary strategies of the Public Health System has been to mainstreaming the AYUSH through revitalizing the local health traditions at the facility level and to reorient medical education to support Public Health issues including regulation of medical care and medical ethics.

The additional strategies of the Public Health System has been to ensure effective and visible risk pooling and social health insurance to provide health security to the poor by ensuring accessible, affordable accountable and good quality hospital care as per needs of the people.

6. Public Health Initiatives

An emphasis of the Public Health System has been on the preparatory activities necessary for laying the groundwork for implementation of the Public Health Services at the facility level.

6.1. *Institutional Framework*

Institutional framework for the Public Health System is as follows:

- To set-up State Health Mission, District Health Mission, Block Health Mission and Village Panchayat Health Mission.
- Institutional framework includes Mission Steering Groups, Empowered Programme Committees at various levels have been put in place.
- State launch of Health Mission has been organized in Uttar Pradesh in which apart from the State level functionaries Chairman, Zila Panchayat, District Collectors and Civil Surgeons of the District Hospitals have been involved. State launches have been doubled up as orientation workshop for the District Level functionaries.
- Mission document guidelines on Indian Public Health Standards, Guidelines for Accredited Social Health Activists, Training Modules for ASHAs, guidelines for State Health Mission, District Health Mission, merger of societies have been shared with the competent authorities.
- Memorandum of Understanding has been signed with the States. Memorandum of Understanding clearly spells out the reform commitments of the State in terms of their enhanced public spending in health, full staffing of management structure, steps for the decentralization and promotion of district level planning and implementation of various activities, achievement of milestones under the leadership of the Panchayati Raj Institutions.
- Task Groups have been fornulated to ensure the goals of the Health Mission — Strengthening of Public Health System Infrastructure, Role of Panchayati Raj Institutions, Accredited Social Health Activists and Technical Support Activities have been completed.
- Task groups on health financing, district planning and Public Private-Partnership are in the process of finalizing their recommendation.

6.2. *Public Health Programmes*

- Reproductive and Child Health Programme-II and Janani Suraksha Yojana have been launched.
- Polio Eradication Programme intensified cases reduced from 134 in 2004-05 to 63 up to now.

- Sterilization compensation scheme has been launched.
- Accelerated implementation of the Routine Immunization Programme has been taken up.
- Groundwork for introduction of Japanese Encephalitis vaccine has been completed.
- Groundwork for Hepatitis Vaccine has also been completed.
- Auto Disabled Syringes have also been introduced.
- State Programme for Implementation of Plans for the Reproductive and Child Health-II, have been appraised by the National Coordination Committee, have been set-up by the government. Funds to the extent of 254.15 per cent, i.e. ₹ 1,811.74 crore have been released under the National Rural Health Mission Outlay.

6.3. *Public Health Infrastructure*

- Facility Survey has been introduced.
- Repair and renovation of Sub-Health Centres under Reproductive and Child Health-II.
- Untied funds of ₹ 10,000 to Sub-Health Centre.
- Selection of 2 Community Health Centres for upgradation as per norms of the Indian Public Health Standards.
- Upgradation of Community Health Centres as First Referral Unit and Primary Health Centres to 24 × 7 units have been taken up.
- Release of funds for upgradation of the Community Health Centres as per guidelines of Indian Public Health Standards.

6.4. *Public Health Planning*

Public Health Planning has been ensured as per the following details:

- Strengthening of planning process in 50 per cent of the districts.
- Selection of Accredited Social Health Activists completed.
- Training of Trainers for Accredited Social Health Activists completed.
- An Empowered Procurement Wing is being set-up in the Government.
- Procurement procedures are being finalized and procedural assistance are being provided for the procurement of equipments, drugs, etc.

6.5. *Technical Support*

- A National Health System Resource Centre has been set-up at the National Level and Planned to set-up State Health System Resource Centre.
- Seven Hundred consultants appointed at the district level programme management units.
- Training Programme has been started for the skilled Birth Attendants.

6.6. *Public Health Priorities*

An unique opportunity for carrying out necessary reforms in the health sector has been prioritized at the facility level. The reforms are necessary for restructuring the health delivery system as well as for delivering better health financial mechanisms. The institutions like Sub-Health Centre/Tehsils/District Hospitals have positive consequences for health programmes, i.e. Tuberculosis, Malaria, HIV/AIDS, Filaria and Family Planning and Welfare, Leprosy, Disease Surveillance, etc. as all programmes are based on the assumption that a functioning of Public Health System actually exists at the facility level.

The submission of Task Group Reports and the recently published reports of the Commission on Micro-Economics and Health and Mid-Term Appraisal by the Planning Commission provides valuable insights on these critical issues. In order to provide health outcomes, it is necessary to give close attention to critical areas like service delivery, finances including risk pooling resources human, physical knowledge, technologies and the leadership at the grossroots level.

The following are identified as some of the critical priority areas for concerted action:

- Well functioning health facilities.
- Quality and accountability in the delivery of health services.
- Taking care of the needs of the poor and vulnerable sections of the society and their empowerment.
- Prepare for health transition with appropriate health financing.
- Pro-people public-private-partnership.
- Convergence for effectiveness and efficiency.
- Response Health System meeting people's health requirements.

7. Implementation of Public Health Programme

National Rural Health Mission seeks to provide accessible, affordable and quality health care to the rural people especially the vulnerable sections of the society. It also seeks to reduce Maternal Mortality Ratio from 407 to 100 per 1,00,000 live births, Infant Mortality Ratio from 60 to 30 per 1,000 live births and the Total Fertility Rate from 3.0 to 3.1 within the seven-year period of the Mission.

The key features in order to achieve the goals of the Mission include making the Public Health Delivery System fully functional and accountable to the community, human resources management, decentralization, rigorous monitoring and evaluation against standards, convergence of health and related programmes from village level upwards, innovations and flexible financing and also interventions for improving the health indicators at various levels.

Given the status of the Public Health Infrastructure, it will not be possible to provide the desired services till the infrastructure is sufficiently upgraded. The Mission seeks to establish health facilities in the public domain through revitalization of the existing infrastructure and fresh construction or renovation wherever required. The Mission also seeks to improve health services delivery by putting in place enabling system at all levels. It involves simultaneous correction in the manpower planning as well as infrastructure strengthening. The Mission would provide priority to both of these aspects at the facility level.

7.1. *Public Health Infrastructure*

Government of India has so far supported only the construction/ upgradation of sub-Health Centre due to their difficult financial conditions because the states have usually not provided sufficient funds for construction/upgradation of Primary Health Centres, Community Health Centres, District Hospitals. As a result health infrastructure is in poor conditions in Uttar Pradesh.

National Rural Health Mission allows the expenditure for construction subject to the conditions that it would not be more than 33 per cent of the total National Rural Health Mission Outlay in the case of high focus areas and 25 per cent in the case of Non-High Focus area. National Rural Health Mission also provides support for upgradation of District Hospitals.

Having Rogi Kalyan Samiti for managing health facilities has already been approved by the Government of India. The funds are released as untied funds to the Rogi Kalyan Samitis as 100 per cent grant.

The National Rural Health Mission also seeks to improve outreach activities in unserved and underserved areas especially inhabited by vulnerable sections of the society through provision of Mobile Medical Units covering all Anganwadi Centres. It also seeks to ensure the availability of requisite equipments and drugs at all public care facilities. Procurement of equipments/drugs would be progressively decentralized at the facility level.

7.2. *Manpower Availability*

The issue of availability of critical manpower in the villages is to be addressed through initiatives like introduction of trained voluntary Community Health Workers (ASHA) in every village and additional Auxiliary Nurse Midwife at each Sub-Health Centre, three staff nurses at the Primary Health Centres to make them operational round the clock and additional specialists and para-medical staff at the Community Health Centres. The conditions of local residency has been proposed to ensure that the staff stay posting of doctors in the rural area, better cadre in management and personnel policies would also help to improve the availability of manpower at the facilities level.

In order to provide managerial support for taking funds and monitoring activities, a provision has been made to set-up Programme Management Units at various levels in which over 500 Professionals have already been recruited.

The successful implementation of the Mission would require health sector reforms and human resources development. Capacity-building at all levels is a huge challenge, hence, it is proposed to set-up National Health System Resource Centre at the State level. It also emphasizes the setting up fully functional Block and District Level Health Management Systems, as under National Rural Health Mission 70 per cent of the resource would be utilized at Block level and below Block level and 20 per cent at the District level.

In view of the given large army of Accredited Social Health Activists, Auxiliary Nurse Midwife and Rural Medical Practitioner requires continuous skill development. Strengthening Nursing Institution, linking with medical colleges for providing skill development support to rural health workers, involving the voluntary sector in skill development are few key interventions to be taken up at the facility level.

To make the health facilities more accountable, the health sector control would be gradually shifted to the Panchayati Raj Institutions and civil society. The sub-centres are proposed to be placed exclusively under the control of Panchayat Samitis and Rogi Kalyan Samitis.

As per approval of the Government one female Accredited Social Health Activist is to be provided for every village with 1,000 population. ASHA would be the link between the community and the health facility and ASHA would be the first Port of Call for any health related demand.

ASHA along with the Anganwadi Workers and Auxiliary Nurse Midwife, Self Help Groups and Community based organization, *Preraks* of continuing education centres through their coordinated action at the Village Level and through combined organization of monthly Village Health Nutrition and Sanitation Day at the Anganwadi Centres would be expected to bring about perceptible changes in the health status of the community.

The Panchayati Raj Institutions and a large range of community based organizations like self-help groups, school, water, Health Nutrition and Sanitation Committee, Mahila Samakhya Groups, Zila Saksharata Samiti provide an opportunity for seeking local levels accountability in the delivery of social sector programmes. Schools and Anganwadi would form the base of these activities. National Rural Health Mission provides for School Health check-ups and School Health Education, to be worked out in consultation with the State Government of Uttar Pradesh. Convergence of programmes would be at the village level and facility level.

7.3. *Decentralization of Public Health Programme*

The indicators of the health depend as much on drinking water, nutrition, sanitation, female literacy, women's empowerment as they do on functional health facilities. National Rural Health Mission seeks to adopt a convergent approach for interventions under the Umbrella of the District Plan which seeks to integrate all the related initiatives at the Village → Block → District levels.

The District Health Plan would be the main instrument for planning, Inter-sectoral convergence, implementation and monitoring of the activities under the Mission. Rather than funds being allocated to the States for implementing programmes and State would be encouraged to prepare their perfective and annual plan which in turn would be based on the District Health Plan.

Even though village is envisaged as the Primary Unit for planning, looking at the extensive capacity building required before it would be in a position to take up the exercise, the Mission would not insist on the village plans at least during the first two years. The District Health Mission under the Zila Panchayat would get the District plan prepared covering health as well as the other determinants of health. Household and facility surveys would define the baseline. Periodic surveys would thereafter be taken up on an annual basis to track the improvements in the facilities as well as in the reduction in the health indicators.

District Health Plans would be collated into State Plan which would be appraised and approved by the Mission at National Level. As far as other determinants of health are concerned, the funds for them would continue to flow through the existing channels but the District Plan would clearly bring out the convergent action being taken at the District Level Plan. National Rural Health Mission recognizes that delegation of financial powers and administrative powers at various levels would be necessary for the successful implementation of the decentralized health action planning at the facility level.

7.4. *Mainstreaming of AYUSH*

Provision has been made for State specific proposals for Mainstreaming AYUSH, including appointment of AYUSH Doctors/paramedics on contractual basis, providing AYUSH wings in Primary Health Centres and Community Health Centres. As envisaged under National Rural Health Mission vision and goals, efforts will be made to integrate AYUSH system of medicines in Primary Health Delivery Services.

The District Health Action Plans would be prepared based on normative framework. The cost norms have been derived from three sources —

- **Firstly,** existing norms of the schemes brought under the umbrella of National Rural Health Mission.
- **Secondly,** norms developed by the National Council of Medical Health.
- **Thirdly,** norms developed and approved as new interventions under National Rural Health Mission.

7.5. *Accountability Framework Programme*

The National Rural Health Mission framework is based on a right based approach. The framework proposes accountability at every level through a three pronged processes of community based monitoring external surveys, household surveys by Accredited Social Health Activists, facility surveys and stringent internal monitoring.

The process of community involvement of the health institutions itself would enhance accountability and the National Rural Health Mission would facilitate this process by wide dissemination of the results. For effective monitoring a strong Management Information System is being put in place.

The citizen charter would help the public to know their rights and entitlements at each facility. The setting-up of Indian Public Health Standards at each level of health delivery system would be instrumental in provision of minimum service guarantees at those levels. Monitoring would also in terms of service guarantees providing by each facility, utilization of such services by the community especially the weaker sections changes in their health seeking behaviour, etc. The facilities survey is expected to create a baseline for each health facilities and assist in monitoring annual progress against the baseline in terms of services guaranteed. Independent evaluation would ensure midcourse corrections at the facility level.

7.6. *Pro-People Partnership in Public Health System*

The investments by Non-governmental organizations are critical for the success of National Rural Health Mission. The Mission provides for partnerships with the voluntary groups/organizations for advocacy, building capacity at all facility levels, monitoring and evaluation of health sectors, delivery of health services and working together with community organization.

It has been proposed to provide people friendly regulatory framework that promotes ethical practices through accreditation, standard treatment protocols and training and upgradation of skills of Non-government Health Providers. Thus, 5 per cent of the total National Rural Health Mission outlay is proposed to be the resource allocation to voluntary organizations on the basis of approved guidelines and norms of the Indian Public Health Standards.

7.7. *Reducing Mortality Rate and Disease Burden*

Reproductive and Child Health Programme (RCH-II) was launched in 2005 as a part of the Mission as the principal vehicle for reducing Infant Mortality Rate, Maternal Mortality Rate and Total Fertility Rate, upgradation of Community Health Centres as First Referral Units for dealing with Emergency obstetric care 24 × 7 delivery services at the Primary Health Centres operationalizing of the Sub-Health Centres multiskilling of doctors contractual appointment of medical officers in Anesthetic skills, training Doctors/ANMs/Nurses as Skilled Birth Attendants, permitting ANMs to administer certain drugs in emergency, partnerships with voluntary organization, IEC Activities are the major interventions in reducing Maternal Mortality Rate.

For reducing Neo-Natal Mortality programmes for Integrated Management of Childhood Illness is being extended at the community can facility levels, Activities of ASHAs, Anganwadi workers, ANMs, *Preraks* of Continuing Education Centres and Self-Help Groups at the village level with focus on both preventive and promotive aspects of health care accelerated immunization programme, advocacy on age of marriage/against sex selection, spacing of births, institutional delivery, breast feeding, meeting, unmet demands for contraception, besides providing a range of Reproductive and Child Health Services are to have impact on reducing the health indicators.

Efforts are being made to integrate HIV/AIDS programmes with Reproductive and Child Health at the facility levels, Convergence of disease control programme, integration of services, combined awareness generation, education and the advocacy at Community and Facility levels, taking care of the preventive, promotive and curative health care are expected to bring down Infant Mortality Rate/Maternal Mortality Rate/Total Fertility Rate and reduce the burden of disease.

National Rural Health Mission recognizes that in order to reduce the out of pocket expenditure of the rural poor, there is an imperative need for setting up effective risk pooling systems as already envisaged. State specific community oriented innovations and flexible insurance policies needs to be developed and disseminated. While the first priority of the Mission is to put the enabling public health infrastructure in place, various innovative models would be pilot tested to assess their utility at the facility level.

7.8. *Public Health Manual*

Public Health Manual is intended to be a user friendly tool to assist range of stakeholders to be engaged in the District Health Action Planning. The intended target group includes the following:

- Members of State and the District Health Mission.
- District and Block Level Programme Managers of line Departments, i.e. Health and Family Welfare, AYUSH women and Child Development including ICDS and Sanitation and Water related Departments.

- State Programme Management Unit and District Programme Management Unit Staff.
- Members of Panchayati Raj Institutions, Non-governmental organizations and Civil Society Groups.

Besides above referred groups this work will also be found useful by Public Health System managers, academicians, faculty from training institutes and people engaged in programme implementation and monitoring and evaluation.

This study needs to be used in conjunction with many other documents. It is highly recommended that the planning team entrusted with the task of developing the plan have access to all the documents as the head of the commencement of planning processes and familiarize themselves with the contents of this study.

8. Public Health Delivery System

The Community Health Centres (CHCs) constitute the secondary level of health care, were designed to provide referral as well as specialist health care to the rural population. Indian Public Health Standards (IPHS) for CHCs have been prescribed under National Rural Health Mission (NRHM) to provide optimal specialized care to the community and achieve and maintain an acceptable standard of quality of care. As setting standards is a dynamic process, the need was felt to update the IPHS keeping in view the changing protocols of existing National Health Programmes, development of new programmes especially for non-communicable diseases and prevailing epidemiological situation in the country and different States of the country; accordingly the revision has been carried out. These standards would act as benchmarks and help monitor and improve the functioning of the Community Health Centres.

8.1. *Public Health Services*

- Unlike Sub-centre and PHCs, CHCs have been envisaged as only one type and will act both as Block level health administrative unit and gatekeeper for referrals to higher level of facilities.
- The revised IPHS (CHC) has considered the services, infrastructure, manpower, equipment and drugs in two categories of Essential (minimum assured services) and Desirable (the ideal level services which the states and UT shall try to achieve).

- All essential services as envisaged in the CHC should be made available, which includes routine and emergency care in Surgery Medicine, Obstetrics and Gynaecology, Paediatrics, Dental and AYUSH in addition to all the National Health Programmes.
- Standards of services under existing programmes were updated and standards added for newly developed non-communicable disease programmes based on the inputs from various programme divisions. Standards for Newborn stabilization unit, MTP facilities for second trimester pregnancy (desirable), The Integrated Counselling and Testing Centre (ICTC), Blood storage and link Anti-Retroviral Therapy Centre have been added.

8.2. *Minimum Requirements for Delivery of Health Services*

The following requirements are being projected based on the assumption that there will be average bed occupancy of 60 per cent. The strength may be further increased if the occupancy increases with subsequent upgradation. With regard to Manpower, 2 specialists, namely, Anesthetist and Public Health Specialist will be provided in addition to the available specialists, namely Surgery, Medicine, Obstetrics and Gynaecology and Paediatrics.

A Block Public Health Unit is envisaged at the CHC having a Block Medical Officer/Medical Superintendent, one Public Health specialist and at least one Public Health Nurse. The support manpower will include a Dental Assistant, Multi-Rehabilitation Worker, Cold Chain and Vaccine Logistic Assistant in addition to the existing staff. The manpower at CHC has been rationalized in order to ensure optimal utilization of scarce manpower

8.3. *Public Health Facilities*

The lists of equipment and essential drugs have been updated; the drug list for obstetric care and sick newborn and child care [for First Referral Unit (FRU)/CHC] has been incorporated.

Physical Infrastructure will be remodelled or rearranged to make best possible use for optimal utilization as per given guidelines in the relevant section.

8.4. *Public Health Accountability*

It is mandatory for every CHC to have functional "Rogi Kalyan Samiti" (RKS) to ensure accountability and also shall have the Charter of Patients'

Rights displayed prominently at the entrance. A grievance redressal mechanism under the overall supervision of RKS would also be set-up.

Standard Operating Procedures and Standard Treatment Protocols for common ailments and the National Health Programmes should be available and followed. To maintain quality of services, external monitoring through Panchayati Raj Institutions and internal monitoring at appropriate intervals is advocated. Guidelines are being provided for management of routine and emergency cases under the National Health Programmes so as to maintain uniformity in Management in tune with the National Health Policy.

9. Public Health Management

The Community Health Centres (CHCs) which constitute the secondary level of health care were designed to provide referral as well as specialist health care to the rural population. These centres are, however, fulfilling the tasks entrusted to them only to a limited extent. The launch of the National Rural Health Mission (NRHM) gives us the opportunity to have a fresh look at their functioning.

In order to provide Quality Care in the CHCs Indian Public Health Standards (IPHS) are being prescribed to provide optimal expert care to the community and achieve and maintain an acceptable standard of quality care. These standards would help, monitor and improve the functioning of the CHCs.

Service Delivery

- All "Assured Services" as envisaged in the CHCs should be available, which includes routine and emergency care in Surgery, Medicine, Obstetrics and Gynaecology and Paediatrics in addition to all the National Health Programmes.
- Appropriate Guidelines for each National Health Programme for management of routine and emergency cases are being provided to the CHCs.
- All the support services to fulfil the above objectives will be strengthened at the CHC level.

10. Minimum Requirement for Health Delivery

The requirements are being projected based on an average bed occupancy of 60 per cent. It would be a dynamic process in the sense that if the utilization goes up, the standards would be further upgraded. As regards manpower, 2 specialists, namely Anesthetist and Public Health Programme Manager will be provided on contractual basis in addition to the available specialists, namely Surgery, Medicine, Obstetrics and Gynaecology and Paediatrics.

The support manpower will include a Public Health Nurse and ANM in addition to the existing staff. An Ophthalmic Assistant will also be needed to be provided in centres where currently there is none.

It is mandatory for every CHC to have "Rogi Kalyan Samiti" to ensure accountability. Every CHC should have the Charter of Patients' Rights displayed prominently at the entrance. A grievance mechanism under the overall supervision of Rogi Kalyan Samitis should be set-up at the facility level. Every CHC shall also have the Standard Operating Procedures and Standard Treatment Protocols for common ailments and the National Health Programmes. Social audit by involvement of the community through Consumer Forum and Rogi Kalyan Samitis is being recommended. To maintain quality of services, external monitoring through Panchayati Raj Institutions and internal monitoring at appropriate intervals will be advocated. Guidelines are being provided for management of routine and emergency cases under the National Health Programme so as to maintain uniformity in management in tune with the National Policy.

11. Choice of the Time Period

The choice of the time period is very much a matter of convenience, as the analysis is based on field observations, filedwork and field survey. Time period for the study has been 2012-13 as the base year for this study for the observation of the temporal variations for the dependent and independent variables. The fieldwork, field observations and field survey has been completed for the recent years to analyze the problems of the year 2013-14 to the critical condition of the Water Contamination causing the water-borne diseases and impact of various rural health services at the grassroots level, i.e. village panchayat level in Bhadainya Block of District Sultanpur, Uttar Pradesh.

12. State Profile

(i) *Geography*

State of Uttar Pradesh is bounded by Nepal on the North, Uttrakhand on the north-west, Haryana on the west, Rajasthan on the south-west,

Madhya Pradesh on the south and south-west and Bihar on the east; Uttar Pradesh is situated between 23°52' N and 31°28' N latitudes and 77°3' E and 84°39' E longitudes. Uttar Pradesh is the fourth largest state in the country. Uttar Pradesh can be divided into three distinct physiographic regions:

(a) Himalayan Region in the north.
(b) Gangetic Plain in the centre.
(c) Vindhyan Hills and Plateau in the south.

(ii) *History*

Major area of the Northern plain or Indo-Gangetic Plain are fertile. This area was occupied by the groups of the referred to as "Dasas" by the Aryans. Agriculture was main occupation of the habitants. Till B.C. 200 the Aryans had not settled in this region. Aryans occupied this area and laid down foundation of the Hindu Civilization. The great war of Mahabharat was said to have been fought here. Besides the *Kauravas* and *Pandavas*, the Kosis, Hosalas, etc. formed the early region of Uttar Pradesh. These areas were called Madhyadesa. During the Aryan's inhabitation of the epics of *Mahabharata*, *Ramayana*, the *Brahamanas* and *Puranas* were written. During the period of Ashoka, works related to public were taken up. There was active trade within and outside the country due to rich sources. The rule of the Magadh empire continued due to rich natural resources. The role of Magadh empire brought Buddhism and Jainism into this region. Administrative and economic advances had been witnessed during this period.

The Kushans exercised their power over this region till 320 AD. The territory passed into the hands of the Guptas during whose rule, the Huns invaded this region. After the decline of the Guptas, the Maukharis of Kannauj gained power. During the rule of Harshavardhana, Kannauj was an important city. After his rule political chaos was set in. It was amidst this confusion that the Muslims invaded into Uttar Pradesh though the society was dominated by the Rajputs, Jats and other local chiefs in Mahmud Ghazni laid his eyes on the wealth of Kannauj. He was followed by Mohammad Ghori. Throughout the rule of the Delhi Sultanate and the Mughals, the territory progressed. After the Mughals, the Jats, the Rohillas, and the Marathas established their rule. By 1803, the British controlled this region and annexed it by 1856. It was in the Uttar Pradesh (The period between 1857-58) that the first struggle for liberation from the British rule was unleashed. The revolt was suppressed and from then till Independence it remained under British dominance. In 1950, the state was organized and named as Uttar Pradesh.

Uttar Pradesh has an area of 2,40,928 sq. km. and a population of 16,620 million. There are 75 districts, 813 blocks and 1,07,452 villages. The State has population density of 689 per sq. km. (as against the national average of 312). The decadal growth rate of the state is not available (against 21.54% for the country) and the population of the state continues to grow at a much faster rate than the national rate.

13. Health Indicators of Uttar Pradesh

The Total Fertility Rate of the State is 3.5. The Infant Mortality Rate is 61 and Maternal Mortality Ratio is 359 (SRS 2007-2009) which are higher than the National average. The Sex Ratio in the State is 908 (as compared to 940 for the country).

14. Geographical Background of the Study Area

District of Sultanpur has been named after its headquarters town. Sultanpur District lies on both sides of river Gomati between 26°58' North and 26°40' North latitudes and 81°32' East and 82°41' East longitudes.

Sultanpur District is bounded by Faizabad and Ambedkar Nagar Districts on the north, the Districts of Jaunpur and Azamgarh on the east, the District of Pratapgarh on the south and south-west, Districts of Amethi and Barabanki are on the north-west respectively. The administrative set-up of Sultanpur is shown in Map 1.1. Total population of the District Sultanpur is 24,07,897 persons. Administratively Sultanpur District has been divided into four Tehsils, *viz.* Sultanpur Sadar, Kadipur, Lambuwa, Jaisinghpur and there are 14 Development Blocks in the District Sultanpur.

14.1. *Historical Background of the Area*

Historically, the past of the District Sultanpur had been extremely famous, honoured and appreciated Archaeologically, Historically, Culturally, Geographically and Industrially, District Sultanpur has very important place. In spite of several continued changes, the identity of the district Sultanpur has been permanent.

District Sultanpur had been the worship place of Saints like Valmiki, Durwasa, Vashishtha, etc. Saint Kanva mentioned in the *Vishnu Purana*

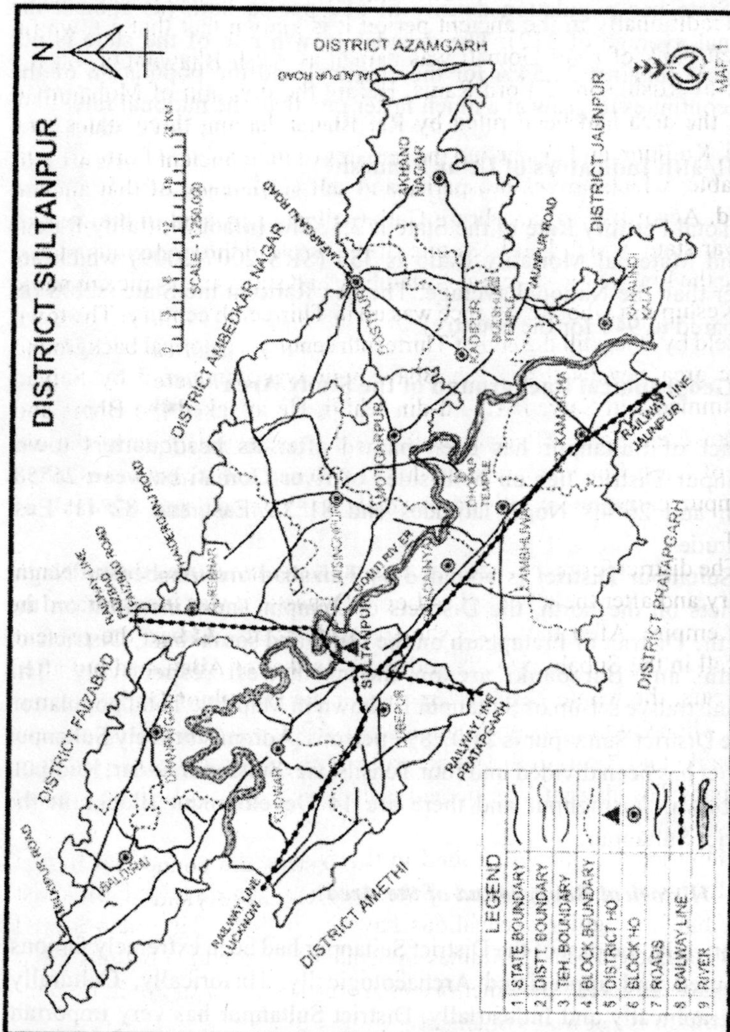

Map 1.1: District Sultanpur.

belonged to this place. In the centre of Ayodhya and Prayag, left and right side of the Gomati river in between Sai and Tamasa rivers, the land was highly unapproachable. The rope developed by Kush and Kash and its famous marketing place known as Badh Mandi is also located here.

Traditionally in the ancient period it is known fact that a town on the left bank of river Gomati was named as Kush Bhawanpur, on the name of Kush, son of Lord Rama. Before the invasion of Mohammad Gori, the area had been ruled by Raj Bharsa having three states, *viz.* Isauli, Koolpur, and Dadar and the remains of their ancient Forts are still available, which proves prosperity and self-sufficiency of that ancient period. According to Janashruti, Garha village is located in the west of Kurwar state, which had been one of the ten Buddhist religious places where the king of the state was Kalambanshi Kshtriya. His ancient name was Keshiputra whose existence was up to Thirteenth century. The town was held by Bhars till the end of Thirteenth century. Historical background of the area reveals that Kush Bhawanpur was conquered by Saiyad Muhammad and Saiyad Ala-ud-din Khilji. He attacked the Bhars and overpowered them. After about one year's unsuccessful seize the old town of Kush Bhawanpur was reduced to ashes and a new town called Sultanpur came up in existence which was named from the rank of victor.

The district formed the part of Jaunpur Kingdom during the Fifteenth century and after the downfall of Lodhi Dynasty, it was incorporated in Delhi empire. After the establishment made by the Akbar, the present area fell in the Subah of Oudh and partly in that of Allahabad but after 250 years, the whole District came under the Nawab of Oudh. During 1856, when Oudh was annexed a district was formed including present Barabanki and Rai Barelli Districts and additions were made to it from Faizabad. The district was named Sultanpur and assumed its present shape in 1869.

Many ancient mounds found in the District are connected by the local tradition with the Bhars. Some of them have yielded Buddhist relics, but no regular excavations have been done. The main sacred places connected with the Ramayana epic are Sitakund, a bathing Ghat on the Gomati river. The other places are the ruins of a fort built by Sher Shah, which is known as Shahgarh.

14.2. *Administrative Set-up of the Study Area*

The administrative set-up of the study area has been adversely affected due to its natural diversity, especially the Gomati River which flows from west to east part of the district has undulated topography due to ravines and sandy soils. The *usar* land and waterlogging in the low-lying areas due to the overflow of the canal irrigation water has also badly affected the socio-economic and adverse health problems among the people surviving the remote villages of the District Sultanpur.

Sultanpur District comprises four Tehsils and 14 Development Blocks which has been depicted in Figure 1.1.

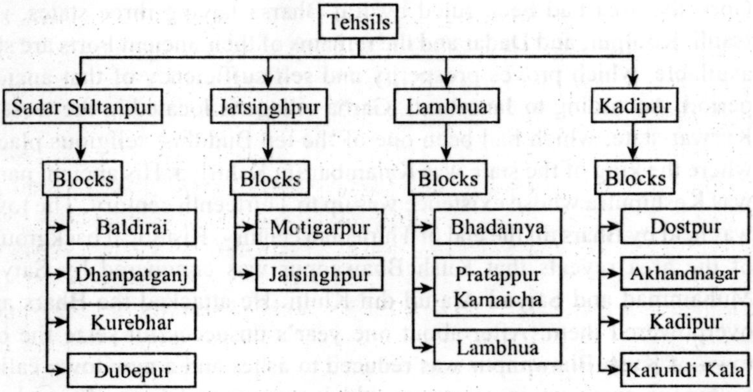

Figure 1.1: Administrative Set-up of Sultanpur District.

The total area of the District Sultanpur has been 2,672.89 sq.km. and the total area of the Bhadainya Block has been recorded 221.23 sq.km. which has been mentioned in Table 1.1. The estimated number of total houses in District Sultanpur has been 5,97,788 of which total number of houses in Bhadainya Block has been 25,354. The total population of the District Sultanpur has been noted 24,07,897 which comprises both males and females of which total population of the Bhadainya Block has been recorded 1,56,601. There are 5,16,928 scheduled caste population in the District Sultanpur while 36,343 scheduled caste population has been observed in the Bhadainya Block.

The literacy of the District Sultanpur has been recorded 53-84 per cent to the total population of which 57.60 per cent literacy has been noted in the Bhadainya Block.

The proportionate distribution of the scheduled caste population to the total population in District Sultanpur has been recorded 22.81 per cent to the total population of the district. It has also been noted that there 23.16 per cent scheduled caste population of the district. It has also been noted that there are 23.16 per cent scheduled caste population to the total population of the Bhadainya Block of the District Sultanpur.

Table 1.1: Demography — District Sultanpur

Sl. No.	*Tehsil*	*Sl. No.*	*Block*	*Area in sq.km.*	*No. of Houses*	*Total Population*	*SC Population*	*Literacy*	*SC %*
1.	Sadar	1	Baldirai	224.18	31431	182455	40841	56.14	22.75
		2	Dhanpatganj	225.20	27774	162765	34577	57.07	21.31
		3	Kurebhar	221.88	32646	194430	39896	57.48	20.18
		4	Kurwar	214.07	32387	203850	30548	57.77	15.21
		5	Dubepur	192.28	39435	244373	41426	59.31	17.14
2.	Jaisinghpur	6	Jaisinghpur	225.75	32558	199942	46195	55.74	22.58
		7	Motigarpur	122.74	16062	99776	25981	56.99	25.72
3.	Lambhua	8	Bhadainya	211.23	25354	156601	36343	57.60	23.16
		9	Lambhua	214.87	29034	176585	43775	55.76	24.11
		10	Pratappur Kamaicha	136.86	20062	129451	28748	57.82	22.82
4.	Kadipur	11	Dostpur	183.93	20016	129040	30893	54.14	23.82
		12	Akhand Nagar	220.51	25112	168686	47608	55.64	27.37
		13	Kadipur	152.85	19846	132880	34812	57.97	26.97
		14	Karaundi Kala	107.47	11418	80171	21885	56.28	25.34
			Total	**2672.89**	**597788**	**2407897**	**516928**	**53.87**	**22.81**

There are 8 Nyaya Panchayats in Bhadainya Block and 63 village panchayats and 149 revenue villages. The details of the revenue villages and village panchayat of the Bhadiayna Block has been mentioned in Table 1.2.

Table 1.2: Nyaya Panchayats, Village Panchayats and Revenue Villages, Block Bhadainya, District Sultanpur

Sl. No.	*Nyaya Panchayat*	*Sl. No.*	*Village Panchayat*	*Sl. No.*	*Revenue Villages*
1	*2*	*3*	*4*	*5*	*6*
1	Barui	1	Jagdishpur	1	Chachpara
				2	Jagdishpur
		2	Pakhrauli	3	Pakhrauli
		3	Babhangawna	4	Babhangawna
		4	Barui	5	Barui
				6	Jhauwara
		5	Belasada	7	Belasada
				8	Shankarpur
		6	Belamohan	9	Belamohan
		7	Sarai Achal	10	Sarai Achal
				11	Bhusaka

(Contd.)

Table 1.2 (*Contd.*)

1	*2*	*3*	*4*	*5*	*6*
		8	Salahpur	12	Salahpur
				13	Badruddinpur
2	Kenaura	9	Asarwan	14	Asarwan
		10	Kenaura	15	Kenaura
		11	Kaima	16	Kaima
				17	Madhopur
		12	Jaddupur	18	Bhagatpur
				19	Jamuwawa Ratan
				20	Jamuwawa Khanpur
				21	Arjunpur
				22	Jaddupur
				23	Chitari
				24	Ram Chandrapur
		13	Jamuwawa Paschim	25	Aujhi
				26	Jamuwawa Paschim
		14	Balampur	27	Balampur
		15	Maheshwa	28	Maheshwa
		16	Lahia Jalpapur	29	Birapur
				30	Lahia Jalpapur
3	Kandhaipur	17	Kandhaipur	31	Paniyarvaisya
				32	Parsipur
				33	Bhadiayana
				34	Kanhaipur
		18	Patipur	35	Jairampur
				36	Amari
				37	Karmisirpur
				38	Patipur
		19	Bajethi	39	Harchandpur
				40	Bajethi
		20	Bokharepur	41	Palepur
				42	Bokharepur
		21	Rudauli	43	Pithipur
				44	Kashipur
				45	Rudauli
		22	Shiripur	46	Shiripur
				47	Khorepur
				48	Aswa
		23	Sakarasi	49	Sakarasi
		24	Semari Purushottampur	50	Semari Purushottampur
		25	Saurai	51	Basantpur
				52	Madapur
				53	Saurai
4	Miranpur	26	Kalyan Patti	54	Khajuri
				55	Kalyanpatti
				56	Judapatti

(*Contd.*)

Table 1.2 (*Contd.*)

1	*2*	*3*	*4*	*5*	*6*
		27	Gyanipur	57	Gyanipur
		28	Daudpatti	58	Kishapatti
				59	Kunaiyapatti
				60	Daudpatti
		29	Dilawalpur	61	Dilawalpur
		30	Belsauna	62	Belsauna
		31	Bhikhampur	63	Bhikhampur
				64	Mahmoodpur
				65	Khalilpur
		32	Miranpur	66	Kodar
				67	Kamapur
				68	Miranpur
				69	Ratanpur
		33	Rampur	70	Baijupur
				71	Karanpur
				72	Rampur
		34	Sansaripur	73	Sansaripur
				74	Sendhuwa
				75	Asrafpur
5	Bikwajitpur	35	Abhiyakala	76	Siktapur
				77	Abhiyakala
		36	Gopalpur	78	Abhiyakhurd
				79	Gopalpur
		37	Judara	80	Ramnathpur
				81	Judara
				82	Maha Anandpur
				83	Harinathpur
				84	Bhagwatgarh
		38	Murarpur	85	Narharpur
				86	Murarpur
				87	Agresar
		39	Bikwajitpur	88	Maheshpur
				89	Laxmanpur
				90	Bikwajitpur
				91	Jalapur
		40	Hanumanganj	92	Mankapur Prasin
				93	Hanumanganj
				94	Shahupur
		41	Haripur Banwa	95	Saraiya
				96	Dubepur
				97	Hari Narayanpur
				98	Haripur Banwa
6	Bhapta	42	Unchhara	99	Unchhara
		43	Gaura	100	Gaura
				101	Pitambarpur
				102	Shivpur

(*Contd.*)

Table 1.2 (*Contd.*)

1	2	3	4	5	6
		44	Narayanpur	103	Great Narayanpur
				104	Naubasta
				105	Narayanpur
		45	Palhanpur	106	Gupsad
				107	Palhanpur
				108	Purekrita
		46	Purebaghrai	109	Purebaghrai
				110	Lodipur
				111	Satanpur
		47	Bhapta	112	Chainpur
				113	Bhapta
		48	Bharthipur	114	Bharthipur
				115	Lakhipur
				116	Sarai Ambarpur
		49	Majhlegaon	117	Arau Paharpur
				118	Majhlegaon
				119	Rampur
		50	Misirpur Puraina	120	Puraina
				121	Misirpur
7	Bhadainya	51	Alipur	122	Bhagwanpur
				123	Bharsare
				124	Alipur
		52	Teranye	125	Teranye
				126	Gopal Patti
				127	Lodhpur
				128	Sultan Teri
		53	Trilok Chandrapur	129	Trilok Chandrapur
				130	Rai Chandrapur
				131	Bhuwapur
				132	Barsara
		54	Panna Tikari	133	Panna Tikari
		55	Bhadainya	134	Bhadainya
		56	Bhairopur	135	Dhanuspur
				136	Bhairopur
				137	Rahayakpur
		57	Ramgarh	138	Ramgarh
				139	Khanipur
				140	Manapur
		58	Sakawa	141	Sakawa
8	Chhatauna	59	Karomi	142	Bhatpura
				143	Karomi
		60	Kuchhmuchh	144	Madhopur
				145	Kuchhmuchh
		61	Chhatauna	146	Chhatauna
		62	Malikpur	147	Malikpur
				148	Jadipur
		63	Vajupur	149	Vajupur

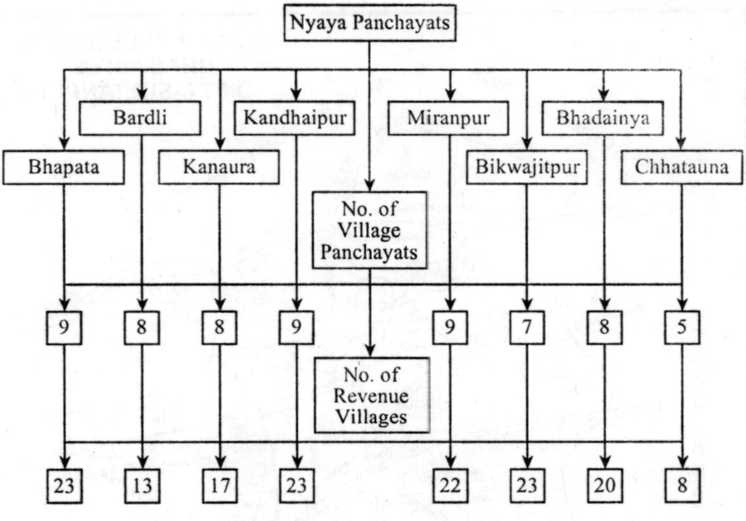

Figure 1.2: Administrative Set-up of Bhadainya Block.

Thus, there are 9 village panchayats and 23 revenue villages in Bhapata Nyaya Panchayat, 8 village panchayats and 13 revenue villages in Barui Nyaya Panchayat, 8 village panchayats and 17 revenue villages in the Kanarua Nyaya Panchayat, 8 village panchayats and 23 revenue villages in the Kandhaipur Nyaya Panchayat, 8 village panchayats and 22 revenuê villages in Miranpur Nyaya Panchayat, 7 village panchayats and 23 revenue villages in the Bikwajitpur Nyaya Panchayat, 8 village panchayats and 20 revenue villages in the Bhadainya Nyaya Panchayat while 5 village panchayats and 8 revenue villages has been recorded in the Chhatauna Nyaya Panchayat of Bhadainya Block of the Sultanpur District.

The location of the village panchayats of the Bhadainya Block has been depicted in Map 1.2.

The number of houses, population and distribution of the scheduled caste population at the village panchayat level has been mentioned in Table 1.3.

The highest number of houses 1059 has been noted in Bhadainya Village Panchayat, having 6904 population and 1809 scheduled caste population. The lowest number of the houses 223 has been recorded in Misirpur Puraina village panchayat and lowest number of population 1380 in Rampur village panchayat and the lowest number of scheduled caste population has been noted 126 in Karomi village panchayat of Bhadainya Block.

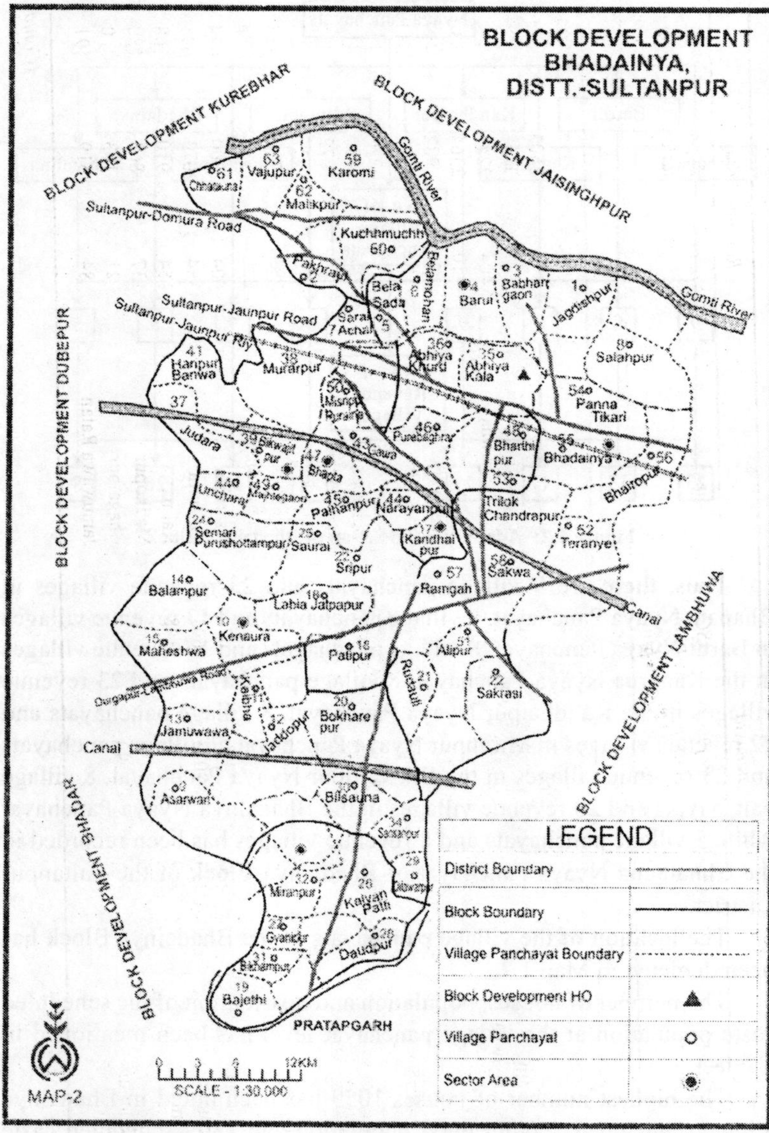

Map 1.2: Village Panchayats of Bhadainya Block, Distrcit Sultanpur.

Table 1.3: Demography — Village Panchayat and Revenue Village-wise, Block Bhadainya, District Sultanpur

Nyaya Panchayat	*Village Panchayat*				*Revenue Village*			
	Name	*No. of Houses*	*Popu-lation*	*SC Popu-lation*	*Name*	*No. of Houses*	*Popu-lation*	*SC Popu-lation*
1	*2*	*3*	*4*	*5*	*6*	*7*	*8*	*9*
Barui	Jagdishpur	456	2930	260	Chachpara	52	427	49
					Jagdishpur	404	2503	211
	Pakhrauli	611	3568	999	Pakhrauli	311	3568	999
	Babhangawna	404	2246	353	Babhangawna	404	2246	353
	Barui	585	3346	727	Barui	410	2364	230
					Jhauwara	175	982	487
	Belasada	257	1445	454	Belasada	174	941	311
					Shankarpur	83	504	143
	Belamohan	284	1480	411	Belamohan	284	1480	411
	Sarai Achal	394	2199	421	Sarai Achal	343	1872	338
					Bhusaka	51	327	83
	Salahpur	673	3312	219	Salahpur	293	1730	181
					Badruddinpur	280	1582	38
Kenaura	Asarwan	404	2300	674	Asarwan	404	2300	674
	Kenaura	354	2073	691	Kenaura	354	2073	691
	Kaima	289	1773	348	Kaima	154	910	168
					Madhopur	137	863	180
	Jaddupur	375	2190	444	Bhagatpur	21	103	0
					Jamuwawa Ratan	84	519	191

(*Contd.*)

Table 1.3 (*Contd.*)

1	*2*	*3*	*4*	*5*	*6*	*7*	*8*	*9*
					Jamuwawa Khanpur	86	496	76
					Arjunpur	69	424	112
					Jaddupur	107	609	42
					Chitari	05	23	7
					Ram Chandrapur	03	16	16
	Jamuwawa Paschim	304	1992	417	Aujhi	170	1040	137
					Jamuwawa Paschim	134	952	280
	Balampur	673	3905	786	Balampur	673	3905	786
	Maheshwa	406	2378	798	Maheshwa	406	2378	798
	Lahia Jalpapur	306	1846	196	Birapur	58	381	56
					Lahia Jalpapur	248	1465	140
Kandhaipur	Kandhaipur	398	2503	641	Paniyarvaisya	25	147	13
					Parsipur	98	542	44
					Bhadiyaanup	15	73	70
					Kanhaipur	260	1641	514
	Patipur	437	2642	660	Jairampur	0	0	0
					Amari	189	1166	384
					Karmisirpur	25	138	8
					Patipur	223	1338	325
	Bajethi	277	1704	264	Harchandpur	39	221	71
					Bajethi	238	1483	93
	Bokharepur	257	1613	313	Palepur	1	8	0
					Bokharepur	256	1605	313
	Rudauli	336	2067	656	Pithipur	138	769	281

(*Contd.*)

Table 1.3 (*Contd.*)

1	*2*	*3*	*4*	*5*	*6*	*7*	*8*	*9*
					Kashipur	0	0	0
					Rudauli	198	1298	375
	Shiripur	427	2563	1124	Shiripur	120	720	217
					Khorepur	143	845	335
					Aswa	164	898	572
	Sakarasi	447	2941	577	Sakarasi	447	2941	577
	Semari Purushottampur	413	2680	510	Semari Purushottampur	413	2680	510
	Saurai	350	1925	546	Basantpur	98	579	144
					Madapur	0	0	0
					Saurai	258	1346	402
Miranpur	Kalyan Patti	392	2740	583	Khajuri	141	1010	171
					Kalyanpatti	75	519	351
					Judapatti	178	1211	61
	Gyanipur	544	3383	970	Gyanipur	544	3383	970
	Daudpatti	370	2271	440	Kishapatti	137	853	408
					Kunaiyapatti	67	387	0
					Daudpatti	166	1031	32
	Dilawalpur	308	2016	181	Dilawalpur	308	2016	181
	Belsauna	308	1989	823	Belsauna	308	1989	823
	Bhikhampur	328	2046	368	Bhikhampur	155	956	224
					Mahmoodpur	127	765	0
					Khalilpur	46	325	144
	Miranpur	260	1731	227	Kodar	11	93	0
					Kamapur	40	288	0

(*Contd.*)

Table 1.3 (*Contd.*)

1	*2*	*3*	*4*	*5*	*6*	*7*	*8*	*9*
					Miranpur	142	919	136
					Ratanpur	67	421	91
	Rampur	237	1380	196	Baijupur	73	403	22
					Karanpur	17	91	0
					Rampur	147	866	174
	Sansaripur	320	2500	761	Sansaripur	233	1733	474
					Sendhuwa	51	350	177
					Asrafpur	76	417	110
Bikwajitpur	Abhiyakala	573	3864	934	Siktapur	137	1047	247
					Abhiyakala	436	2817	687
	Gopalpur	287	1736	387	Abhiyakhurd	137	805	155
					Gopalpur	150	531	232
	Judara	397	2354	422	Ramnathpur	14	73	0
					Judara	158	876	237
					Maha Anandpur	72	483	128
					Harinathpur	44	278	59
					Bhagwatgarh	109	644	0
	Murarpur	376	2181	859	Narharpur	98	536	177
					Murarpur	178	991	507
					Agresar	102	854	175
	Bikwajitpur	309	1692	656	Maheshpur	61	441	153
					Laxmanpur	8	62	62
					Bikwajitpur	228	1126	441
					Jalapur	12	63	0

(*Contd.*)

Table 1.3 (*Contd.*)

1	*2*	*3*	*4*	*5*	*6*	*7*	*8*	*9*
	Hanumanganj	598	3796	484	Mankapur Prasin	123	844	89
					Hanumanganj	459	2666	395
					Shahupur	16	86	0
	Haripur Banwa	357	2396	587	Saraiya	47	288	149
					Dubepur	5	38	0
					Hari Narayanpur	166	1029	314
					Haripur Banwa	139	1041	124
Bhapta	Unchhara	253	1694	581	Unchhara	253	1694	581
	Gaura	261	1664	532	Gaura	191	1172	336
					Pitambarpur	28	196	196
					Shivpur	42	296	0
	Narayanpur	282	1848	412	Great Narayanpur	28	170	0
					Naubasta	88	644	117
					Narayanpur	166	1114	295
	Palhanpur	314	1752	626	Gupsad	99	516	375
					Palhanpur	146	817	162
					Purekrita	69	419	89
	Purebaghrai	472	3063	1103	Purebaghrai	194	1292	494
					Lodipur	111	716	168
					Satanpur	167	1055	441
	Bhapta	307	1847	437	Chainpur	49	319	75
					Bhapta	258	1528	382
	Bharthipur	328	2033	617	Bharthipur	165	1017	194
					Lakhipur	75	440	270
					Sarai Ambarpur	88	563	153

(*Contd.*)

Table 1.3 (*Contd.*)

1	2	3	4	5	*6*	7	*8*	*9*
	Majhlegaon	325	1818	484	Arau Paharpur	61	314	43
					Majhlegaon	132	775	324
					Rampur	112	729	117
	Misirpur Puraina	223	1517	291	Puraina	142	986	110
					Misirpur	81	531	181
Bhadainya	Alipur	376	2111	225	Bhagwanpur	111	621	15
					Bharsare	122	687	130
					Alipur	143	903	80
	Teranye	522	3426	874	Teranye	476	3151	851
					Gopal Patti	1	7	7
					Lodhpur	0	0	0
					Sultan Teri	45	268	17
	Trilok Chandrapur	487	2895	989	Trilok Chandrapur	130	726	200
					Rai Chandrapur	121	695	201
					Bhuwapur	20	159	39
					Barsara	216	1315	549
	Panna Tikari	552	3138	882	Panna Tikari	552	3138	882
	Bhadainya	1059	6904	1809	Bhadainya	1059	6904	1809
	Bhairopur	387	2556	339	Dhanuspur	95	737	57
					Bhairopur	189	1059	178
					Rahayakpur	103	760	104
	Ramgarh	387	2677	729	Ramgarh	193	1262	486
					Khanipur	116	797	126
					Manapur	78	458	117

(*Contd.*)

Table 1.3 (*Contd.*)

1	*2*	*3*	*4*	*5*	*6*	*7*	*8*	*9*
	Sakawa	333	2187	446	Sakawa	338	2187	446
Chhatauna	Karomi	351	2207	156	Bhatpura	95	533	0
					Karomi	256	1674	156
	Kuchhmuchh	736	4594	658	Madhopur	92	482	94
					Kuchhmuchh	644	4112	564
	Chhatauna	586	3892	597	Chhatauna	586	3892	597
	Malikpur	419	2770	976	Malikpur	254	1564	388
					Jadipur	165	1206	588
	Vajupur	393	2534	100	Vajupur	393	2534	100
	Total	**25299**	**156601**	**36343 (23.16%)**		**25299**	**156601**	**36343 (23.16%)**

The distribution of number of houses, population and the scheduled caste population at the revenue villages level has been mentioned in Table 1.3. There is no house and population in the Lodhipur, Kashipur, Madapur, Jairampur revenue villages while 3 houses and 5 houses are found in Ramchandrapur and Chitari revenue villages of Bhadainya Block.

The highest number of the houses having 1,059 houses and 6,904 population and 1,809 scheduled caste population has been noted in Bhadainya revenue village of the study area. Thus, the distribution of houses, population and the scheduled caste population are diversely distributed at the revenue village level. The revenue villages located on the road side and dominated by the general caste population are concentrated with the number of houses and population as well as the scheduled caste population. The revenue villages located in the remote areas are having low number of houses, population and scheduled caste population and these villages are earmarked as revenue villages on the revenue records for the collection of Mal Gujari.

It has been noticed that the natural infrastructure of Bhadainya Block of Sultanpur District has been adversely affecting the socio-economic and health status of the people living below poverty line in the remote villages. The sandy ravines of the Gomati River, *usar* land, water-logging caused through excessive irrigation water has been the major source of water pollution and contamination of the water at the grassroots level which has been causing for the growth of the various water-borne diseases among the common people of the study area. The growth of the various water-borne diseases has adversely affected the life of the people and created the loss of the life of the human being, animal, flora and fauna of the study area. It has also created economic loss including the poverty to save the life of the suffering patients from such water-borne diseases.

Therefore, it has become an important challenging task to prevent the Water Pollution and control the contamination of the water through standard safe supply of the drinking water at the village level with the view to control the occurrence of different water-borne diseases. To train and demonstrate the common people of the study area to prevent the Water Contamination and check the growth of the water-borne diseases through appropriate medical care and medical treatment to save the life of suffering people from various water-borne diseases, communicable diseases and non-communicable diseases at the village panchayat level in Bhadainya Block of Sultanpur District.

14.3. *Physiography*

Physiographically, the district may be divided into two main physical divisions such as — Northern Tract which lies to the north of the river Gomati running from west to east and comprised the development Block of Baldirai Dhanpatganj, Kurebhar, Jaisinghpur, Dostpur, Akhandnagar, Motigarpur, and Kadipur and Southern tract, lying to the south of the river Gomati comprising Bhadainya, Lambhua, Dubepur, Pratappur Kamicha Development Blocks.

The plain is characterised by an unrelieved monotony of alluvial deposits which completely shroud the old land surface to a depth of several thousand metres. The solid geology of the plain is totally obscured underneath the mantle.

The *Kankarili* land is found in the northern part, where some *usar* lands are also observed. The soils are mainly sandy-loamy and clayey and sub-divided, into *Khadar* or newer alluvium. The whole plain of the area is formed of rich alluvial soil which is of great agricultural importance but *Kankar* or calcarious limestones are common. Various hypotheses have been put forward to explain the geological evolution of this plain.

Geologically, the district Sultanpur does not reveal anything striking except the ordinary Gangetic alluvium. The *Kankar* is only the mineral found along the bed of the Gomati. It lies at depth up to about one metre from the surface. *Reh* and *Multani Mitti* known as clay is also found in some parts of the District which are used for washing and pottery respectively. Older alluvial and saline and saline alkali are the soils found in the district Sultanpur.

14.4. *Geology*

There are no noteworthy feature in the physiognomy of the district Sultanpur. Thus, geologically Sultanpur District can be divided in three tracts —

(a) Ravine tract of the Gomati,
(b) Central tract, and
(c) Lake tract.

The slope of the District runs from the north-west to south-east. The rivers which flow in the District are Gomati, Majhuai and Mangar.

The physiography of the area is gradual with a scarcely perceptible slope from north-west to south-east. The surface of the area is generally plain. The average height of the area is 110 metres. Heterogeneity of the physical landscape is caused actually by local eminences. These are the perceptible notches of *banjar* tracts. In real sense, the scenery is of varied character.

Sultanpur District lies in the Ganga-Yamuna Doab which is part of the Indo-Gangetic Plain. The plain is a depression between the Himalayas in the North and the Deccan plateau in the South. This plain has been filled by the alluvium brought down by the Himalayan rivers. The composition of this alluvium commenced after the upheaval of the mountain and has continued all through the Pleistocene up to the present.

Accurately, the depth of the plain is not known. Boring down mainly for artesian wells has penetrated only up to 1.606 metres is the recent alluvium strata. Geologists differ in their estimates of the thickness of the alluvial deposits on the basis of observations. It has been estimated about 1.950 metres thickness of alluvial deposits.

14.5. *Drainage System of the Area*

The rivers which flow in the District are Gomati, Majhuai and Mangar. The general characteristic features throughout the plains are that the rivers meet at acute angles and several *nalas* from parallel or sub-parallel lines to the mainstream. There are several tanks, *jhils* and lakes. There are number of shallow *Jhils*, or swamps, but none of them is of any considerable size or importance.

14.6. *Climate of the Area*

The study area experiences a rhythm of seasons with reversal of prevailing winds. The reversal is regularly felt twice during the year. From November to May winds blow from the west and are of the continental character, whereas from June to October, they are of oceanic origin and come from the east. The complete reversal of direction of winds on a gigantic scale between summer and winter is responsible for the monsoon.

Sultanpur District experiences typical tropical climate with distinctive summer, rainy and winter seasons. The mean daily maximum temperature rises to 40.6 °C and mean daily minimum temperature drop to 8.6 °C on an average. The average annual rainfall is 1005 mm occurring of dust-storm and thunder-storms in the hot season is the special phenomena of the local climate in the District. The relative humidities rise to 85 per cent during south-west monsoon and decreases to 30 per cent in the summer season. The climate of the area is normal and suitable for agricultural activities.

(i) *Temperature*

The changes in the temperature are the outcome of the monsoon currents. It tends to set up surface pressure differences, resulting in a low pressure over the land and high pressure over the adjoining areas. May and June are the hottest months of the year. The mean temperature during these months are 32.3 °C and 31.7 °C respectively. The extreme maximum temperature in the month of June is 45 °C. It is due to the sun's rays falling almost vertically. Conversely, the extreme minimum temperature occurring in the month of December is 4.4 °C, since the sun is low during this month owing to the earth's position during winter solstice.

(ii) *Pressure and Winds*

The pressure is 985 millibars during the month of June, July and August. It rises 1,004 millibars during the month of December. A shallow cell of high pressure with sea-ward gradient develops over the land in December and January. In summer the pressure gradient is towards the land. The shallow depression visits the district in a cyclonic form ascending from the Bay of Bengal, but the high pressure winds in December and January reach here from west causing rough weather and little rain.

(iii) *Moisture and Humidity*

The principal factor which determines the potentiality of rainfall is the humidity level in the atmosphere. Humidity is high in the months of June, July, August and September. The winds are dry during the months of March, April and May. The temperature during these months is also high and the pressure is subsequently low and the relative humidity is comparatively low.

(iv) *Rainfall*

The annual rainfall in Sultanpur District is received within short period of four months, i.e. mid-June to October.

Rainfall during the other months is scanty and sporadic. The annual rainfall for the area is 1,005 mm, but it is unevenly distributed over the year —

(a) *Annual Variability of Rainfall:* The prosperity of the farmers depends largely on the uniform distribution of annual rainfall. An annual variability of 12 per cent or more makes an area susceptible to famine. In this regard Amethi stands very often in the danger of super-abundance or deficiency of rainfall. Some areas of the district experience drought conditions, while other areas are liable to face serious flood and waterlogging due to heavy rain.

(b) *Seasonal and Monthly Variability of Rainfall:* Seasonal and monthly variability of rainfall is rather more significant than the annual variability from the point of view of agricultural activities. If the rainfall in the month of June is insignificant or excessive, it can delay the sowing of the early Kharif crops and thus reduces the production. If the rainfall is heavy and alternates with long intervals, floods and droughts are experienced simultaneously. The state of abnormality frequently causes havoc and the whole cropping pattern is affected seriously. Early or late retreat of the monsoon in September and October affects maturing of the Kharif crops. On the other hand heavy rainfall may cause postponement of sowing of Rabi crops.

Thus, the weather elements together and considering the variations in their incidence, the year is divided into three distinct seasons:

I. *The rainy season* — mid-June to October.
II. *The cold weather season* — November to February.
III. *The hot weather season* — March to mid-June.

Thus, the climate of the area is mild and healthy. Westerly winds prevail from October to June gradually increasing in strength as the hot season approaches. The northern part of the district receives more rainfall than the southern part.

14.7. *Soils*

Older alluvial and Saline and Saline-alkaline are the soils found in the District. Soils of the area are transported from sedimentary rocks of the Himalayas and the product of decomposition of these rocks have been deposited over the tract through water action. Therefore, the soils of the District fall under the alluvial group of the Indo-Gangetic plain. Scientific data regarding the soils of the District are not available.

A brief account of the soils and land classification based on the texture of the soil is, however, prepared by the revenue authorities to assess the land revenue. The main factors governing the system of classification are texture, colour, availability of water and the level of the land. On the basis of texture, the soils of the district have been sub-divided into the following groups:

(i) *Bangar Soil:* Bangar (upland plain) soils vary from sandy loam to stiff clay, depending upon topography and drainage. Bangar land arise on the basis of the principle that when a river grows older, its deposits subsequently occupy a lower position along its basin and the terraces and the flood plain are gradually left free by the spreading action of water during the old age of river. These raised uplands, which are called *bangar*, are again eroded by the newer channels, but they always remain above the flood plain and are never affected.

(ii) *Loamy Soil:* Loamy soil is locally called "Domat Soil". It is extensively distributed over the *bangar* or upland plain. Patches of loamy soils are found in the District Sultanpur. The patches of Domat soil are very well drained. Sand and clay are present in this soil which is almost equal in proportions, therefore, it can easily be recognized. Depending on the fertility, *Domat* soil has been further divided into:

- *Domat Awal,*
- *Domat Doam,* and
- *Domat Soam.*

Depending upon the percentage of sand the colour varies from yellow to brown. The sub-soil is brownish and yellow, sometimes mixed together and sometimes with alternating layers. The water holding capacity also varies according to the texture. Loamy soil is preferred by the cultivators, since it can be used for double and multiple cropping.

(iii) *Clayey Loam:* Clayey loam soil is locally known as *Matiyar* Soil and it has grey or yellowish grey colour at the surface. The sub-soil in the lower horizons is dark grey in colour. In comparison to the *Domat* Soil, the percentage of clay in it is high, its water retention capacity is also very high. It has been observed that almost in every village *Matiyar* Soil is seen to occupy low level areas which results in accumulation of rainwater. Consequently, the soil responds well to paddy crop. Sometimes clayey loam soil is characterised by the pressure of calcareous concretions which are leached from the surface and get accumulated at various depths in the form of *Kankar*.

(iv) *Clayey Soil:* The Clayey Soil is locally known as "*Dhankhar* Soil" and it is grey to dark grey colour. *Dhankar* Soil as its name indicates, is largely used for growing *Dhan*, i.e. paddy. It has compact and cloudy structure and becomes sticky when wet and very hard when dry. It is mostly used for raising single crop of late paddy while during other parts of the year it is almost left idle. The villagers call such fields with the clayey soil as "*Jadhan Khet*" (type of Paddy land). In fact, ploughing and sowing are almost impossible when this land is dry. Clayey soil is found only in small patches. It mostly lies in the vicinities of *Tals* and *Jhils* and occasionally near low-lying areas.

(v) *Khadar Soil:* Khadar Soil is mainly confined to the flood plains of rivers and *jhils*. *Khadar* soil is generally light, but it is rich in calcareous matter. Beds of sand and clay are deposited as alternate layers. The soil in the vicinity of rivers has more sand in comparison to soil lying away from river beds. In various areas of the district soil is loamy and makes cultivation non-profitable. *Khadar* soils are found in relatively low-lying areas which are subject to occasional flooding, and therefore, get freshly deposited silt, which enhances their fertility and allows growing of excellent Rabi crops in the Sultanpur District.

(vi) *Saline and Alkali Soils:* Soils which have excessive proportions of soluble salts and/or exchangeable sodium, due to which crop production is seriously hampered are locally known as "*Reh/Usar*". They have a high soil *p*H value. There is a deficiency of calcium, nitrogen and micro-nutrients like zinc, extremely low water intake rate and hydraulic conductivity, resulting in poor moisture transmission characteristics. The presence of calcium carbonate nodules, called *Kankar*, often occurring at almost one metre depth and poor physical condition lead to hindrance in root penetration.

14.8. *Natural Vegetation*

The area has an almost inhabited human occupance for over three millennia and centuries of plough and pastoral culture has reduced the natural vegetation, except in pockets of *Tarai* and some river banks, with a moderate and healthy climate and fertile soil, the district flora presents no peculiarities. Patches of *Dhak* (*Butea frondosa*) are found here and there. The district in general, well wooded and contains magnificent groves of Mango, *Jamun* (*Eugenia Jambolana*) and *Mahua* (*Bassia Latifolia*) trees.

14.9. *Religious Importance*

Religious, historical and archaeological importance can be obtained from the museum established in the super market in the city of Sultanpur, in which various important photos and other materials can be seen. Religiously, District Sultanpur has been very important and the various religious places make it clear that District Sultanpur had very important role in the ancient historical periods. Important religious places of District Sultanpur are as follows:

1. *Bijethua Mahaviran:* It is one of the famous religious picnic spots known as 'Bijethua Mahaviran' located in Kadipur Tehsil of the District Sultanpur. There is beautiful temple of Hanumanji. Local fair/Mela is being organized in the Shravan Month on every Tuesday. Makari Kund is also located at Bijethua Mahaviran.
2. *Pancho-Piran:* Very famous Pancho-Piran Mazar of Muslim saints/Fakirs are located at the North and South of the Gomati river. Religiously Pancho Piran Mazar is famous for the sacrifice and peace of the five Fakir brothers whose Mazars known as Sultan Shah Mazar, Sarmad Shah Mazar, Pancho-Piran Mazar, Danka Shahid Baba Mazar and Gaus Baba Mazar. Every Thursday the interested people visit these Mazars to pray the saints and local fair on the Urs day is also organized.
3. *Dhopap:* Dhopap is religiously famous place located in Lambhua Block of the District Sultanpur. Many religious people used to take bath on Jyeshtha Shukla Dashmi and Ram Navami. It is the feeling of the local people that the soul of the people gets peace in heaven whiie taking bath at Dhopap.
4. *Sitakund:* Sitakund is located at the bank of the river Gomati in the Sultanpur city. Chait Ram Navami Magh Amavasya, Kartik Purnima are the important occasions when the maximum people take bath in the Gomati River. According to the common people's version, lastly Sita Ma took place in the earth, due to which it is famous and known as Sita Kund.
5. *Loharamau:* Loharamau is a religious place located adjacent to the Sultanpur District. Big fair is being organized on Shivratri and in the month of Savan to worship Maa Durga.
6. *Pahalwan Bir Baba:* Famous saint's Mazar known as Pahalwan Bir Baba is located at Payagipur. People use to worship Pahalwan Bir Baba on every Thursday and local fair is also being organized.

7. *Gadha:* Village Gadha is one of the ten states as mentioned in the Buddhist religious Book located in Kurwar Block of Sultanpur District. The king of Gadha was Kalam vanshi Kshatriya whose ancient name was Keshiputra, whose existence was up to Thirteenth century.

15. Demographic Profile of Uttar Pradesh

It has been recorded that the total population of Uttar Pradesh is 20.39 crore and there are 75 districts, 773 Community Health Centres and 3,692 Primary Health Centres in Uttar Pradesh.

Demographic Profile of Uttar Pradesh has been illustrated in Table 1.4.

Table 1.4: Demographic Profile of Uttar Pradesh

Infrastructure	*Number*
Population of the State	20.39 crore
District	75
Community Health Centres	773
Primary Health Centres	3,692
Sub-Health Centres	20,521
Village	1,07,452
Filaria Control Unit	29
Urban Malaria Unit	14

Source: State Programme Management Unit, National Rural Health Mission, Uttar Pradesh.

There are 4,207 Microscopic Centres, 20,521 Sub-Health Centres, 1,07,452 villages, 29 Filaria Control Units and 14 urban Malaria Control Units in Uttar Pradesh.

In view of the above, an attempt has been made in this study to analyse the various public health programmes and Progress of the Public Health Activities and Management of the Public Health Programme at the facility level.

16. Conclusion

There is a significant progress in improving the life expectancy at birth reducing the mortality due to Malaria, as well as reducing infant and maternal mortality over the last few decades in India. In spite of the progress made, a high proportion of the population especially the remote villages continue to suffer and die from preventable diseases, pregnancy and child birth related complications as well as malnutrition.

In addition to the old unresolved problems the health systems in our country are facing an emerging threats and challenges. The rural health care system in many areas is an unsatisfactory state leading to pauperization of poor households due to excessive extensive private sector health care.

Our country is in the midst of an epidemiological and demographic transition with the attendant problems of increased chronic disease burden and a decline in the mortality and fertility rates leading to an ageing of the population.

Premature morbidity and mortality from chronic disease has been a major loss of economic and human resources. The large disparity across different places the burden of these conditions mostly on the poor and on women scheduled castes, backward castes especially those who are living in the remote villages. The inequity has also been reflected in the skewed availability of public resources between the advanced and less developed villages.

Most of the Public Health determinants are correlated to high levels of poverty and to degradation of the environment of the villages. It has been noted that state of Uttar Pradesh has to deal with multiple health crisis, rising costs of health care and mounting expectations of the people.

It has been visioned to ensure effective integration of health concerns through decentralized management of District, Block and Village Level with the determinants of health, like sanitation, hygiene, nutrition, safe drinking water, gender and social concerns.

It has been viewed to provide universal access to equitable, affordable and quality health care which is accountable at the same time responsive to the requirements of the village people and reduction of child and maternal deaths as well as stabilization of population, gender and demographic balance.

It has been strategically viewed to develop a framework for promoting inter-sectoral convergence for ensuring promotive, preventive and curative public health care system at the facility level.

An important objective of the Public Health Programme has been to ensure reduction in Maternal and Child Mortality Rate to ensure universal immunization, family planning prevention and control of communicable and non-communicable diseases including locally endemic diseases and to mainstream AYUSH health system for promotion of healthy life-styles and implementation of various National Disease Control Programmes at the facility level.

It is being expected that outcomes from the public health systems will be helpful in reducing the Infant Mortality Rate to 30/1000 live births by 2012 and Maternal Mortality Rate reduction to 100/1,00,000 live births of 2012 and reduction in the Total Fertility Rate to 2.1 by 2012 and Maternal Mortality Reduction Rate — 50 per cent up to 2010 additional 10 per cent by 2012. It has also been planned to reduce Kala-Azar Mortality Rate — 100 per cent by 2012 and substantial elimination until 2012 and Filaria/Micro-Filaria Reduction Rate — 70 per cent, by 2010 and 80 per cent by 2012 and elimination by 2015, Dengue Mortality Reduction Rate — 50 per cent by 2010 and sustaining at that level until 2012.

It has been planned to provide improved access to universal immunization through induction of Auto-Disabled Syringes, alternate vaccine delivery and improved mobilization services and to provide improved facilities for institutional deliveries through provision of referral transport escort and improved hospital care under Janani Suraksha Yojana and Janani Shishu Suraksha Karyakram.

The Core Strategy of public health system includes strengthening of the existing Primary Health Centres through better staffing and development of human resources, health policy clear quality standards, better community support and untied funds to enable the local management committee to achieve the norms of Indian Public Health Standards.

The supplementary strategy of the Public Health System has been to mainstream the AYUSH system of Medicine through revitalizing the local health traditions at the facility level and to reorient the medical education to support Public Health issues including regulation to medical care and medical ethics.

An unique opportunity for carrying out necessary reforms in the health sector has been prioritized at the facility level. The reforms are necessary for restructuring to health delivery system as well as for delivery of better health financing mechanisms. The strengthening and effectiveness of health institutions, like Sub Health Centres/Primary Health Centres/Community Health Centres/Taluka/District Hospitals have positive consequences for all health programmes, i.e. Tuberculosis, malaria, HIV/AIDS, Filaria, Family Planning and Welfare, Leprosy, Disease Surveillance Project, etc. as all programmes are based on the assumption that a functioning of Public Health System actually exists at the facility level.

The key features in order to achieve the goals of the Mission include making of the Public Health delivery system fully functional and accountable to the Community, human resource management, decentralization, rigorous monitoring and evaluation against standards, convergence of health and related programme from village level upwards innovations and flexible funding and interventions for improving the health indicators at the various levels.

Public Health System seeks to improve outreach activities in unserved and underserved areas especially inhabited by vulnerable sections of the society through provision of Mobile Medical units covering all Anganwadi Centres. It also seeks to ensure availability of requisite equipment and drugs of all Public Health care facilities. Procurement of equipments/ drugs should be progressively decentralized at the facility level.

In order to provide managerial support for tracking funds and monitoring activities, a provision has been made to setting up Programme Management Units at facility level, over 500 professionals have already been recruited.

In view of the given large army of Accredited Social Health Activists, Auxiliary Nurse Midwife, Nurses and Rural Medical Practitioners require continuous skill development. Strengthening nursing institutions, linking medical colleges for providing skill development support to rural health worker involving the voluntary sector in skill development are few key interventions to be taken up at the facility level.

To make the health facilities more accountable the health sector control would be gradually shifted to the Panchayati Raj Institutions and civil society. The sub-centres are proposed to be placed exclusively under the control of Panchayat Samitis and Rogi Kalyan Samitis.

The District Health Plan would be the main instrument for planning, inter-sectoral convergence, implementation and monitoring of the activities under the Public Health System.

Provisions has been made for state specific proposal for main-streaming AYUSH including the appointment of AYUSH doctors/ paramedics on contractual basis, providing AYUSH Wings in the Primary Health Centres.

The process of community involvement of health institutions itself would enhance the accountability and the National Rural Health Mission would facilitate this process by wide dissemination of the results. For effective monitoring, a strong Management Information System is being put in place.

The citizen charter would help the public to know their rights and entitlements at each facility. Efforts are being made to integrate HIV/ AIDS programmes with Reproductive and Child Health at the facility levels. Convergence of Disease Control Programme, integration of service, combined awareness generation, education and advocacy at community and facility levels, taking care of the preventive, promotive and curative health care are expected to bring down Infant Mortality Rate/Maternal Mortality Rate/Total Fertility Rate and reduce the burden of diseases.

Public Health Manual is intended to be a user friendly tool to assist range of stakeholders to be engaged in the District Health Action Planning at the facility level. The Community Health Centres constitute the secondary level of health care which has been designed to provide referral as well as specialist health care to the rural people. Indian Public Health Standards for Community Health Centres have been prescribed under National Rural Health Mission to provide optimal specialized care to the community and achieve and maintain an acceptable standard of quality health care.

To maintain quality of services, external monitoring at appropriate intervals has been advocated. Guidelines are being provided for management of routine and emergency cases under the National Health Programme so as to maintain uniformity in Management in tune with the National Health Policy.

The minimum requirements are being projected based on an average bed occupancy of 60 per cent. It would be a dynamic process in the sense that if the utilization goes up the standards would be further upgraded. As regards to manpower, 2 specialists, namely Anesthetist and Public Health Programme Manager should be provided on contractual basis in addition to the available specialists, namely Surgery Medicine, obstetrics and Gynaecology and Paediatrics. The support manpower will include a Public Health Nurse and Auxiliary Nurse Midwife in addition to the existing staff. An ophthalmic Assistant will also be required to be provided in the centres where currently there is none.

It is mandatory for every Community Health Centre to have "*Rogi Kalyan Samiti*" to ensure accountability. Every Community Health Centre will have the charter of Patients' Rights displayed prominently at the entrance.

A grievance mechanism under the overall supervision of Rogi Kalyan Samiti should be set-up at the facility level. Each Community Health Centre should have the standard operating procedure and standard treatment protocols for common ailments social audit by involvement of the Community through Consumer Forum and Rogi Kalyan Samiti has been recommended and to maintain quality of services external monitoring through Panchayati Raj Institutions and internal monitoring at appropriate intervals are being advocated. Guidelines are being provided for management of routine and emergency cases under the National Health Programme so as to maintain uniformity in management in tune with the National Health Policy.

Strengthening of Public Health System including First Referral Units achieving 24 × 7 public health care facilities and improved quality of health care and access to safe delivery of the health services and Disease Control Programme and Medical Education strategies, regularly and Community Process, Training Programmes for staff for the skill upgradation to ensure need based appropriate health delivery services at facility level.

Bhadainya Block of the Sultanpur District has been selected for analyzing the delivery of the health system at the village panchayat level because most of the population of the area are suffering from the various communicable and non-communicable diseases.

The total fertility rate of the Uttar Pradesh is 5.3, the infant mortality rate is 61 and the maternal mortality rate is 259 which are higher than the National average.

Historical background of the study area has been extremely famous, honoured and appreciated Archaeologically, Historically, Culturally, Geographically and Industrially District Sultanpur has very important place. In spite of several continued changes, the identity of the Sultanpur has been permanent.

There are four Tehsils and fourteen Blocks in the Sultanpur District. There are 8 Nyaya panchayats and 63 Village Panchayats and 149 revenue villages in the Sultanpur District.

Physiographically Sultanpur District has been divided into two main physical divisions such as Northern Tract and Southern Tract. The plain is characterized by unrelieved monotony of alluvial deposits which completely should be old land surface to a depth of several thousand metres. The solid geology of the plain is totally obscured underneath the mantle.

There are no noteworthy features in the Physiognomy of the Sultanpur District. Geologically Sultanpur District has been divided into the ravine tract of Gomati River, central tract and the lake tract.

The Rivers which flow in the district Sultanpur are Gomati, Majhuai, and Mangar, Sultanpur District experience a rhythm of seasons with several of prevailing winds. The several of its regularly felt twice during the year. The rainfall during the months is scanty and sporadic. The annual rainfall of the study area is 1005 morbidity and mortality but it is unevenly distributed every year.

The older alluvial and saline and alkaline soils are the main soils found in the study area. The soils of the District are transported from the sedimentary rocks of the Himalayas and the products of decomposition of the rocks have been deposited over the tract through the water erosion. On the basis of the texture of the soils of the District the soils have been sub-divided into *Bangar*, Loamy soils, clayeye loam, clayey soil, *Khadar* soils, saline soils, saline and alkaline soils.

District Sultanpur has an almost inhabited human occupancy for over three millennia and centuries of plough and pastoral culture has reduced the natural vegetation except in the Pocket of Tarai and some river banks with a moderate and healthy climate and fertile soils, the District's Flora presents no peculiarities.

District Sultanpur has very important role in the ancient, historical periods. Important religious places of the District Sultanpur are Bijethua, Mahaviran, Pancho-Piran, Sultan Shah Sharmad Shah Baba, Dhopap, Sitakund, Loharamau, Pahalwan Bir Baba and Gadha.

In view of the above an attempt has been made in this study to explain the public health programme related to Maternal Health, Child Health, Family Planning, Routine Immunization and National Disease Control Programme at Sultanpur District. An effort has also been made to explain the progress of the public health system and also to analyse the management of the Public Health Programme related to Maternal Health, Child Health, Family Planning, Routine Immunization and implementation of various Disease Control programmes at the grassroots level and to progress of the public health system at the facility level and need based management of the public health system has been analyzed at the health facility level.

2

PUBLIC HEALTH PROGRAMMES

1. Introduction

There is a significant progress in improving the expectancy at birth, reducing mortality due to Malaria as well as reducing infant and maternal mortality. In spite of the progress made, a high proportion of the population, especially in the rural areas, continues to suffer and die from preventable diseases, pregnancy and child birth related complications as well as the malnutrition.

In addition to old unresolved problems, the health system is facing emerging threats and challenges. The rural Public Health Care System in the remote rural areas are in an unsatisfactory state leading to pauperization of poor households due to expensive private sector health care.

Our country is in the midst of an epidemiological and demographic transition with the attendant problems of increased chronic disease burden and a decline in mortality and fertility rates leading to an ageing of the Rural population.

Since independence, of our country 5 million people are living with HIV/AIDS, a threat which has the potential to undermine the health and development gains. Non-Communicable diseases such as cardio-vascular diseases, cancer, blindness, mental illness and tobacco use related illness have imposed the chronic disease burden on the already overstretched health care system.

Pre-mature morbidity and mortality from chronic disease can be major loss of economic and human resources for the rural people. The large disparity across the rural areas, the burden of these conditions mostly on the poor and on women scheduled caste and downtrodden sections of the society especially those who are living in the remote rural areas. The inequity is also reflected in the skewed availability of public resources between the advance and less developed areas.

The public spending on the prevention health services has a low priority over curative health. Indian Public Spending on Health is amongst the lowest in the world whereas its proportion of private spending on health is one of the highest. The private sector health care is unregulated pushing the cost of health care up and making it unaffordable for the rural poor.

Thus, it is clear that maintaining the health system in its present form will become untenable in the rural areas. Persistant malnutrition, high levels of anaemia amongst children and women, low age of marriage and first child birth, inadequate safe drinking water round the year in many villages, overcrowding of dwelling units, unsatisfactory state of sanitation and disposal of wastes constitute major challenges for the public health system in the rural areas.

Most of the public health determinants are correlated to high levels of poverty and to degradation of the environment in our villages. Thus, the rural areas have to deal with multiple health crisis, rising costs of the health care and mounting expectations of the people.

The challenge of the quality health services in the remote rural areas has to be met with a sense of urgency, given the scope and magnitude of the problems, it is no longer enough to focus on narrowly defined programmes. The urgent need is to transform the public health system into an accountable, accessible and affordable system of health services in the remote rural areas.

2. Objectives of the Rural Health Programmes

The important objectives of the rural health programmes are as follows:

- Reduction of child and maternal mortality.
- Universal access to public services for food, nutrition, sanitation, hygiene, and universal to Public Health care services with emphasis on services addressing women's and children's health and universal immunization.
- Prevention and control of Communicable and Non-Communicable Diseases including locally endemic diseases.
- Access to integrated comprehensive Primary Health.
- Population stabilization, gender and demographic balance.
- Revitalize local health traditions and mainstream AYUSH.
- Promotion of Healthy Lifestyle.

3. Rural Health Programmes

Important rural health programmes are as follows:

- Reproductive and Child Health Programme-II and Janani Suraksha Yojana launched.
- Polio eradication programme intensified cases reduced from 134 in 2004-05 to 62 up to now.
- Sterilization Compensation scheme launched.
- Accelerated implementation of the Routine Immunization Programme taken up, catch up rounds initiated.
- Ground work for introduction of Japanese Encephalitis vaccine completed.
- Auto Disabled Syringes introduced.
- State Programme Implementation Plans for Reproductive Child Health-II appraised by the National Programme coordination committee set up by the Ministry of Health and Family Welfare, Government of India.

❑ *Infrastructure*

- Facility survey introduced.
- Repair and renovation of Sub-Centre under Reproductive Child Health-II.
- Untied funds for ₹ 10,000 to each Sub-Health Centre.
- Selection of two Community Health Centres in each state for upgradation to Indian Public Health Standards.
- Upgradation of Community Health Centre as First Referral Units and Primary Health Centres to 24 × 7 units taken up.
- Release of funds for upgradation of two Community Health Centres per District to Indian Public Health Standards.

❑ *District Plans*

- Strengthening of Planning Processes.
- Accredited Social Health Activists selected.
- Training of the State/District level trainers of Accredited Social Health Activists completed and District level training taken up.

❑ *Procurement*

- An Empowered Procurement Wing is being set up in the Ministry of Health and Family Welfare.
- Procurement of procedures are being finalized and procedural assistance being provided to the state in the procurement activities.

❑ *Technical Support*

- A National Health System Resources Centre set up at the National Level.
- 700 consultants (MBA/CA) appointed for State/District Level Programme Management Units.

❑ *Training*

- Comprehensive Training strategy finalized.
- Training started on skill Birth Attendant.

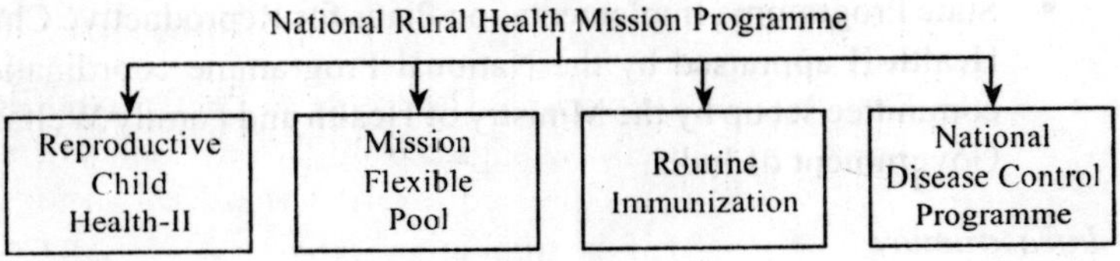

4. Reproductive Child Health Flexible Pool

Reproductive Child Health Flexible Pool Programmes under the National Rural Health Mission (NRHM) are as follows:

4.1. *Maternal Health*

The programme on the maternal health under the National Rural Health Mission are as follows:

4.1.1. *Key Maternal Health Indicators*

- An Ante Natal Care.
- 3+ Ante Natal Care.
- Registration with 12 weeks.
- Institutional Delivery.
- Safe Delivery (Home by Skill Birth Attendant).
- Home Delivery.
- C-Sections out of institutional deliveries —
  - At Public
  - At Private
- Anaemic women and severely anaemic and Pregnant Women.

To ensure appropriate Maternal Health System fully functional First Referral Unit and fully functional First Referral Unit 24 × 7 at

Primary Health Centres and functional licensed Blood Banks and licensed Blood storage units. Village Health and Nutrition Doctors and Trained Skilled Birth Attendants and other trained personnel should be employed with the view to provide appropriate maternal health services at the village level.

4.1.2. *Janani Suraksha Yojana*

I. *Home Deliveries:* The estimated live births for the 2013-14 has been 51 lakhs in Uttar Pradesh under the Janani Suraksha Yojana for the home deliveries (Number of Below Poverty Line Home Deliveries by skilled Birth Attendants has been kept at 15,000).

II. *Institutional Deliveries:* The target of institutional deliveries has been reduced as suggested by Government of India. The budget has been estimated for the target 25 lakh for 2013-14 year. The ratio of the rural/urban deliveries has been maintained as planned by the district, i.e. 89 per cent rural and 11 per cent urban deliveries.

III. *Budget Estimates:* Revised budget for Janani Suraksha Yojana has been ₹ 47,124 lakh inclusive of 5 per cent administrative cost and 1 per cent administrative budget are being spent on the State level information, education and communication activities under the maternal health and strengthening of the maternal health cell at the State Programme Management Unit and Janani Suraksha Yojana cell at the Directorate of Family Welfare.

4.1.3. *Janani Shishu Suraksha Yojana*

An appropriate budgetary provision has been made to ensure free drugs and consumables which include outreach support.

State of Uttar Pradesh has proposed free diagnostic services through Village Health and Nutrition Days (VHNDs). It has been proposed that rapid diagnostic test kit will be used for VHNDs and diagnostic equipments will also be provided from the budget. As per approval of the Government of India, the cost of rapid diagnostic kits and diagnostic equipments has also been covered.

An appropriate budget has been allocated for free diet to the women beneficiaries in which provision of free diet at the rate of ₹ 100 per beneficiary per day has also been included.

Requisite budget has also been allocated for free drop back. The 102 and 108 ambulance services are being operationalized fully. It has been believed that the Referral Transport are being provided to more number of beneficiaries.

4.1.4. *Operationalization of Comprehensive Abortion Care Services*

The Safe abortion care services has been planned and strengthened at the District level. The activities and budget has been planned to promote proper functioning of District level committee:

— Regular inspection and review to register new facilities.
— Monitor equality of services in all register of site.
— Strengthen record keeping and reporting from all the service sites at the District Level Committee and from District Level Committee to the State Level is planned to be undertaken in the forthcoming year. The operationalization of comprehensive abortion care services are as follows:
  - Strengthening of District Level Committees.
— Contingency support for District Level Committees, Printing of facility log books, Printing of Certification booklet, consent forms facility reporting system to be institutionalized.
— Quarterly Meeting of District Level Committee with certified service providers.
— State level reviews are being ensured with comprehensive Maternal Health Review.

4.1.5. *Maternal Death Review*

The close monitoring is being ensured for the implementation of the maternal death reporting and review programmes.

1. *Old Activities:* It has been estimated that 80 per cent deaths will be reported and 60 per cent will be audited by block teams and facilities. Quarterly reviews and media workshops will be conducted at quarterly basis at each division to spread messages for maternal death reporting from all quarters.
   District will conduct one day orientation of Maternal Death Review team from each facility and conduct monthly review.
   The contingency support at the Block level has been proposed for printing of all forms.
   Audit by independent Audit Teams have been planned in the high focus district under 5 divisions with Maternal Mortality

Rate > 400 lakh live births. A sum of ₹ 3000 per team has been budgeted for each review visit. Thus, an 80 per cent of total expected 6,980 maternal deaths, i.e. 5,584 maternal death has been expected to be done by them.

II. *New Activities:* An incentive for primary informers for reporting a maternal death has been increased to ₹ 200 per case. The New Activity has been budgeted under the Accredited Social Health Activists incentives.

The orientation of Primary Informers — Accredited Social Health Activists/Anganwadi Workers/Panchayati Raj Institutions and other with appeal to Pradhans has been proposed at each Block level by the Medical Officer Incharge. Budget has also been planned @ ₹ 50 per person. Number has been decided based on the number of functional Accredited Social Health Activists × 3 in the District for ease of calculation.

Support for analysis of Data and its dissemination has been provided by United Nations Children Education's Fund. Therefore, no budgetary proposal has been made for this activity.

4.1.6. *Maternal Health Review Workshops/Meeting*

State of Uttar Pradesh has proposed 9 review workshops/meetings at various levels in which 4 quarterly review workshops/meetings would be organized at the State Level and 4 Zonal Level review workshops/ meetings at 4 zones and one National Level review/workshop/meetings.

4.1.7. *Human Resources*

The human resources has been proposed at various levels under the Maternal Health Programmes.

4.1.8. *Training*

Training programmes have been proposed at various levels under maternal health programmes.

MTP Training under MTP Act has been proposed to be provided to MBBS doctors. It has been proposed that 100 doctors should be trained and certified by the District Level Centres. No additional budget has been planned for this training activity.

Thus, 5 days training of 90 doctors and nurses has been planned under the training activity by State Institute of Health and Family Welfare.

4.1.9. *Information, Education and Communication*

Information, Education and Communication activities have been carried out under the Maternal Health Programme which includes printing of "Safe Motherhood Booklets".

Further, two campaigns — *chance kyo lena Hai* and *Chaar Gaanth* has also been proposed to promote maternal health services.

Additionally there are some other activities like wall writing 10 × 8 sq.ft. @ ₹ 10.00 per sq.ft. at block level. One wall painting in each block and sub-centre and Natal Care and Pre Natal Care and Stay at 48 hours in the Hospital which will be met from village Health Nutrition and Sanitation Committee, Untied Fund. It has also been proposed for hoardings 4 per district and 2 per block at the size of 20 × 10 sq.ft. of Janani Suraksha Yojana and Janani Shishu Suraksha Yojana which will be met from 1 per cent Janani Suraksha Yojana Administrative Budget.

4.1.10. *Procurement*

The procurement of Drugs, equipments and consumables under the Maternal Health Programmes are as follows:

I. Equipments Cost for Maternal Health

Sl.No.	*Name of Equipment*	*No. of Proposed Equipments*	*Unit Cost*	*Total Budget (lakh ₹)*
1.	MVA/EVA for safe Abortion Services	866	2500	21.65
2.	Establishment of New Sub-Centres	1,000	—	450.00

Thus, a total budget of ₹ 471.65 lakh has been proposed for the procurement of equipments for the Maternal Health.

II. Drugs and Supplies for Maternal Health

Sl.No.	*Name of Equipment*	*Quantity*	*Unit Cost*	*Total Budget (lakh ₹)*
1.	Drugs for safe abortion	2,500	200	50.00
2.	RTI/STI Drugs	75	—	1,259.09
3.	RPR Kits	75	—	22.66

Thus, a total budget of ₹ 1,331.75 lakh has been proposed for the procurement of drugs under Maternal Health.

4.2. *Child Health*

Infant Mortality Rate has been declining very slowly and the State of Uttar Pradesh has initiated to celebrate the year 2013-14 as a year of *Navjat Shishu Suraksha Varsha*.

Trained Accredited Social Health Activists at the community level are paying home visits 6/7 times to each of the mother up to 42 days after delivery, so as to provide care to the mother and Neonate and accordingly action has been suggested by the Accredited Social Health Activists including referral services.

4.2.1. *Facility Based Interventions*

- *Sick New Born Care Units (SNCUs)* — Institutional deliveries in Uttar Pradesh are increasing at various facilities. Sometimes, there is a need of emergency care of the Neonates. To reduce the Neonatal and Pre-Natal deaths, all facilities of level-III type should be made available for sick new born care units in the hospital.
- *New Born Stabilization Units (NBSUs)* — Where there is no sick New Born care units at the level-III health facilities, 4 bedded New Born Stabilization Units have been established to stabilize sick neonates and to work as referral units for level-II and level-I facilities.
- *New Born Care Corners (NBCCs)* — New Born Care Corners have been established in each labour room of L-3 and L-2 facilities to prevent birth, asphyxia, hypothermia and infections. The staff members working in the labour rooms have been trained in the Navjat Shishu Suraksha Karyakarm and equipment handling skills. This year onwards L-1 facilities (Primary Health Centres and Accredited Sub-Centres) will be strengthened and New Born Care Corners will be established along with Navjat Shishu Suraksha Karyakarma and equipment handling training.
- *Nutrition Rehabilitation Centres (NRCs)* — To manage Service Acute Malnutrition (SAM) cases 26 Nutrition Rehabilitation Centres, including 5 in the Medical Colleges, have been established and made operational by March 2013. Additionally, 2 Nutrition Rehabilitation Centres have been proposed for establishing in the District Male Hospital during the year 2013-14.

Details of the above functional units in Sultanpur District are as follows:

4.2.2. *Status of SNCUs, NBSUs, NBCCs and NRCs in Sultanpur*

It has been observed that there is no Sick New Born Care and Nutrition Rehabilitation Centre in Sultanpur District while 2 New Born Stabilization units and 12 New Born Care Corners are functional in Sultanpur District.

Status of SNCUs, NBSUs, NBCCs and NRCs in Sultanpur District

Name of the District/State	*SNCUs*	*NBSUs*	*NBCCs*	*NRCs*
Sultanpur	0	2	12	0
Uttar Pradesh	27	110	996	26

4.2.3. *Priorities to Reduce Neonatal Deaths*

Priorities to reduce Neonatal deaths are as follows:

- *Sick New Born Care Units:* It has been planned to establish 27 Sick New Born Care Units out of which 15 Sick New Born Care Units have been made functional and 12 are under progress.
- *New Born Stabilization Units:* There are 92 New Born Stabilization Units. Where there was no Sick New Born Stabilization Units will soon have these units. Therefore, the target of 117 units have been prioritized.
- *New Born Care Corners:* There are 996 New Born Care Corners established in all labour rooms in the District Women Hospital, Community Health Centres and Primary Health Centres. The target for New Born Care Corners is 1430 units and the accredited centre will also be covered during the year.
- *Nutrition Rehabilitation Centres:* There are 26 Nutrition Rehabilitation Centres made functional out of which 24 Nutrition Rehabilitation Centres are made functional this year.

4.2.4. *Human Resource*

Required human resources for the child health are as follows:

I. *Sick New Born Care Units:* Presently, there are 27 Sick New Born Care Units in the District Women Hospital of 3 Paediatricians (MD/DCH) and 6 staff nurses at the District level Sick New Born Care units.

II. *New Born Stabilization Units:* The Doctor and the staff working in the Hospitals are managing the New Born Stabilization Units. They are being trained for Navjat Shishu Suraksha Karyakrama.

III. *New Born Care Corners:* The Doctor and the Staff Working in the hospitals are managing the New Born Care Corners. They are also being trained for Navjat Shishu Suraksha Karyakrama and equipment handling. The human resources are being proposed at various levels under Child Health Programme.

4.2.5. *Training*

Various training programmes have been proposed at different levels under the Child Health Programme. The present status of the training under Child Health Programme is as under:

- *Navjat Shishu Suraksha Karyakrama Training:* The staff posted at the delivery points are trained for Navjat Shishu Suraksha Karyakrama. Training programme for 2 days was arranged. The Medical Officer/Staff Nurse/Auxiliary Nurse Midwife posted at Level-2 and Level-3 have been trained.
- *Essential New Born Care Equipment Training:* All the staff trained for Navjat Shishu Suraksha Karyakrama working at delivery points has been provided one day equipment handling training for the use and maintenance of equipment.
- *Home Based New Born Care (Community Based Inventions):* It has been proposed to provide 10 days training to Accredited Social Health Activists. An incentive of ₹ 250 is being provided to Accredited Social Health Activist after providing the following services —
    - Ensuring Birth Registration.
    - Ensuring BCG and Zero Dose Polio.
    - Ensuring Recording of Birth Weight.
- Conducting 6/7 Post Natal Visits for Mothers and Neonates and ensuring baby alive up to 42 day.

It has been recorded that up to March 2013 about 50,000 Accredited Social Health Activists are trained and during the year 2013-14 about 15,000 Accredited Social Health Activists are being trained. An incentive of ₹ 250 per child for 12 months to already trained has been provided. ASHAs and for those ASHAs who are being trained the incentive is for 9 months only.

4.2.6. *Home Based New Born Care Drug Kits*

The provision of Home Based New Born Care Drug kit is to ensure availability of the basic medicines at the level of ASHAs like Syrup Paracetamole, Syrup Contrimoxazole and Gentian violet, so that she can provide basic community care to the New Born. These drug kits are provided to trained ASHAs who have undergone training of Navjat Shishu Suraksha Karyakrama.

4.2.7. *Printing of Formats*

Printing of Home Based New Born Care Formats has been proposed for the Post Natal Visits. The printing of Job aids and tools has also been ensured.

4.2.8. *Infant Young Child Feeding*

It has been established that 13 per cent Infant Mortality Rate can be reduced only by exclusive breast feeding and if timely complementary feeding initiated, then 6 per cent deaths may be reduced. Hence, to create awareness and promote Infant Young Child Feeding practices, World Breast Feeding Week is being celebrated every year from 1st to 7th August for this funds have been asked but Government of India has not approved and kept it as pending.

The key features of Infant Young Child Feeding as per operational guidelines of the Government of India are as follows:

- Development of State Plan of Action and its release during breast feeding week.
- Breast feeding week celebration across 75 districts and 820 blocks.
- Orientation of Child Medical Officers on the IMS Act.
- Skill based training on Infant Young Child Feeding in 10 high priority districts using existing master trainers available in the State.
- Information, Education and Communication activities during breast feeding week and in institutions.

4.2.9. *Management of Diarrhoea*

The diarrhoea is one of the major causes of the Child Death. There is National Policy for Management of Diarrhoea among children less than 5 years which recommends the use of Zinc tablets along with ORS in the treatment of diarrhoea as per the Ministry of Health and Family Welfare, Government of India directive dated 2nd November, 2006.

The Revised Diarrhoea Management Policy recommends for every case of diarrhoea, a dose of Zinc 20 mg/day for 14 days (even if diarrhoea has stopped) for children above age 6 months to 5 years and 10 mg/day for 15 days old for 2-6 months. However, the ORS use rate is only 17.3. as compared to the National Average of 34.2. The Zinc use rate is very minimal.

The development patterns like Micro-Nutrition Initiative are providing active support in this programme. A detailed guideline of the treatment protocol and implementation strategy of childhood diarrhoea and shared with health and Integrated Child Development Scheme Counterparts. The guideline emphasizes on capacity building of functionaries (Medical Officers/Incharges, ANMs, Supervisors, ASHAs, AWWs of departments, timely procurement and usage of supply, intensive monitoring and promoting use of Zinc and ORS for treatment of Diarrhoea.

4.2.10. *Bal Swasthya Poshan Mah*

The Vitamin A supplementation programme in Uttar Pradesh is in the line with Government of India, policy of ensuring I doses of Vitamin-A supplementation for children between 9 months to 59 months age groups. The strategy for administering Vitamin-A is to provide first dose along with the measles in the age group of 9 months. The second dose onwards Vitamin-A supplementation has to be done through a bi-annual exercise at a six months interval.

- *Bi-annual Bal Swasthya Poshan Mah*

State of Uttar Pradesh is implementing bi-annual strategy in the form of bi-annual Bal Swasthya Poshan. Under the Bio-annual Bal Swasthya Poshan Strategy, two months, *viz*. June and December, six months apart have been identified as health and nutrition months. During these months, health sector is assigned with the task of providing immunization and other services to the beneficiaries by organizing intensive social mobilization and information, education and communication activities. These bi-annual months have been linked to village-wise routine immunization sessions organized as per the immunization/outreach sessions micro plan of Auxiliary Nurse Midwife.

The Programme is being implemented jointly by the Directorate of Family Welfare and Integrated Child Development Scheme with the support of development partners mainly UNICEF and Micro nutrient initiative.

During the Bi-annual rounds, vitamin-A is administered along with other high impact interventions, which are crucial for child survival and development. Package of these services include immunization catch up, advice on breast feeding and complementary feeding, screening and referral for severely malnourished children and education and demand generation for iodized salt.

The Bi-annual Bal Swasthya Poshan Programme focuses on strengthening joint health and ICDS Planning and interrupted supplies. It has been observed that the coverage has been on decline since last one and half years due to supply bottleneck.

4.2.11. *Information, Education and Communication Activities*

Under the child health programme, to carry out Information, Education and Communication activities a budget of ₹ 18.69 lakh has been proposed for 2013-14 year.

4.2.12. *Procurement*

Under the Child Health Programme, a total budget of ₹ 200.52 lakh has been proposed for the procurement of equipments and ₹ 1415.13 lakh has been proposed for the procurement of drugs and supplies.

4.3. *Family Planning*

"The Population Policy looks at the issues related to population stabilization and improvement of the health status of the people, particularly women and children in a holistic manner."

Total fertility rate of Uttar Pradesh has declined from 4.1 to 3.8 as per National Family Health Survey 2 and 3. However, compared to the National average of 2.7, the rates are still very high. To enhance the performance of Family Planning, it is important to meet the desired unmet needs. The unmet need for spacing method has increased from 9 per cent to 1998-99 to 12 per cent in 2005-07. As per the projections in the Population Policy of Uttar Pradesh (2000) to reach the policy objectives of a replacement level of total fertility rate of 2.1 by 2016, 12.1 lakh couples should be provided for limiting method of family planning.

4.3.1. *Family Planning Management Activities*

Regular review of Family Planning performance is being done at State/ District/Divisional level review meetings on monthly basis. District performance reports are reviewed in detail special attention is given to discuss the problems and issues leading to low/poor performance in the Districts. The measures are taken to resolve the issues of poor performing districts.

In view of the frequent transfers and change of district's functionaries, it is important to conduct dissemination workshop at the various levels. It has been proposed to conduct one state level workshop and 4 batches in one workshop per district.

4.3.2. *Terminal/Limiting Method (Providing Sterilization) Services*

Two fixed day services "under fixed day sterilization service" (Legation/ abdominal/Tubectomy) has been continued at all District Women Hospitals/Combined Hospitals/Community Health Centres having either a surgeon or Gynaecologist.

Preferably, Tuesdays and Fridays have been fixed for such service. However, any other day may be fixed as per suitability in consultation with the Chief Medical Officer. Wide publicity of fixed days would be ensured through wall writing, leaflets, brouchers, etc.

A separate register would be maintained to record number of sterilizations conducted on the fixed days, including the details of the clients and the surgeon conducting the sterilization.

The provision of fixed day for NSV (Non-Scalpel Vasectomy) Service at each district Male Hospital/Combined Hospital and First Referral Units will continue. Any day may be fixed in consultation with the Chief Medical Officer. Wide publicity of the fixed days would be ensured through wall writing, leaflets, brochures, etc.

In order to achieve the target of sterilization, each district organizes sterilization camps at Block or Tehsil level on regular basis. Expenditure on these camps relating to compensation money to client and medicines, etc. is borne by the compensation head for female sterilization.

In view of the low performance (still shortage of service providers, so the fixed day/daily services are not available at every facility) of sterilization, it is now proposed to provide funds for Female Sterilization Camps.

Besides providing Non-Scalpel Vasectomy (NSV) Services on regular basis, it is proposed that each district hospital will organize at least 2-12 NSV camps per year depending on their performance and client load.

4.3.3. *Accreditation of Private Centre's/Non-Governmental Organizations for Sterilization Services*

It has been noticed that there are certain hindrances because of which private nursing homes and centres have not been accredited. For this purpose a budget of ₹ 1.00 lakh is required for organizing a state level workshop in 2 batches at State level to address the issues in Accreditation of Private Centres/Nursing Homes to increase the sterilization services. At the district level one workshop per district with private nursing homes, has been proposed for offering Family Planning services and increase the acceptance of family planning services through private sector.

4.3.4. *Plans for Post Partum Sterilization*

Family Welfare counsellors have been deployed. Taking the large number of institutional delivery under Janani Suraksha Yojana scheme the Family Planning Counsellors are being deployed. They will have the opportunity to reach all the mothers and they will counsel the women and address their concern for small family norms. They will also counsel for adaptation of Post Partum Family Planning method. It has been proposed to deploy 1 family welfare counsellor at those facility centres where more than 150 deliveries are being done during two months. Thus, the number of the required counsellors will be 345.

4.3.5. *Spacing Method*

The expected number of cases of IUD insertion are 14,35,044 for which budget of ₹ 287 @ ₹ 20 is required. During this year fixed days for services are being proposed at the L-1 Centres (1563) @ ₹ 5,000 per year to meet logistic supplies to organize these fixed days.

4.3.6. *Performance Based Rewards to Institutions and Service Provider*

To encourage the service providers and for better community mobilization for family planning services, it has been proposed to give performance based rewards to the facility service provider, Auxiliary Nurse Midwife, Accredited Social Health Activists. This will help to enhance acceptance of programme in the community along with motivation of the service providers and boosting up their performance level.

4.3.7. *Incentives for ASHA*

To promote permanent method of Family Planning after only 2 children

@ ₹ 1,000 per case incentive for ASHA has been provided for 13,268 cases in Uttar Pradesh.

4.3.8. *Social Marketing of Contraceptives*

Social marketing of contraceptives has been implemented. Under this, condom promotion and oral contraceptive pills, are being made available through conventional and unconventional retail outlets and community based depot holders.

4.3.9. *Other Strategies/Activities*

Two strategies/activities have been proposed —

I. Orientation of District Nodal Officers for change in Family Planning Beema Policy.
II. Family Planning Indemnity Scheme.

4.3.10. *Human Resources*

Human Resource has been proposed under Family Planning at various levels for which an amount of ₹ 2147.46 lakh has been proposed.

4.3.11. *Training*

Various training programmes have been proposed under Family Planning Programme. For clinical Family Planning Training, SIFPSA has been designated as nodal agency. The requirement of funds for NSV, Laparoscopic, Abdominal Tubectomy, IUCD Training, PPIUCD for Medical Officer Training and FWC Training for meeting the set objectives will be required.

4.3.12. *Information, Education and Communication*

Under the family planning programme child health, three information, education and communication campaign have been proposed. These campaigns are proposed by UNFA/USAID "Ek Teen Do". Information, Education and Communication activities under the family planning are proposed in order to promote spacing and small family norms demand generation for IUCD/PPIUCD and other spacing methods. "World Population Day" is being celebrated in Uttar Pradesh for which a sum of ₹ 159.0 lakh budget has been proposed.

4.3.13. *Procurement*

The following procurement has been proposed under the family planning programme:

- *Procurement of Drugs Materials:* It has been planned to procure IUD Kits, NSV Kits and Minilap kits for which total sum of ₹ 119.04 lakh has been proposed.
- *Maintenance of Laparoscopes and Annual Maintenance Cost:* Uttar Pradesh State has approximately 1,500 laparoscopes out of which 20 per cent expected to need repairing, etc. At average rate of ₹ 40,000 per unit has been proposed for the year 2013-14.

4.3.14. *Public Private Partnership Activities Under Family Planning*

Clinical outreach model for strengthening sterilization services — Mostly all sterilization services are provided by the government sector. However, still there is an unmet need that exist compounded with a serious need for quality of Care. In order to supplement a state government's efforts to provide quality family planning service State has proposed to take help of Marie Stopes India on the same model as they are helping Government of Rajasthan.

Marie Stopes India's clinical outreach model is a combination of Marie Stopes International Mobile Clinical Services delivery team approach quality improvement team approach and mobile community outreach worker approach.

The Partnership with the government happens in two years —

I. Logistic and Demand Generation support's India's Team provides logistic and demand generation to the government technical team to conduct sterilization with quality of care on sterilization days.
II. Service Provision along with logistic support: Marie Stopes India's Clinical Outreach Team conducts the procedures too in facilities which do not have the requisite providers, especially in the remote area.

On the predetermined days Marie Stopes India's Team not only provides the logistics support as above but also the services.

In addition to the above, the support also includes:

- Setting up the facility especially the operation theatre.

- Provide all equipments, consumables and medicines.
- Arrange post-operative hardware, like beds, mattresses, quilts, pillows, etc.
- Complete all documents as per the government norms.
- Provide the financial compensation to the clients and the motivators as per Government of India norms.
- Provide ambulance as per requirement.
- Completed documents will then be presented to the concerned District Chief Medical Officer for reimbursement as per Government norms, i.e. ₹ 1,500 per case in case of any complication. Marie Stopes will treat the patient on their own cost.

Thus, all these facts are included in the form of Memorandum of Understanding between State Government and Marie Stopes India. Hence, no additional expenditure/budget are required for the same activity.

4.4. *Adolescent Reproductive and Sexual Health (ARSH)*

It has been proposed to appoint Health Counsellor in the District Male and Female Hospitals at the rate of ₹ 12,000 per month per honoraria.

Training of the Health Counsellor has been conducted by State Institute of the Health and Family Welfare.

It has been proposed to give basic salary of ₹ 10,000 per month to all the counsellors with a mobility support of about ₹ 4,000 per month/ per counsellor as an incentive and mobility to visit one school of the vicinity per day for 20 days in the month which has not been approved. Hence, this proposal is being sent to the Government of India for consideration.

- *Training* — To identify, diagnose and treat various diseases of adolescent age group include ASHAs, AWWs, ANMs and Medical Officers are being trained under Adolescent Reproductive and Sexual Health.
- *Menstrual Hygiene* — In school going adolescent girls, problems during menstrual period and lack of knowledge constraints school attendance and possibly contribute to infections related issues of the personal hygiene. Weekly Iron Folic Acid and bi-annual de-worming tablet is also being provided to the non-school going adolescent girls by ASHAs in the rural areas in

addition to provision of subsidized sanitary napkins by Government of India.

To address the issue of anaemia in adolescent age group, weekly, bi-annual De-worming tablets are being provided for non-school going girls covered by Integrated Child Development Schemes. ANM and Health Volunteers/AYUSH Lady Doctors address issue of health, personal hygiene and nutrition arising in adolescent age group during monthly meeting organized by ASHA for Kishories with the support of Anganwadi workers.

4.4.1. *Rashtriya Bal Swasthya Karyakrama*

An expanded scheme for School Health Programme has been launched to cover health examination, treatment and referral of all the children of age 2-19 in the rural areas of the State. The scheme is being implemented in a phased manner.

❑ *Ist Phase*

Initially, the scheme is being implemented through covering school going children of all Government Schools from Class 1 to 10.

The Health examination are being conduced through a dedicated Medical team consisting of one Doctor, one Female Nursing Staff and one Paramedical Personnel. Two such Teams are being recruited on contact in each Block to visit pre-decided school as per micro plan prepared at the Block level and general examination of each child is being done with a focus on 3Ds — Disease, Deficiency and Disability. Even child is being provided with bi-annual de-worming tablets and weekly, bi-weekly IFA tablet syrup to prevent Anaemia.

❑ *IInd Phase*

School children of the Government schools up to class-12 and Government Aided Schools like Madarasas, Sanskrit Schools, Schools of Informal education are covered under the scheme along with children below 6 years of age attending Anganwadi School.

As per the guidelines of the Government of India, children of six weeks onwards are being screened for birth defects, diseases, deficiencies and disabilities by ANMs/ASHAs and Anganwadi Workers. Such children are referred to *District Early Intervention Centres* which has to be established at District level Hospitals. One paediatrician, one medical officer, one dentist, one audiologist, one optometrist, nutritionist and counsellors are the core team of District Early Intervention Centres.

To have real time reporting system it is proposed to make use of Information Technology and implement the best technology options available for Daily Monitoring Framework:

(i) An automated call shall be generated to Head Master or the nodal teacher incharge in each school.
(ii) Head Master or teacher incharge will punch the relevant information on the keypad of his/her mobile.
(iii) The information is passed on the Daily Monitoring Framework.
(iv) The analysis reports are made available on Internet Portal.
(v) SMSs will be sent to concerned CMOs, Medical Officer Incharges, District Project Manager, Divisional Project Manager, District Magistrate, Programme Officer, Mission Director at the State level.

The Daily monitoring system would use the following technologies —

- Telephony Cluster without bound dialling.
- SMS gateway (supporting incoming and outgoing Messages).
- Daily Monitoring Portal Framework.
- Call Centres (7 seats) for the Project to Handle information requirements of the stakeholders.
- Three Tier Data centre and disaster recovery site as part of Disaster Recovery Mechanism.

The functionalities/features of the Daily Monitoring System will be flexible and will have provision for multiple tries for contacting head master/teacher, will have provision for teacher to inform that he/she is on leave to receive automated call to report data. The Daily Monitoring System will be designed to schedule the visit of Medical Team to each school for 15 days.

4.4.2. *Human Resource*

Under the Adolescent Reproductive and Sexual Health Programme, Human resource has been proposed at various levels.

4.4.3. *Training*

Under the Adolescent Reproductive and Sexual Health Programme, various training programmes have been proposed at various levels.

4.4.4. *Information, Education and Communication*

Under the Adolescent Reproductive and Sexual Health Programme to carry out Information, Education and Communication activities a budget of ₹ 40.79 lakh has been proposed and for the school health programme ₹ 502.96 lakh has been proposed.

4.4.5. *Procurement*

Under the Adolescent Reproductive and Sexual Health Programme a total budget of ₹ 23.80 lakh has been proposed for the procurement of equipments and ₹ 247.09 lakh has been proposed for the procurement of drugs and supplies.

4.5. ***PCPNDT and Sex Ratio***

The sex ratio is an important indicator to measure gender equity. The rapidly increasing sex ratio in Uttar Pradesh is likely to create severe gender imbalance that can destroy thé social fabric. It should also be viewed both as child right issues (girls are killed either through sex selective abortions or die prematurely due to violence and neglect).

The 'Civil Registration' data clearly indicates that the sex ratio is declining in most of the commonly viable areas where sonography centres are in abundance indicating a direct correlation. Nearly about 4,430 centres have been registered under the PCPNDT Act in Uttar Pradesh.

It has been well known fact that it is difficult to regulate the private sector and therefore, initiatives to monitor the implementation of the PCPNDT Act together with social reform efforts including enhancing the value of a daughter is a significant step towards the prevention of female foeticide.

— A PCPNDT Cell has been established at the Directorate of Family Welfare.
— A separate divisional level PCPNDT Cell is being established at the Divisional Additional Director's office.
— It has also been planned to establish a separate District level PCPNDT Cell at the office of the Chief Medical Officer. The cell will work on line data reporting on web portal of PCPNDT on regular basis.

❑ *State Inspection and Monitoring Committee*

The Inspection and Monitoring Committee at State level has been established which will undertake inspection of Ultrasound centres in the

10 worst districts. It has been estimated that for each inspection visit around ₹ 10,000 would be incurred for one visit per district.

❑ *Divisional Level Inspection and Monitoring Committee*

A separate divisional level inspection and Monitoring Committee is being constituted which will ensure inspection and monitoring of the centres in the districts of the division.

❑ *Review Meeting at the State Level*

It has been proposed to review the activities conducted by the district for implementation of the PCPNDT Act, District Nodal Officer would participate in these meetings. Two batches of meeting would be required to be conducted to cover all the districts.

❑ *State Level Meeting of Committee*

Three committees have been constituted at the State level under the PCPNDT Act. These Committees would meet at Regular intervals to review the activities under PCPNDT and suggest necessary actions to be taken, if required.

❑ *State Level Orientation Workshop*

It has been proposed to conduct State level orientation workshop involving different stakeholders including different doctors, District Magistrates, Divisional Assistants, representatives from Non-Governmental Organizations from the legal field, social welfare departments, women and child welfare departments, District Administration and Panchayati Raj Institutions. Other participants will be members from Indian Medical Association, Nursing Home Association, Gynaecologists, Radiologists, Ultrasonologists.

❑ *Gender Sterilization Workshop*

Considering the state need of gender mainstreaming and PCPNDT Act owners, it has been proposed that one day's sensitization workshop should be organized in the high focus areas.

❑ *State Level Information Education Communication Activities*

To create awareness about the decreasing sex ratio and PCPNDT Act to the masses, state of Uttar Pradesh proposed to conduct Information, Education and Communication activities through electronic media

(Doordarshan and Akashvani) and advertisement in Newspapers. Other Information, Education and Communication activities like print media (wall painting, hoardings, banners, posters, display boards, etc.) are being ensured by the Districts.

❑ *Training/Capacity Building of Inspection Teams*

Appropriate training capacity building of the Inspection Team are conducted regarding the processes of inspections and record keeping and filing of the cases has been planned.

❑ *Orientation of Members of the District Advisory Committee*

District level Advisory Committee has been constituted. The Members of the Committee are required to be oriented regarding their role and responsibilities. Accordingly, it has been proposed to conduct one day orientation meeting of the functionaries.

❑ *District Level Inspections and Monitoring*

The inspection of centres are being done at district level on regular basis. In this activity registration/renewal fees can be utilized.

❑ *District Level Sensitization Workshop*

One day District Level workshop would be organized for creating publicity regarding need to address discrimination against girl child and creating awareness regarding the provisions of PCPNDT Act and its enforcement. Various stakeholders in the District would be sensitized through organizing two sessions of the sensitization workshop:

I. *First Session* — For Medical Officer, NGOs officials from the Department of Women and Child Development, Social Welfare, Panchayati Raj, Human Rights Commission.
II. *Second Session* — For Representatives of Indian Medical Association, Nursing Home Association, Gynaecologist, Radiologist, Ultrasonologist, etc. To conduct these activities an amount of ₹ 10,000 has been allocated to each District.

4.5. *Infrastructure and Human Resources*

Human Resources for Maternal Health, Child Health, Family Planning, Adolescent, Reproductive and Sexual Health/School Health, Routine Immunization, Dental Doctors, Para Medical and others have been analyzed in details.

4.5.1. *Human Resource—Maternal Health*

Under Maternal Health there is requirement of human resources at delivery points with the following details:

(i) *Contractual ANMs on Vacant Posts for Outreach Services:* The extra support of contractual ANMs for level-I sub-centre. Level-I facilities availability on Auxiliary Nurse Midwife is necessary for all 24 hours to look after women in labour and outreach or delivery care services do not get neglected. Additional ANMs are required to be placed at Level-I delivery points based on their delivery load on contract from the National Rural Health Mission to facilitate outreach as well as delivery and sub-centre clinic (services).

(ii) *Proposal for Human Resources at Level-2 (24 × 7) Delivery Points:*

- **Staff Nurse** — It has been proposed by the Government of Uttar Pradesh that at least 3 staff nurses are required to operationalize a 24 × 7 delivery point and at least 9 staff nurses required at Functional First Referral Units. A total of 1,319 staff nurses have been proposed to be hired on contract to maintain quality of services at functional Level-2 delivery points during the year 2013-14 @ ₹ 18,000 per month.
- **MBBS Lady Doctors** — 100 functional 24 × 7 centres in Uttar Pradesh get referral from sub-centres and now catering to maximum load of normal deliveries under Janani Suraksha Yojana. It has been proposed to have at least one MBBS Lady Doctor to supervise Out Patient Department, Indoor Patient Department and Labour Room services. State has been continuing efforts towards regular deployment of MBBS Lady Medical Officers through Commission but 296 MBBS Lady Medical Officers are required at on contract @ ₹ 40,000 per month.

(iii) *Proposal for Human Resources at Level-3 First Referral Units) Delivery Points*

- **Staff Nurses** — Staff Nurses are crucial for proper functioning of Level-3 delivery points, therefore, it has been proposed that 658 staff nurses are required on contract at designated Level-3 centres.

- **MBBS Lady Medical Officer** — A Community Health Centre only one post of Gynaecologist has been sanctioned by the State whereas they have to cater to heavy load of OPD Labour Room and Operation Theatres. In such cases usually Labour Room and OPD gets neglected. It has been proposed to hire 152 MBBS Lady Medical Officers to support quality of services at 161 functional First Referral units.

(iv) *Specialist on Call* — The specialists on call are proposed only for Gynaecologist/Paediatrics/Anesthesia/General Surgeons which will be monitored against performance/complications managed/lives saved at the rural facilities, i.e. Community Health Centre only. Chief Medical Officer are asked to submit utilization with justification note and status of regular or contractual specialists available at the facility centres. On call Gynaecologist are allowed at those for Community Health Centre, first referral units to maintain continuity of services if gynaecologist posted there are on leave.

- Any surgeon/gynaecologist/anesthetist on administrative posts at District level — government sector is encouraged to attend specialist calls on potential First Referral Units — Community Health Centre facility and club a supervisory visit with that call. The specialists are proposed to be paid ₹ 1500 per call and can be able to use transport provided for supervisory visit.
- Any regular surgeon/gynecologist/anesthetist government sector posted at functional First Referral Units and they are willing to perform at other First Referral Units where no regular or full time contractual specialists of that specialty is available and club a supervisory visit with that call, has been proposed to be paid ₹ 1,500 per call and be able to use transport provided for supervisory visit.
- On call surgeon/gynaecologist/anesthetist from private sector has been proposed to be paid ₹ 2,000 per call, if no regular or full time contractual specialist of that speciality is available.

(v) *Auxiliary Nurse Midwife: Tracking of Severe Anaemia* — All the ANMs who show 80 per cent of expected Pregnant Women registered and 80 per cent registered women getting 4 Ante

Natal Care Check-ups. It has also been proposed that ANMs to be paid an incentive of ₹ 10,000 of Safe Motherhood Day.

4.5.2. *Human Resource — Child Health*

Under the Child Health Programme, there is requirement of human resources especially staff nurses, medical officers, child health specialists, nutritionist — Child health and support staff for Health facilities at the various facility level.

4.5.3. *Human Resources — Family Planning*

Family Planning Counsellors are provided in those delivery units where delivery load is more than 150 per month. These counsellors are being contracted @ ₹ 10,500 per month, in which ₹ 500 is included as communication support. Further staff nurses @ ₹ 18,000 month and medical officers @ ₹ 40,000 per month has been allocated to the districts as per actual need of the blood banks.

4.5.4. *Human Resource — Adolescent Reproductive and Sexual Health/ School Health*

There is requirement of the human resource under Adolescent Reproductive and Sexual Health/School Health Programme. It has been proposed to recruit 2 teams per block with 5 members in each team. Efforts are being made to recruit at least One MBBS Doctor in each Block because most of the Anganwadi Centres are functional in the School Premises. Already recruited Dental Doctors are being posted in the school going teams where their expertise are being utilized. The Team has dedicated members consisting of one Doctor (MBBS/BDS/AYUSH), one Nursing Staff (GNM/ANM) and one paramedical (Optometrist/ Dental/Hygienist/Physiotherapist/Pharmacist) in each team will be hired on contractual basis for each Block. These teams will be visiting the schools and outreach areas for about 25 days per month for the purpose of health check-up of children to be covered under the scheme.

The MBBS Doctors are hired on contract @ ₹ 40,000 per month, BDS Doctors @ ₹ 38,000 per month, while AYUSH Doctors @ ₹ 30,000 per month and the nursing staff are being hired on contract for GNM @ ₹ 18,000 and ANMs @ ₹ 11,000 per month. The paramedics are being hired on contract @ ₹ 13,500 per month. The remuneration of counsellors are being proposed @ ₹ 10,000 per month are basic pays and for mobility support ₹ 200 per visit has been provided approximately for 20 days in a month.

4.5.5. *Human Resources — Routine Immunization*

To support routine immunization programme in the state, there was a position of regular state cold chain officer who retired in 2011-12. Uttar Pradesh is a large state and there is an urgent need of an Assistant Cold Chain Officer for proper maintenance of Cold Chain.

- There is a need of semi-skilled person (Cold Chain handlers) to be available for 24 hours for electricity backup, contingency plan and loading and unloading of vaccine and logistic. These cold chain handlers have been hired on contractual basis at the State/Division and District Level.
- Apart from government persons additional Technicians (Refrigerator Mechanics) have been hired on contractual basis in vacant position to repair cold chain equipment to reduce sickness rate.
- Apart from Government Vaccine Store-keepers have been hired at Division level in Vacant position for proper maintenance of Cold Chain emergency plan and smooth flow of vaccine and logistic.
- Driver for vaccine van have been hired.

4.5.6. *Human Resource — Dental Doctors*

It has been proposed by the State Government to deploy Dental Doctors on contractual basis. The contractual Dental Doctors are being placed at Rural Health Facilities where dental chairs are available and the regular posts of dental doctors are vacant.

Out of 382 dental Units, 172 Units having dental chairs and Doctors are being placed Remaining 200 Units, budgetary provision for procurement of dental chairs and basic instruments are being made under procurement head. An approval has been given for placement of dental doctors in rural area @ ₹ 35,000 per doctor per month. This year approximately 10 per cent hike in monthly remuneration is being proposed for the dental doctors.

4.5.7. *Human Resource — Para Medicals*

It has been observed that there are vacancies against sanctioned posts of Lab-Technicians, operation theater Technicians/Assistant, Pharmacists, Radiographers/X-Ray Technicians, etc. Regarding their regular appointments, efforts are being made but there are certain legal issues, which are under the jurisdiction of the court and the decisions are still pending. Thus, there is requirement of Laboratory Technician, OT Technicians/Assistants, Pharmacists and Radiographers and other paramedical staff to be hired on contractual basis at the facility level.

4.5.8. *Human Resource — Others*

The Districts have proposed various human resources. These human resources are pooled here and will be provided to the Districts as per the actual needs of the districts.

Other human resources include Staff Nurses, Medical Staff, Pathologists, Radiologists, Surgeons, etc. which has been proposed by the districts for their deployment at various facilities levels.

4.6. *Training*

Training is an important component of capacity building of the personnel to provide quality services. Training providers and Community level volunteers also become essential to ensure that consistent message reach communities and the community volunteers are able to follow up the health need of the community.

The Training Policy of the State is to enhance the knowledge and skills of each and every category of health personnel as per the latest technology to enable them to provide quality and efficient health services as well manage health programmes.

State Institute of Health and Family Welfare has been the collaborating Training Institute for the Uttar Pradesh and conducts clinical as well as management related trainings. The State Innovations in Family Planning Services Agency (SIFPSA) conducts family planning related training in the state. Both agencies and concerned departments also collaborate with National Institutions, Medical Universities and Medical Colleges as training sites for conducting clinical training.

It has been noted that there are 87 Government Training Facilities in the State of which State Institute of Health and Family Welfare is the apex Institute at the State Level, 11 are Regional Health and Family Welfare Training Centres, 40 are ANM Training Centres, 30 are Actual Prashikshan Kendras (DPTT), 4 are health school (LHV) training centres and one Primary Health Centre. Each of these facilities are located in the state owned buildings which include class rooms, hostels, furniture and audio-visual equipments.

The State Institute of Health and Family Welfare has been contributing a lot in state training activities under National Rural Health

Mission. Several training courses have been proposed to be organized at the State Institute of Health and Family Welfare level for capacity building including. Managerial, Administrative and Financial Training for the Chief Medical Officer, Chief Medical Superintendents, equivalent and National Rural Health Mission Programme management unit officers, programme based training for medical and paramedical personnel as well as training course related to Inter-sectoral convergence.

Most of the training courses are ongoing activities from previous year but apart from those activities some new programmes have been proposed like Ward Management, Infection Prevention and Patient Care Training for nursing staff.

In inter-sectoral convergence programme training of District Ayurveda and Homoeopathy Officers, Principals of Government Inter College, Child Development Programme Officers, Integrated Child Development Scheme Department and District Development Officer/ Project Director of District Rural Development Agency has been included in the Training plan.

Apart from the State Level Training Activities State Institute of Health and Family Welfare has been implementing various training projects in different fields:

- Life Saving Anesthesia Skill Training.
- Emergency Obstetrics Care Training.
- Skill Birth Attendant Training.
- RTI/STI Training
- Adolescent Reproductive and Sexual Health Training.
- MTP Training.
- Skill upgradation (Logistic Management Training and Sub-centre Management Training).
- Accredited Social Health Activists Training.

4.6.1. *Maternal Health Training*

Various training programmes have been planned. A comprehensive training plan has been illustrated in Table 2.1.

4.6.2. *Skill Lab Training*

As per the operational guidelines of the Government of India for skill labs, comprehensive skill labs with skill stations are to be established with the aim of acquisition and upgradation of skills of health care providers to enhance their capacity to provide good quality RMNCH

Table 2.1: Comprehensive Training Plan

Area and Name of Training	*Trainer's Category*	*Duration*	*Details of Training*	*Comments*	*Total Batches*
1	*2*	*3*	*4*	*5*	*6*
Skilled Birth Attendant's Training	One of the most crucial objectives of the National Rural Health Mission is to reduce maternal mortality. Skilled Birth Attendant Training is one of the important Training to achieve these objectives. Training of ANMs/Staff Nurses posted at First Referral Units and Accredited Sub-Centre. Training is conducted at District Women Hospital and District Combined Hospital.				
Strengthening of Skilled Birth Attendant's Site	—		25 (DFH/CH/FRUS	—	72 Units
Training of Trainers Reorientation	CMS (DFH) Gynae, Paed Staff Nurse Dir, PMS/DPMS	2 Days	State Institute of Health and Family Welfare, U.P.	Trainers of District Female Hospital and FRUs who import training of field operatives	15
Training of Staff Nurse/ ANM/LHV/SBA	ANM/LHVs Staff Nurses	21 Days	District Female Hospital and First Referral Units	It provides knowledge and skill about safe delivery with introduction of AMTSL Partographs and use of Mag. Sulphmeso Prestol, etc.	450
Life Saving Anesthesia Skills	For effective functioning of the FRUs, C-Section Delivery at the nearest place of the pregnant women is essential to this and training for supporting C-Section delivery is very important. Training is being continued at 5 Medical Colleges of U.P. with target of 40 Medical Officers.				
Training of Trainers	Anesthetists	2 days	Medical College of Lucknow, Agra, Meerut, Kanpur, Jhansi	This training is for Anesthetists of District Female Hospitals who will work as Trainers	10
Life Saving Anesthesia Skill (Field Training)	MBBS Medical Officers	18 Weeks	Medical College	Training is provided at respective Medical College and then Trainees are attached to DFH for practical Training	10

(*Contd.*)

Table 2.1 (*Contd.*)

1	*2*	*3*	*4*	*5*	*6*
Emergency Obstetrics Care Training	For effective functioning of the FRUs, C-Section delivery at the nearest place of the pregnant women is essential. To this Emergency Obstetrics Care Training is very important. This Training is being continued in two Medical Colleges with a target of 32 Medical Officers.				
Training of Medical Officer in Emergency	Gynaecologists	11 days	Medical College such as Vellore Gandhi Gram Surat Bangalore, etc.	Training for Emergency obstetrics care and short term Emergency obstetrics care	1
Field Training	MBBS Medical Officer	11 days	Medical College Lucknow and Aligarh have been included	Out of 16 weeks 6 weeks EM OC Training, 9 weeks practical training in DFH and last week to their respective Medical College	4
Centre Running Cost Certification Monitoring	Centre running cost, Monitoring Certification	One year	Medical College of Lucknow and Aligarh have been included		1
Field Training	Medical Officers of L-2 Centres	10 Days	7 Medical Collegees of U.P.	10 Days Practical Training regarding Maternal and Child Health	50
MTP Using MVA	MTP refreshers training plan includes training of 60 service providers from all districts on MTP skills with MVA Method.				
Training of Trainers	Pool of Trainers from Distt. Male and Female Hospital and Training Centres	5 days	SIHFW in Collaboration with Female Hospital	20 Trainers are available and 30 new trainers will be trained	2
Field Training	Medical Officer Female	5 days	District Female Hospital	Refresh Training with MVA Method	20
RTI/STI Training	Medical Officers and Lab Technicians are provided RTI/STI Training. It is planned to train 1230 Medical Officers and 60 LTs posted at the functional FRUs				
Induction Training of Medical Officers	Medical Officers	2 days	District Hospitals/District Women Hospitals/Head Quarter	Latest Knowledge about Case management regarding RTI/STI has been given to medical officers	105
RTI/STI Training for LTs	Lab Technicians	2 days	SIHWW and KGMU, Lucknow	Lab Technician of CHC will be trained on RTI/STI at Medical College.	2

services. As per operational guidelines skill labs have to be established at State Division and district levels.

It has been proposed to establish one skill lab at the state level and 11 skill labs at Regional Health and Family Welfare Training Centres.

The Lucknow District Regional Health and Family Welfare Training Centre located within the campus of State Institute of the Health and Family Welfare and the proposed skill lab shall be located within this campus. Therefore, the district level skill lab of Lucknow is proposed at Avanti Bai Hospital which is a district level female hospital of Lucknow. As the establishment of skill lab, procurement and recruitment of staff shall be a time consuming process in the first year, therefore, the state has proposed only six month salaries for Doctors and nurse trainers and 3 batches of Training per centre.

4.6.3. *Child Health Training*

The following trainings have been proposed at various levels under Child Health Programme which has been mentioned in Table 2.2.

Table 2.2: Child Health Training

Sl. No.	*Training Details*	*Unit*	*Physical Target*
1	*2*	*3*	*4*
	Integrated Management of Neonatal and Childhood Illness Training (IMNCI) (Pre-Service and In-Service)		
1.	Training of Trainers on IMNICI (Pre-Service and in-Service)	No. of Batches	14
2.	IMNCI Training for ANMs/LHVs	No. of Batches	714
3.	F-IMNCI Training for Medical Officers	No. of Trainees	48
4.	F-IMNCI Training of Staff Nurses	No. of Trainees	384
	Home Based New Born Care (HBNC)		
5.	Training of Trainers on Home Based New Born Child Care	—	—
6.	Training on Home Based New Born Child Care for Accredited Social Health Activists	No. of Batches	233
7.	Navjat Shishu Suraksha Karyakram Training for Medical Officers	No. of Batches	233
8.	Other Child Health Training		
	10 days Physician Training on IMNCI Plus (Pre-Service and in-service) Physicians at State Level in Medical College	No. of Trainees	578
	Sick New Born Care Unit Equipment Handling Training	No. of Batches	23

(Contd.)

Table 2.2 (*Contd.*)

1	*2*	*3*	*4*
9.	Printing of Training Modules of Navjat Shishu Suraksha Karyakram	No.	4697
10.	Printing of 3 Formats (No. of ASHAs for Incentives)	No.	59261
11.	Auxiliary Nurse Midwife/Local Health Volunteers/ Accredited Social Health Activists, Printing of Training Modules of CCSP and Printing of set of Job aid and tools	No.	20000

4.6.4. *Family Planning Training*

Following Training have been proposed under the Family Planning Programme which has been illustrated in Table 2.3.

Table 2.3: Family Planning Training

Sl. No.	*Training Details*	*Unit*	*Physical Target*
	Laparoscopic Sterilization Training		
1.	Training of Trainers on Laparoscopic Sterilization	No. of Batches	6
2.	Laparoscopic Sterilization Training for doctors (team of doctors, staff nurse and DT Assistant)	No. of Batches	21
	Mini lap Training		
3.	Training of Trainers of Minilap	No. of Batches	3
4.	Mini Lap Training for Medical Officers	No. of Batches	13
5.	Non-Scalpel Vasectomy Training of Medical Officers	No. of Batches	32
6.	Training of Trainers for IUD Insertion	No. of Batches	5
7.	Training of Medical Officers in IUD Insertion	No. of Batches	215
8.	Training of ANMs/LHVs in IUD Insertion	No. of Batches	344
9.	Training of Family Planning Counsellors	No.	435
10.	Training/Orientation on Technical Manual	No.	150

4.6.5. *Adolescent Reproductive and Sexual Health Training*

Adolescent Reproductive and Sexual Health/School Health Training Programmes have been proposed and mentioned in Table 2.4.

Table 2.4: Adolescent Reproductive and Sexual Health Training

Sl. No.	*Training Details*	*Unit*	*Physical Target*
1.	Adolescent Reproductive and Sexual Health Training for ANMs/LHVs	No. of Batches	225
2.	School Health Training — Training of Team — Technical and Managerial	No. of Batches	274
3.	Training of Nodal Teacher	No. of Batches	274
4.	One day orientation for programme managers/medical officers	No. of Participants	7500
5.	Training/Refresher Training of Auxiliary Nurse Midwife	No. of Batches	820

4.6.6. *Programme Management Trainings*

The Programme Management Training, other trainings — Integrated skill upgradation training for Paramedicals, Training for inter-sectoral convergence, etc. has been illustrated in detail in Table 2.5.

Various trainings related to programme management and others (like-finance, administration, and inter-sectoral convergence, etc.) have been proposed at various levels.

4.6.7. *Clinical Establishment Act*

Various activities have been proposed under the Clinical Establishment Act at the State and District level.

A. State Level

Sl.No.	*Name of Posts*	*Units*
1.	State Coordinator	2
2.	Administrative Assistant-cum-Data Entry Operator	2
3.	Computer and Printer	2 Sets
4.	State Level Meetings	6
5.	Workshop and Capacity Building	12

B. District Level

Sl.No.	*Name of Posts*	*Units*
1.	Coordinator	1
2.	Administrative Assistant-cum-Data Entry Operator	1
3.	Computer and Printer	1 Set
4.	District Level Meetings	6
5.	Workshop and Capacity Building	5

4.6.8. *PC and PNDT Training*

Training/Capacity Building of Inspection Team — The processes of inspection, record keeping and filing the cases have been planned and inspection teams of the state are not very clear about the process and records to be ceased. Therefore, to update inspection teams, this training has been proposed at the state level.

4.6.9. *Strengthening of Existing Training Institution*

The following activities have been planned as a measure for strengthening of State Institute of Health and Family Welfare:

Table 2.5: Programme Management Training

Sl. No.	*Area and Name of Training*	*Category of Training*	*Duration*	*Details of Training sites*	*Comments*	*Total Batches*	*No. of Trainees*
1	*2*	*3*	*4*	*5*	*6*	*7*	*8*
Programme Management Training							
	Programme Management, Human Resource Development and Capacity Building Training.	NRHM is an area which is to be understood in depth by different levels of Health functionaries. Besides this the managerial and administrative skill enhancement of the functionaries are required. To this end the capacity development training will be provided to different health functionaries.					
1.	Material and Administrative Skill Development Training	CMO/ACMO/ Dy. CMO	5 days	SIHFW	Training of NRHM Related programme and activities	4	25
2.	Hospital Management Training	M.S. Male and Female	5 days	SIHFW	Giving knowledge and skills about effective management of hospital related services	4	25
Other Training Related Programme Management, Finance Administration and Inter-sectoral Convergence							
3.	Programme Management Training	Sr. M.Ds. and Supdtt. of CHCs	5 days	SIHFW	Training of NRHM related activeness and programmes	4	25
4.	Administrative and Financial Training for CMS	CMS Male and Female	5 days	SIHFW	Administration and Financial Rules and Regulations, office management, etc.	4	25
5.	Monitoring and Evaluation Training for Programme	CMO/ACMO/DPM (NHRM) Dy.CMO	5 days	SIHFW	Gender planning, gender budgeting and knowledge about PCPNDT Act	4	25
6.	Gender Sterilization Training	PNDT Nodal Officers and SMOs	5 days	SIHFW	Gender Planning, Gender Budgeting and Knowledge about PCPNDT Act	4	25
7.	Disaster Management Training	Medical Officer	3 days	SIHFW	Preparedness in Hospital/PHC/CHC in case of Disaster and to make them aware to prepare village level disaster plan	4	25

(*Contd.*)

Table 2.5 (*Contd.*)

1	*2*	*3*	*4*	*5*	*6*	*7*	*8*
8.	Ward Management and Patient Care	Matrons/Sister incharge/Sr. Staff Nurse	5 days	SIHFW	To provide knowledge and skill on house keeping, record keeping, infection prevention and Public relations for better functioning of hospital	5	25
9.	Foundation Training	HEOs	12 days	SIHFW	Training on roles and responsibilities of Govt. Servant, conduct rules, financial rules, etc.	4	25
				SIHFW	To sensate district training programme under NRHM and their Monitoring work	4	25
10.	Monitoring of Training	Principals/JD of AD Office	3 days	SIHFW	To sensate District at Training Programme under NRHM and their monitoring work	4	25
11.	Training Skill Development	RHFW,TC Faculty ANMTC Tutors/ DPHN/DHV		SIHFW	To train field training methodology and development of trainers' skill. These trainers will impart training to basic health workers	4	25
12.	NRHM Financial Management	DAM and Account Officer	3 days	SIHFW	NRHM Financial Manual and Guidelines	6	25
13.	NRHM Financial Management	Block Manager and Data Entry Operator	3 days	SIHFW	NRHM Financial manual and guidelines	66	25
14.	IEC/BCC Training	Different levels of Health Functionaries involved in communication activities are trained for 5 days communication package. This training includes all the interventions planned under State BCC strategy. The Counsellors manning ICTC and PPTCT bring run UPSACS.					
15.	Family Welfare Counsellors' Training	Family Welfare Counsellors	7 days	SIHFW	Family Welfare Counsellors to be appointed at DFH will be given training on counselling and communication	5	50

(*Contd.*)

Table 2.5 (*Contd.*)

1	*2*	*3*	*4*	*5*	*6*	*7*	*8*
16.	BCC training for District Programme Management Units	DPMs/ DCMs/HEO and NGO Personnel	5 days	SIHFW	Knowledge about Behaviour change communication for implementation of NRHM Programme	6	25
17.	HIV/AIDS Counselling	Counsellors of ICTC/PPTCTs	3 days	SIHFW	There are new development in the area of HIV/AIDs. The counsellors of ICTC/PPTCT would be updated about new developments	6	25
18.	Adolescent Health Training	The Adolescent of group age which is vulnerable to various problems like Anaemia, Pregnancy, Malnutrition for which a large section of health functionaries has to be trained to handle the people in this age group very sensitively. The ARSH Training will achieve this goal.					
19.	Adolescent Health Training	ANM LHV	3 days	District Level Training Centres/Facility	Adolescent Health Component as per GOI Module	75 × 3 = 225	30
Integrated Skill upgradation Training for Para-medical		NRHM is an area which is to be understood in depth by different levels of health functionaries. The IST Training will define the roles of different levels of Health functionaries to understand their roles under NRHM.					
20.	Skill upgradation	Statistical Officers, ARO and ICC	5 days	RHFWTC	Their role and responsibilities in NRHM different formats regarding HMIS	22	25
21.	Skill Upgradation	Store keepers and Pharmacists	3 days	RHFWTC	Their roles and responsibilities in NRHM and logistic management	44	15
22.	Foundation of Pharmacists	Pharmacists	12 days	RHFWTC	Focus on their role and responsibilities NRHM activities, government servant rules, office procedure, financial procedure, etc.	55	30
Management of Sub-Centres		To streamline all the activities on the sub-centre by providing knowledge about the new roles and responsibilities and record keeping under NRHM and other National Programmes.					
23	Training of Trainers	District Level Trainers	3 days	SIHFW	Development of skills for operationalization of sub-centre	8	25

(*Contd.*)

Table 2.5 (*Contd.*)

1	*2*	*3*	*4*	*5*	*6*	*7*	*8*
24.	Field Training	ANM/LHV	6 days	District Level	Development of skills for operationalization of sub-centres	184	25
	Training of Inter-sectoral Convergence	NRHM is an area which is to be understood in depth by other departments this will help to convergence and inter-sectoral coordination. The departments like ICDS, Education, Rural Development and Panchayati Raj are involved in this training programme.					
25.	NRHM Sensitization Training	District Ayurved Officers and Homoeopath Officers	5 days	SIHFW	To sensitize the principals of GICs about NRHM activities to propagate the issues in their college and civil societies	4	25
26.	Family Life Education	Principles and Teachings of GICs — Girls and Boys	5 days	SIHFW	To sensitize the principals of GICs about NRHM activities to propagate the issues in their college and civil societies	4	25
27.	Management of Public Health Activities	CDP of ICDS	5 days	SIHFW	To sensitize the officers of the ICDS department about public health NRHM related activities	4	25
28.	Management of NRHM Programmes	DDO/PD	3 days	SIHFW	To sensitize the officers of RC Deptt. about public health and NRHM related activities	3	25
29.	Pre-Services Training BHW Female	Health Workers	5 days	SIHFW	One and half year's Training	3	25
30.	Training of Trainers BCPM	BCPM Training	2 days	SIHFW	Orientation of Trainers of 11 RHFWTC	1	50
31.	DCPM Training	DCPM Training	3 days	SIHFW	To orient DCPM	2	40
32.	Distance/E-learning, capacity Building, Programme from SIHFW in coordination with NIHFW for 1 batch.						

Source: National Rural Health Mission, State Programme Implementation Plan-2013-14, Uttar Pradesh.

- To ensure quality of training activities monitoring is necessary from the State Institute of Health and Family Welfare, Directorate of Health and Family Welfare and State Programme Management Unit officers at the state level.
  A provision is being made in the Programme Implementation Plan for organizing study tours, meetings, and seminars and facilitate exposure visits for programme managers and planners. A provision for operational research, ongoing activities under NRHM and RCH-II interventions has also been included.
- Furnishing of new class rooms, tea lounge, recreation rooms, Reception Lounge, Furniture, Mess, Lenin and CTVs for hostel are required.
- There is a need for contractual manpower for security class rooms and hostel attendants, support staff consultants and other support staff for the smooth conduct of training. For various field visits transportation support in the form of fuels, maintenance of vehicle, communication is also required. There is a need of a bus on contract basis for field training of the trainers.
- There is a need to strengthen the library and computer lab so that trainers can get hands on training HMIS, MCTS, etc.
- State Institute of Health and Family Welfare building is very old which requires maintenance of conference room and meeting hall, etc. There is also need for repairing of roads, water facility, fire extinguishers and rain water harvesting and drainage facilities. To ensure regular supply of electricity, a provision for purchase and installation of generator set has also been made. The manpower strengthening and other activities of the State Institute of Health and Family Welfare has been mentioned in Table 2.6.

Table 2.6: State Institute of Health and Family Welfare — Manpower Strengthening and Other Activities

Institute	*Activities*
1	*2*
State Institute of Health and Family Welfare (SIHFW) Manpower Strengthening and other activities	State Institute of Health and Family Welfare, U.P. is working as collaborating training institute for the state to conduct and co-ordinate several clinical training activities as well as management related trainings. Therefore, a plan to provide additional human and monitoring of training activities has been approved under National Rural Health Mission Programme. Implementation Plan Required Manpower support is as follows:

(Contd.)

Table 2.6 (*Contd.*)

1	2
	Consultant — Gynaecologist, Paediatrician, Public Health (2 each) Security Guard and other support staff — classroom hostel, Mess Attendant *Contingency Support* — Library, Communication, Transportation, etc. *Monitoring and Evaluation of different* training programmes by SIHFW and RHFWTCs. *Training designing* related workshops, seminars, Review Meeting and study tours of NRHM/Directorate/SIHFW Official, etc.
State Institute of Health and Family Welfare Strengthening (include Renovation)	For Renovation work of State Institute of Health and Family Welfare under NRHM has been carried out which is incomplete. A total amount sanctioned in different years was ₹ 6.6 crore out of which PACFED had carried out the work of ₹ 3.10 crore. The sanctioned work is incomplete amount is still lying with CHART. If this amount is surrendered an amount of ₹ 5.0 crore shall unfinished task.
Strengthening and Renovation of ANMTC	There are 40 ANMTCs in the state. The capacity of Hostels in the ANMTC is limited (approximately 30 students). Extension of Hostel Rooms is essential to fulfil the capacity of sixty students per ANMTCs. 15 more rooms with furniture and linen in the hostel of each ANMTC is required. Therefore, a sum of ₹ 75 lakh (15 × 5) is required for each ANMTC.
Strengthening and Renovation of RHFWTC	There are 11 RHFWTC, a new hostel and class room have been constructed are essential to utilize these available facilities. Therefore, ₹ 11.0 crore for each RHFWTC is required.

Source: National Rural Health Mission, State Programme Implementation Plan, Uttar Pradesh.

4.7. *Programme Management*

To ensure effective management of activities under NRHM, the State Programme Management Unit has been established in which government doctors designated as General Managers have been deployed as head of various divisions.

Each division has Deputy General Manager, Technical Consultants and Programme Coordinator, etc. Most of the staff has been hired on contract, some have been posted on deputation from relevant Government departments and some staff is on loan basis from SIFPSA. Programme Management Unit have also been established at Divisions, Districts and block programme management units.

Apart from different Programme Management Units, SIFPSA HQ. Directorate of Family Welfare, Directorate of Medical Health and

Additional Directorate, Ministry of Health and Family Welfare are also involved in effective programme management. Therefore, support has to be extended to these units also for their smooth functioning.

Government of India has accorded approval for establishment of 18 cells at State Programme Management Unit.

In view of the quantum of work in various sections of SPMU, Directorate of Family Welfare, Directorate of Medical Health and SIHFW, etc. a senior officer retired from the post of Joint Director level for establishing convergence with different partner departments, it has been proposed to create a position of NRHM coordinator at SPMU.

Cells at State Programme Management Unit:

- Administrative/Human Resource/Legal Cell.
- Construction of Infrastructure Cell.
- Maternal Health Cell.
- Child Health Cell.
- School Health and Adolescent Health Cell.
- Routine Immunization Cell.
- Maternal Mortality Unit Cell.
- National Disease Control Programme Unit.
- Monitoring and Evaluation Cell for quality assurance.
- Planning Cell.
- AYUSH Cell.
- EMTS (108)/Ambulance Service (102).
- Information, Education and Communication.
- Finance Cell.

4.7.1. *Strengthening of Divisional Programme Management Units of SIFPSA*

Uttar Pradesh being a large state of 75 districts is divided into 18 divisions. U.P. State needs special arrangement programme. Therefore, Divisional Programme Management Units of SIFPSA have been established in 18 divisions are being utilized for management of NRHM Programmes and schemes for which operating expenses are being borne by NRHM, Uttar Pradesh.

Apart from SPMU team, Divisional PMUs are filed level extended team of Mission Director NRHM. Divisional PMUs are responsible unit for hand holding, guiding and day to day monitoring of district level programmes and supporting district PMUs.

Divisional Units of SIFPSA are exclusively working for NRHM. All Divisional Project Management Units personnel are having experience in health sector for more than 10 years and working solely for NRHM.

4.7.2. *Strengthening of District Programme Management Units*

At the District level the programme management unit (DPMU) work closely with the Chief Medical Officer of the District.

The District Programme Manager (DPM) is responsible for preparation of district annual action plan, obtain approval for plans, coordinate district health society meetings, supporting CMO in contractual appointment of staff monitoring implementation of programme in field conduct review meetings, facilitate audits monthly, launch new programmes/scheme in the District with CMO and liaise and coordinate between different departments.

The District Community Mobilizer is responsible for Coordination and monitoring of community level activities such as ASHAs, Rogi Kalyan Samiti, Village Health and Sanitation Committee and Village Health and Nutrition Days and is also responsible for assisting District Programme Manager in overall operation of the District Programme. However, with large number of ASHAs, the monitoring of other programme of NRHM is not practically possible by District Community Mobilizer.

District Programme Manager and District Community Mobilizer are overloaded and monitoring of all the activities is not feasible. Hence to support the monitoring, evaluation and reporting additional hands are required at district level for which at least 4 programme coordinators and 2 District Data Assistants are required.

As such, the National Programmes like tuberculosis, leprosy, malaria, blindness control, vector-borne diseases, etc. are presently not being monitored regularly apart from the other NRHM programme. Hence recruitment of 4 programme coordinators and 2 District Data Assistants will necessitate day-to-day monitoring of the above activities and timely feedback to CMO and SPMU resulting in the smooth functioning of the programme.

Key responsibilities of the District Programme Manager are to assist CMOs in effective implementation of NRHM at District level. DPM is responsible for the District Planning, providing support for programme implementation, periodic monitoring and reporting and provide feed-back for evolving programme design and to provide overall leadership and guidance at Block Programme Management Units Assist the CMO in co-ordinating in the functioning of the District Health Society.

Table 2.7: District Programme Management Units

I. ***Descriptive Role of District Programme Manager***

Sl. No.	*Key Role Activity*	*Detailed Activity*	*Key Performance*	*Inter-dependencies*
1	*2*	*3*	*4*	*5*
1.	Administration	◆ Administrative Incharge of the office of DPMU ◆ Drawing and disbursing officer of DPMU ◆ All Procurements for the Office as per functional delegation ◆ Ensure appropriate work allocation between PMU Staff and their performance management of contractual staff ◆ Coordinate with Block PMUs through District Programme Coordination and their administrative requirement and report to Divisional PMU/SPMU ◆ Coordinate visits of review mission in the district ◆ Facilities for smooth conduct of concurrent, internal and external audits at district. Finalization and submission of annual budget for DPMU	◆ Timely submission of monthly expenditure reports for DPMU experience ◆ Staff discipline ◆ Establishment matters are disposed of timely and as per rules ◆ Periodic inspection of work of reporting staff ◆ Appropriately maintain works of records ◆ Expenditure of DPMU is within budget and properly audited	◆ CMO Office ◆ Block PM ◆ District PMU Staff
2.	Planning	◆ Brief and consult CMO in various planning related activities ◆ Coordinate with respective Monitoring Division at SPMU and Conduct Field level studies to identify gap for ascertaining intervention requirement and district action plan scope ◆ Coordination with stakeholders for preparation of district level implementation plans (PIPs) and approval by District Health Society	◆ Timely completion of field study ◆ Timely completion of field study ◆ Timely Development of Block implementation plans for each block in the District and their approval by the DSH	◆ BPM ◆ Monitoring Division for region

(*Contd.*)

Table 2.7 (*Contd.*)

1	2	3	4	5
		◆ Support Block Programme Managers in preparation of the Block action plan in line with district action plan		
3.	Programme Implementation Support Liasing and Coordinating	◆ Coordinate implementation of activities in District according to PIP ◆ Support Block Programme Managers in development of plans for all NRHM intervention ◆ Assist CMO in coordinating District Health Society Meetings ◆ Provide periodic feedback to Chief Medical Officer and regional monitoring Division on quality of services and status of implementation of programme activities ◆ Coordinate survey and research activities at Block level ◆ Dissemination of guidelines of schemes intervention to Block Programme Management Unit and Medical Officers Incharge ◆ Liaise with district level stakeholders to disseminate information and mobilize support for programme activities	◆ In-depth understanding of proposed intervention ◆ Strong working relations with CMO, District Magistrate, Members of District Health Society and other stakeholders at District Level ◆ Monthly implementation progress report submitted to respective monitoring Division by approved timeline of every month ◆ Timely implementation of field level activities and plan	◆ District Community Mobilizer ◆ Programme Coordinator ◆ Block PM ◆ Divisional Programme Manager ◆ District Level Stakeholders ◆ District Health Society ◆ State Programme Management Unit
4.	Quality Assurance	◆ Provide Periodic Feedback to Monitoring Division and Quality Assurance Division on guidelines provided ◆ Support and coordinate research/evaluation being conducted in the district	◆ Localized Interventions designed	◆ Divisional PMU ◆ SPMU ◆ CMS of the District

(*Contd.*)

Table 2.7 (*Contd.*)

1	*2*	*3*	*4*	*5*
5.	Monitoring and Reporting	◆ Independently undertake monitoring of intervention implementation in the District and providing feedback to CMOs/Divisional PMUs/SPMUs ◆ Undertake periodic monitoring of implementing agencies NGOs in line with their implementation plans ◆ Undertake random monitoring in selection stances as directed by MD/DM/CMO ◆ Ensure completion of monitoring progress/ performance reports in the requisite format on a monthly basis ◆ Ensure completion of field visit reports (random and planned)	◆ Submit reports to the Monitoring Division of region in the required formats by approved time line of every month ◆ Submit field visit reports to regional Monitoring Division within 5 days of visit ◆ Submit analysis of financial reports by approved time line of every month ◆ Conduct at least 2 random visits on routine and sporadic activities across the block	◆ BPM ◆ DAM ◆ Finance Division ◆ Respective Regional Monitoring Division
6.	Financial Management	◆ Processing release of funds to various units at district and block level under Part-A, B and C and other National Programme of financial guidelines to personnel in PMUs and CMOs officers	◆ Timely release of funds at District and Block level ◆ Submission of monthly account reconciliation report to SPMU	◆ CMO ◆ SPMU ◆ Finance Division
7.	Financial Monitoring and Reporting	◆ Ensure appropriate receipt and disbursement of funds in accordance with district PIP ◆ Monitor funds received from state from Part-A, B and C and other national programmes of NRHM as per the implementation plan and utilization at Block/District level and request for next trance of funds in time ◆ Ensure appropriate utilization of funds by implementing partners in coordination with District Account Manager	◆ Submit financial reports in requisite format for finance division by the approved timeline	◆ DAM ◆ Finance Division ◆ Respective regional monitoring division

(*Contd.*)

Table 2.7 (*Contd.*)

1	*2*	*3*	*4*	*5*
		◆ Obtaining timely statement of expenditure utilization reports, from different levels and District Programme Officers and submission to SPMU ◆ Provide timely and accurate utilization reports, statement of expenditure and utilization reports to Finance Division in the requisite format		
8.	Convergence	◆ Coordinate programming with other development departments in the District ◆ Coordinate with development partners/aid agencies (UNICEF, WHO etc. and other NGOs) in the field and ensure convergence of programming	◆ Report on inter-sectoral workshop in field ◆ Any funds leverage from other departments and partners	◆ Divisional PMU/ SPMU ◆ Other Department Heads ◆ Development Partner representatives

II. *District Community Mobilizer*

Key Responsibilities	Responsible for coordination and monitoring of community level activities such as ASHAs, Rogi Kalyan Samitis, Village Health and Sanitation Committee and Village Health and Nutrition Days		
District Supervisor	District Programme Manager	Functional Reporting	Divisional, PMU and GM (Community Processes), SPMU, Chief Medical Officer
Direct Reports		Indirect Reports	Block Programme Manager

III. *District Account Manager*

Key Responsibilities	Responsible for overall financial management of NRHM funds release to district. Responsible for maintaining and updating all the required data bases and generating MIS reports. Discharge functions of DPM, in his absence from the District. Responsible as the Data Manager for the district.		
District Superviser	District Programme Manager	Functional Reporting	SPMU-Finance Division
Direct Reports	Data-cum-Accounts Assistant at District and Block District Data-cum-Account Assistant	Indirect Reports	Accountant from CMO's office

IV. *District Data*-cum-*Accounts Assistant*

District Data-*cum*-Account Assistant is responsible for maintaining books of accounts and managing other finance related aspects at District. They are also responsible for maintaining and updating of all the required data base and generating MIS reports and work in the direct supervision of the District Programme Manager and District Account Manager.

V. *District Programme Coordinator*

District Programme Coordinator is responsible to visit and hold monthly meetings at least once in each of the assigned blocks. The block coordinator will be in the field for about 15 days in a month and sort out problems at Block and District level issues.

The District Programme Coordinator has to coordinate with Block Programme Management Unit and their administrative requirements and reports to DPM and ensure conduct of the concurrent, internal and external audits and support in the implementation of plans for all NRHM intervention, including timely reporting and feedback. To undertake monitoring of interventions implemented in the Blocks and provide feedback to DPM/CMO/Divisional PMUs/SPMU and to ensure completion of monitoring progress/performance reports in the requisite format on a monthly basis. To coordinate programming with other development departments in the Block and ensure convergence programme.

VI. *District Data Assistant*

Key role of District Data Assistant is to collate and compile data and prepare reports in prescribed format and maintain an accurate inventory of the assets, equipments and ensure appropriate PMU housekeeping and to undertake day-to-day maintenance of office computer and related accessories and coordinate logistic for meetings.

4.7.3. *Strengthening of Block/Programme Manager Units*

Block is the lowest unit which functions as a referral unit for the common masses where the Primary Health Centres/Community Health Centres exists. At Block level, the Programme Management Unit (Block PMU) has only one BPM and one Data-cum-Account Assistant which is not sufficient looking at the quantum of work. The BPMU works closely with the Medical Officer (Incharge) of the Block. The Block Programme Manager is responsible for preparation of Block Annual Action Plans obtain approvals for plants, facilitate in organizing regular monthly Rogi Kalyan Samiti (Advisory and Executive Committee) meetings, monitoring implementation of programmes in field, conduct review meetings facilities audits duties, monthly reporting to District PMU, launch new programme/schemes in Block with Medical Officer Incharge and liaise and coordinate between different departments as per instructions of CMO/District Programme Management Unit.

❑ *Role and Responsibilities of Block Programme Managers*

- Assist the CMOs/Superintendent/ MO I/C and District Programme Manager in effective implementation of NRHM at Block level.
- Responsible for Block Planning, providing support in Programme implementing, monitoring and reporting and provide feedback for evolving programme designs.
- Provide overall leadership and guidance to Block PMU.
- Supervision and monitoring of the ASHA support system.
- Visit Rogi Kalyan Samiti and Village and Village Health Sanitation and Nutrition Committees and understand their capacity building needs, prepare capacity building plans and implement with support of DPM.
- Facilitate preparation of Village Health Plans and proper timely utilization of the Village Health Sanitation and Nutrition Committee funds.
- Timely Development of Block Health Plans.
- Attend Auxiliary Nurse Midwife-ASHA meetings in their block to overcome bottlenecks.
- Assist in timely payment of Janani Suraksha Yojana and ASHA under various heads.
- Developing plans for Village Health and Nutrition Developments with Medical Officer Incharge and monitoring their implementation.
- Monitoring of School Health Programme.
- 8 to 10 days monitoring in the field.
- Assist Medical Officer Incharge in maintaining books of accounts as per financial guidelines.
- Timely submission on monthly expenditure reports for Block expenditure.
- Expenditure of BPMU within budget and properly audited.
- Monitoring of all programmes of the concerned Block.
- Monthly implementation progress report submitted to DPM within approved time line of every month.
- Submit block financial reports within approved time lines of every months.
- Establishment matters are disposed of timely and as per rules.

The *Block Data-cum-Assistant* is responsible for maintaining data and books of accounts at the block level. Timely monitoring, reporting and implementation of the programmes require additional man-force for which a Block coordinator and Data Assistant is proposed one in each block.

Block coordinator in guidance of Block Programme Manager will coordinate with all stakeholders at the Block level for successful implementation of various programmes.

The Data Assistant shall be primarily responsible to collect, collate, and analyse various reports generated from the field of prescribed formats and put up to BPM and Medical Officer Incharge regularly. The Data Assistant will also be responsible for managing, analyzing Health Management Information System Data, Janani Suraksha Yojana, and Web based reporting regularly on monthly basis. The Block unit will also be fully responsible for any deficiencies in the programmes as well as inappropriate data reporting.

3.7.5. *Supportive Supervision/Mobility Support/Field Visits*

Recognizing the importance of supervision and monitoring is key to reap the fruit of tremendous Investment under National Rural Health Mission. The state has started to develop a comprehensive and integrated supportive supervision and monitoring system for optimum utilization of the limited resource and to ensure delivery of quality health care.

Thus, the goal of supportive supervision is to promote efficient, effective and equitable health care. The check-lists help to organize the work of supervisors to make it regular and reliable. The supervisers find this objective process motivating, because it helps them to identify and address the highest priority problems. They know what is expected of them and when they have met those expectations.

Supportive supervision has also been lead to ensuring maintaining a minimum quality standard and improvement in the service delivery.

The supervision activities may strongly focus on facility operationalization for full range of integrated and quality services.

Quality assurance network will be linked to this monitoring plan and standard monitoring formats for field visits are being developed for all levels by Quality Assurance Working Groups and approved by the state government.

The monitoring visits have to holistically plan to cover all programmes and intervention State level → Divisional → District Block level monitoring teams should be formed. The mobility support for the

State level officers, Divisional Level Officers, District Level Officers and Block Level Officers should be provided to ensure adequate mobility for supervision and monitoring. The details of the Monitoring Team has been depicted in Figure 2.1.

Monitoring Teams

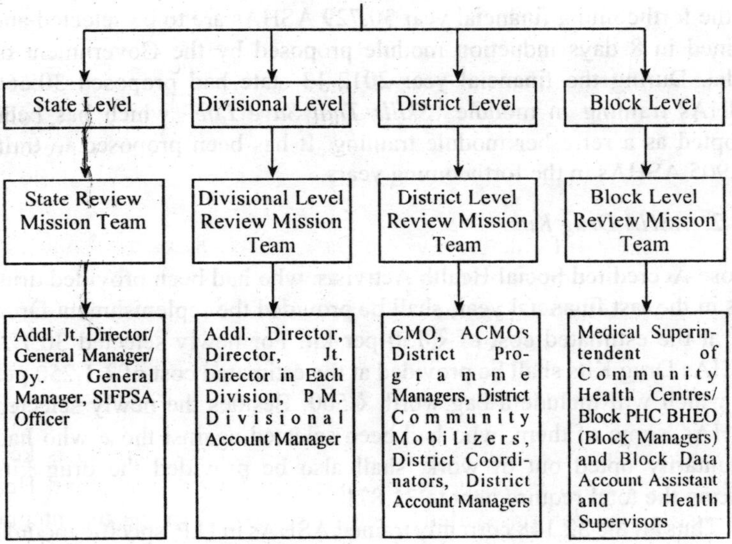

Figure 2.1: Monitoring Teams.

5. Rural Health Mission Flexible Pool

The Rural Health Mission Flexible Pool includes Accredited Social Health Activists, untied funds, Annual Maintenance Grant, Hospital, Strengthening, New Construction, Renovation and setting up, Main-streaming of AYUSH, Information, Education and Communication and Behaviour Change Communication, Medical Mobile Unit, Referral Transport/Patient Transport System, Innovation, Planning Implementation and Monitoring, Procurement, Drug Ware Houses, Health Insurance Scheme, Research/Studies/Analysis, State Health Resource Centre/State Public Health Resource Institute, support services and other expenditure (power backup, convergence), etc. The details of the rurai health mission flexible pool has been described below.

5.1. *Accredited Social Health Activists (ASHA)*

There are 1,36,094 Accredited Social Health Activists against target number of 1,59,482 in Uttar Pradesh as per 2011 population census. Out of 1,36,094 selected ASHAs about 7,341 have either resigned or are not working and 1,28,753 ASHAs are currently engaged. Therefore, state has fixed a target of selection of 30,729 ASHAs in the next financial year.

5.1.1. *Status of ASHA Training*—

In the forthcoming financial year 30,729 ASHAs are to be selected and trained in 8 days induction module proposed by the Government of India. During the financial year 2012-13 state had proposed 30,660 ASHAs training in module "*Skills That Save Life*" which has been adopted as a refresher module training. It has been proposed to train 64,905 ASHAs in the forthcoming years.

5.1.2. *ASHA Drug Kits*

Those Accredited Social Health Activists, who had been provided drug kits in the last financial year, shall be provided the replenishment Drug Kit at the estimated cost of ₹ 750 per kit. For newly selected 30,729 ASHAs Drug Kits shall be provided at the estimated cost of ₹ 1,250 per kit which will include a bag worth ₹ 500. Besides the newly selected ASHAs, some of them, who had been selected against those who had voluntarily opted out of work, shall also be provided the drug kits making the total requirement to 31,871.

Thus all the 32,148 currently trained ASHAs in U.P. specific module skills, that save lives shall be provided Home Base New Care replenishment Drug Kit @ ₹ 300 in the current financial year. Thus, for the estimated number of 64,905 ASHAs who shall be trained Modules 6 and 7 in the round one and two during the next financial year, the Home Based New Care Drug Kit is budgeted at ₹ 1,300 per ASHA which will include ₹ 300 for Home Based New Care medicines and ₹ 1,000 for Home Based New Care equipment kit.

A. Asha Drug Kits

Sl.No.	*Name of Drug in Drug Kit*	*Quantity*
1.	D.D.K.	
2.	IFA Tablets (large)	
3.	ORS Packet (WHO)	
4.	Tablet Paracetamole	
5.	Tab. Dicyclomine	
6.	Providine Ointment	
7.	Cotton Absorbent Roll (500 gm)	
8.	Bandage (4 cm × 4 cm)	
9.	Tab.-Chloroquine*	
10.	Condoms	

* From Existing Stock at Sub-Centre/PHC under Malaria and FW Programmes.

B. Name of Instrument/Drug/Communication Material in Home Base New Care Kit

Digital Watch; Digital Thermometer, Weighing Scale, Baby Blanket and Kit bag, Paracetamol Syrup, Contrimoxazole, Gention violet

5.1.3. *Incentive for ASHAs*

Various incentives for ASHAs are as follows:

Sl.No.	*Incentives*	*Unit Cost (₹)*
(i)	*Incentive under maternal Health:* (ANC/PNC) for mobilizing at laest 5 ANCs for Counselling, Birth Planning and Complete ANC	150
(ii)	*Incentive under Child Health (Home Based New Care):* Incentive for ASHAs for XI and VII module trained ASHAs @ ₹ 250 per Child per month (no. of month)	250
(iii)	*Incentives for Family Planning:* Incentive for ASHA @ ₹ 1,000 is coupled other permanent method after 2 children	1,000
(iv)	Spacing for 2 years after marriage	500
	Spacing for 3 years between 2 children	500
	Other Incentives	
(v)	On taking complicated Pregnancy Cases or New Born cases to the health facility (up to 3 cases per year)	200
(vi)	Completion of Village Health Information Report	750
(vii)	Incentive for conducting one Community Meeting lactating mothers and the other for adosescent girls and for Adolescent Reproductive and Sexual Health/month of village	150
(viii)	Birth and Death Registration (for 30 Births and 9 Deaths/ASHA)	
(ix)	TA/DA for attending monthly meeting	100
(x)	Maternal Death Audit Information	200
(xi)	Facilitating conduction of Village Health Sanitation and Nutrition Committee Meeting for a maximum of 4 meetings/VHSNC	100
(xii)	Mobilization of PW for HIV testing incentive for ASHA facilitators	100

5.1.4. *Annual ASHA Sammelan/Diwas*

Accredited Social Health Activists Scheme has been launched in Uttar Pradesh on 23rd August, 2005. An annual programme for ASHA is organized in each district on the same date that is on 23 August. It is proposed to continued the activity every year. It is an informative programme where ASHA from allover the District interact with each other become motivated and encouraged to perform even more better to get benefited from the speeches of the experienced and important officials of the District and feel a sense of unity and togetherness.

5.1.5. *ASHA Uniform*

As a non-monetary incentive to ASHAs, it has been proposed to distribute uniform to all ASHAs in Uttar Pradesh to enhance their level of motivation and to create a sense of unity and belonging among them.

5.1.6. *ASHA Payment Vouchers and Registers*

Accredited Social Health Activists payment voucher have been in use in Uttar Pradesh since 2009-10. These vouchers are submitted in duplicate by the ASHA and duly verified by the Area Auxiliary Nurse Midwife to be submitted to the Medical Officer in the monthly ASHA Block level meeting further for better monitoring of ASHA's functioning and their payment a master payment register at the block level has been introduced. In this register all types of monthly payments made to ASHA are recorded.

5.1.7. *Newsletter for ASHAs*

Newsletter for ASHA is being published and distributed every quarter. The Newsletter depicts their roles, success stories, Government scheme, progress under various components of NRHM interventions, etc. The copies of the Newsletter are distributed apart from ASHAs among district officials as well as the Pradhan to have a wide dissemination of the magazine. It has been proposed to print 2 lakh copies of the Magazine per quarter.

5.1.8. *ASHA Award Scheme*

A reward scheme for best performing ASHA for their motivation in each block has been proposed. The District Health Society would make for final selection of the best performer based on the evaluation of activities conducted by them during the whole year. The winners would be facilitated publicly on the occasion of the ASHA Sammelan on 3rd August and would be given a certificate of appreciation and a prize of ₹ 5,000.

5.1.9. *ASHA Monitoring Group*

An ASHA Monitoring Group has been constituted at the State and District level. Group at the State level meets quarterly to discuss feedback received from District AMG Meetings, major feedback and decisions are conveyed to the District and this feedback forms the agenda for their next quarterly AMG meeting.

State level AMG finalizes a 15 days time frame within which all districts are required to conduct their AMG Meetings. Minutes of the District Meetings, are compiled and sent to the state for analysis which among others form the agenda for the next state level meetings. For meeting of this group and field visit a provision of ₹ 10,000 per district is being made and an amount of ₹ 2.00 lakh has been provided for the state level meetings.

5.1.10. *Village Health Index Register*

A Village Health Index Register has been developed and provided to most of the ASHAs Training on filling up and maintenance of records on the same has also been conducted. The register included, apart from basic family details, utilization of RCH and other health services, status of nutrition, water supply and sanitation. It is continuously updated for vital events, disease status, services and other health related inputs and services utilization and it can be used for annual planning.

5.1.11. *State Specific Innovation under ASHA Programme*

Uttar Pradesh Government has initiated two innovation-organization of District level ASHA Sammelan every year on 23rd August, in commemoration of the launching of ASHA Scheme in the state on 23rd August and would be given certificate of appreciation and cash prize of ₹ 5,000 as certificate of appreciation. Apart from providing an opportunity to meet ASHAs from other Blocks, the Sammelan serves as refreshing break of the ASHAs from the routine tests, various cultural programmes are also organized by ASHAs themselves on the basis of which best performances are awarded with both cash and kind prices.

The second innovation is the publication of "ASHAYEIN" news magazine for ASHAs on a quarterly basis which is distributed among all the stakeholders of the National Rural Health Mission including ASHAs.

Detailed information regarding any new scheme or programme are covered in the magazine apart from carrying informative article on subject matters related with the topics in which ASHAs have previously been trained.

The newsletter depicts their role, success stories, Government scheme and progress under various components of National Rural Health Mission interventions.

The "ASHAYEIN" magazine serves as an interactive medium through which ASHAs interact with the concerned authorities at the

State Project Management Units. The quaries of the ASHAs are addressed as also refreshment of their learning is attempted through the medium of this magazine.

5.1.12. *ASHA Support System*

Government of India has recommended setting up of ASHA support system in Uttar Pradesh at the State, District and Block levels for facilitating streamlining and supporting the functioning of ASHA scheme. At the State level technical support are being provided by National Health Resource Centre in the form of the development of one state consultant and two regional consultants for better functioning of community processes in general.

Thus, the ASHA scheme in particular is highly appreciable. The State strongly recommends for the continuation of professionals keeping in view a multifold increase in the number of interventions, some of which are currently being implemented and some planned for the next financial year.

An important intervention includes:

- Selection and Development of ASHA facilities.
- Selection and supportive supervision of Block Community Mobilizers in all 820 Blocks of the State.
- Selection and Training of additional 30,729 ASHAs as per the rural population of the state.
- Launching of ASHA Programme Monitoring Mechanism in the entire State.
- Apart from the ongoing training of ASHAs in Uttar Pradesh specific Module-skills that save lives in 17 first phase of the training of all ASHAs.
- Launching of the scheme "Reaching the Unreached" through orientation of all ASHAs Village Health Sanitation and Nutrition Committee.
- Capacity building and implementation of the Home Based New Born Care programme.

District Community Mobilizers have been positioned. At the Block level Community Process Managers are being proposed in the next financial year to provide supportive supervision and monitoring to the ASHA scheme in particular and community process managers activities in general at the block level besides these activities, he will also act as pivot for community monitoring process at the village and block level which has been planned to be initiated in the forthcoming financial year.

There are 4-layer ASHA support system in Uttar Pradesh:

I. State ASHA Resource Cell.
II. District ASHA Community Process Manager.
III. Block ASHA Community Process Managers.
IV. ASHA Facilities.

As the immediate supervisors of ASHA, Facilitators shall be Block level Community Process Managers, their deployment is strongly required, otherwise the purpose of the deployment of the ASHA Facilitators shall be defeated.

In view of the above, a 3-day orientation training of District Community Process Managers in two batches at the State level has been proposed. Similarly, two days orientation programmes for all Block Community Process Managers have been proposed at Regional Health Family Welfare Training Centre level.

Performance based incentive @ ₹ 36,000 per ASHA Facilitators per year (₹ 150 per day × 20 days/months × 12 months). Furthermore ASHA facilitators are planned to be selected in the forthcoming financial year @ ₹ 27,000 per ASHA facilitator per year ₹ 150 per day × 20 days/ month × 8 months.

5.2. *Untied Funds*

Government of India has approved provision of Untied grant @ of ₹ 0.50 lakh per year per facility for Community Health Centres @ ₹ 0.25 lakh per Primary Health Centre and above sub-centre through Rogi Kalyan Samiti and @ ₹ 0.10 lakh for each sub-centre through village Health Sanitation Committee and @ ₹ 0.10 lakh for Village Health Sanitation and Nutrition Committee. To engage these Village Health Sanitation and Nutrition Committee, meaningfully, it is planned to orient the committee village health, need identification and local action proposed under the National Rural Health Mission.

5.3. *Annual Maintenance Grants*

Government of India has approved of Annual Maintenance of Grant @ ₹ 1 lakh per year facility for Community Health Centres @ ₹ 0.50 lakh per facility below Primary Health Centres and above sub-centre through Rogi Kalyan Samiti and ₹ 0.10 lakh for each sub-centre through Village Health Sanitation and Nutrition Committee.

5.4. *Hospital Strengthening*

Strengthening of Hospital should be ensured at the facility levels:

5.4.1. *Trauma Wings*

Trauma Wings (Additional Building) have been proposed in the District Hospitals. In view of the day-to-day increasing population and patients due to accidents in the State and the increasing load of patient in the District Hospital ten high accident prone areas of the State have been identified and is being proposed for construction of Trauma Wings (additional building) in the District Hospitals.

The main aim of the strengthening of hospital is to construct a trauma wing to provide quick and better treatment to the accidental cases.

5.4.2. *Spillover Maternity Wings in District Women Hospital*

It is well known fact that Uttar Pradesh is a very densely populated state with a population of > 20 crore, which is highest in the country with geographical area less than Madhya Pradesh and about 25 lakh Institutional deliveries are being conducted at the Government facilities every year with a bed occupancy of more than 100 per cent in peak season in most of the District women hospitals. It is essential to provide quality services to Janani Suraksha Yojana beneficiaries and comprehensive reproductive maternal new born child services in the Hospitals.

It has been proposed to expand maternity wing at District Women Hospital where Janani Suraksha Yojana load is very high and the land for the construction of additional maternity wing is available in some premises. In some districts, land is not available but some old buildings are available in dilapidated condition. It has been proposed that after demolition of these structure a multi-storied maternity wing will be constructed at the same place.

The maternity wing will include Ante-Natal Wing room, labour room, emergency new born care room, sick new born care unit, operation theatre, Post-Natal Ward, toilet facilities (attached with ward and separate common toilet) Nursing Station, Doctor's Duty Room, Store Room, Kitchen along with provision of Ultra Sonography Machine, Radiologist on contract, R.O. Water System with Cooler, Air Conditioner, Electricity Backup, etc. Facility of the Patient Relation Shed and Canteen is also being provided in the proposed project.

For the construction of maternity wings (100 bedded) in the District Women Hospital, Sultanpur and amount of ₹ 1,000 lakh has been proposed.

5.4.3. *Community Health Centres (30 Bedded, 50 Bedded and Construction)*

During the year 2012-13, state had proposed 30 bedded maternity wings in Community Health Centres and 50 bedded maternity wings in the Community Health Centres and construction of buildings.

It has been proposed to construct 30 bedded Maternity Wings at the two Community Health Centres in Sultanpur District for which a sum of ₹ 400.00 lakh has been proposed by the State Government.

5.4.4. *Spillover Primary Health Centres*

State Government of Uttar Pradesh had proposed construction of buildings in the Primary Health Centres. It has been planned to complete the construction within the scheduled time and Primary Health Centres may function in its own building and quality services may be provided as per norms and guidelines of the Indian Public Health Standards.

5.4.5. *Repair/Renovation of State Drug Warehouse*

The State Drug Warehouse was built about 30 years ago at Amausi. It has low height boundary wall which is also damaged at various places. Besides this the electrical wing is also damaged. In the State Drug Warehouse various costly equipment and medicines are stored.

Owing the incidence of theft in the State Drug Ware House during the last year ₹26.56 lakh (out of which ₹19.98 lakh pertains to boundary wall and ₹6.54 lakh pertains to electricity works) was proposed for electrical works and boundary wall.

5.4.6. *Spillover District Drug Warehouse*

Government of India has approved 22 District Drug Warehouses in Uttar Pradesh during 2012-13 Programme Implementation Plan. The District Drug Warehouse Unit cost approved in the Programme Implementation Plan has been proposed ₹ 50.53 lakh at Gautam Budh Nagar which falls under National Capital Region, so there is acute shortage of government land. The land available for construction of Drug Warehouse is in the filled up area having a filling of 2 to 9 metres, necessitating provision of raft foundation and framed structure for construction of Drug Warehouse. Owing to the above fact the cost for the construction is expected to be ₹ 74.16 lakh. Thus, an additional amount of ₹ 23.63 lakh is required for construction of Drug Warehouse at Gautam Budh Nagar.

5.4.7. *Patient Relation Shed/ASHA Grah*

The motto for construction of patient relation sheds/ASHA Grah is to provide shelter to the patients/relatives, who are coming from backward/ remote areas. Presently, there is no shed/shelter exists in hospitals for staying of relatives of patients as well as ASHA workers. It has been proposed to construct Patient Relation Shed ASHA Grahs to provide meeting halls, living space for patients' relatives and ASHAs.

It has been proposed to construct one Patient Relation Shed/ASHA Grah at Community Health Centre, Lambhua where 30 bedded facility is already available. A sum of ₹ 55.0 lakh has been proposed for the construction of Patient Relation Shed/ASHA Grah at Community Health Centre, Lambhua, District Sultanpur.

5.4.8. *Third Party Evaluation of Construction Work*

During the financial year 2011-12, Government of India has decided to ensure third party Evaluation of Construction Work under the National Rural Health Mission should be done to ensure the quality of construction work *vide* decision dated 12.9.2011 that third party Evaluation of small Work such as sub-centre and Janani Suraksha Yojana (Primary Health Centres Level) should be done by the task force working under District Magistrate. The big works like Community Health Centres and hospitals, etc. should be evaluated by Government Engineering College of the State.

5.4.9. *Sub-Centre Rent and Contingencies*

There are total 20,521 sub-centres in the State, out of which 15,570 sub-centres are operating from Government buildings and 5,027 in rental buildings. Accordingly, a provision of rent @ ₹ 250 per month for 5,027 sub-centres, amounting to ₹ 150.81 lakh was proposed for the year 2012-13 under Mission Flexible Pool. Additionally for the year 2013-14, 1,000 new sub-centres have been proposed to be established based on the population. For these sub-centres, rent is being booked for 6 months @ ₹ 250 per month.

5.5. *New Constructions, Renovation and Setting-up*

The new construction, renovation and setting up includes construction of maternity wings in the Community Health Centres, construction of sub-centres and setting up of Emergency care learning centres.

5.5.1. *Construction of Maternity Wings in Community Health Centres*

It has been noticed that due to the increasing case load/Bed occupancies in the proposed Community Health Centres is very high. To reduce the delivery load in these district hospitals, during the 2013-14, state proposed 50 bedded maternity wings in 30 Community Health Centres.

It has been proposed to construct maternity wings in the 30 bedded Community Health Centres Akhandnagar and Jaisinghpur in which additional 30 bedded maternity wings construction have been initiated which will be completed within two years.

5.5.2. *Construction of Sub-Centres*

There are 20,521 Sub-Centres in the State of Uttar Pradesh, out of which 16,470 sub-centres have been constructed so far and 3,262 are under construction, sanctioned under various schemes. It has been proposed to construct 350 sub-centres out of which 325 are already established and 25 sub-centres are in the process of establishment. Unit cost of the sub-centres as per the prevailing plinth area rates of Public Works Department as on 1.11.2011 is ₹ 10.20 lakh.

Additional sub-centres at Sodhanpur in Sultanpur District has not been established at present.

5.5.3. *Setting-up of Engineering Wings*

The implementation and monitoring of the various construction and renovation works under National Rural Health Mission has been very important task. Thus, the implementation and monitoring of the above works is being carried out by Engineering of Directorate of Family Welfare. It has been proposed to strengthen the Engineering Unit of Family Welfare through the following infrastructure:

	(*₹ in lakh*)
Computer (Desktop and laptops both)	1.00
Printer and UPS	0.50
Data Entry Assistant @ ₹ 0.20 lakh per month for 12 months	2.40
Total	3.90

5.5.4. *Setting-up of Emergency Care Learning Centre*

The Emergency Medical Transportation Services are being provided since 14th September, 2012. The sixth Common Review Mission (November, 2012) referred that in Uttar Pradesh 633 Emergency Ambulance Services are deployed and one form of Public Private Partnership has been unquestionably worked well across state is the dial 108 Emergency response service. In order to achieve 12th Five Year Plan Goals, plans should specify public facilities where emergency and trauma services would be made available to match the growing presence of emergency response services. Development of training capacity in high focus states like Uttar Pradesh should leverage partnerships and creation of new institutions should be the main focus of the first two years of the 12th Five Year Plan.

With the ultimate aim of moving towards universal Health Coverage and focus on scale of referral transport services that the Universal response time does not exceed 30 minutes, augmentation of facilities with special attention to nurses and other allied health care professionals is identified in the Programme Implementation Plan Guidelines by the Ministry of Health and Family Welfare.

The guidelines also specify the need for estimating of training load for the skills based training. Further expansion of training capacities through partnership with Non-governmental organizations/Institutions and developing highly skilled and specialized nursing cadre has been emphasized.

5.5.5 *Establishment of Emergency Medicine Learning Centre*

In the 1st Phase, the following infrastructure requirements are required to conduct the training programmes —

I. *Infrastructure*

◆ Lecture Halls with 80 seats capacity (American Chairs)	4 rooms
◆ Skill stations (20 × 20 feet 9 with 25 stakeholder chairs)	4 rooms
◆ Mankins, medical equipment store room (14 × 12 feet)	1 room
◆ Facility room with a cabin for team lead (20 × 20 feet)	1 room
◆ Hostel Facility for 100 boys and 50 girls	1 hostel

II. *Educational Equipment and Material in all Lecture Halls and Skills Stations*

- LCD Projector, Screen, P.C. Public Address System with collar and lapel mikes.

- White board in each lecture hall and skill stations.
- One Table and a chair for faculty in each lecture hall and skill stations.

III. *Additional Requirements*

- Projector lamps — 2 in numbers should be available in spare.
- One digital camera.

IV. *Basic Expectation*

- Every batch will have minimum of 40 participants.
- Every month should have at least 20 training days.
- Annual training calendar should be finalized in advance.
- Training fee and other budget expenditure should be given as quarterly advance.

5.6. *Rogi Kalyan Samiti*

As per the approved norms and guidelines of the Government of India, @ ₹ 0.50 lakh per year facility for the Primary Health Centres and @ ₹ 1.0 lakh per Community Health Centre and @ ₹ 5.0 lakh for District Hospital through District Health Society has been allocated.

Thus, eight Bal Mahila Chikitsalaya in Lucknow District and one 50 bedded hospital in Bhadohi district has also been included in the list of Community Health Centres for Rogi Kalyan Samiti financial budget.

5.7. *Health Action Plan*

The decentralized planning to formulate State Programme Implementation Plan is an elaborate process for the State of Uttar Pradesh, which has a population of 20 crore, 75 districts, 820 blocks and more than one lakh revenue villages. The detailed guidelines have been received from Government of India regarding preparation of Programme Implementation Plan.

The State level consultative meeting with senior officers of State Headquarters, Divisions and Districts have been organized. The important points relating to schemes have been discussed and consensus have been made.

A consultative meeting with representative of Development Partners and other Government Department has been organized to get their valuable inputs.

During the 1st and 2nd week of January 2013 district teams have been invited for day long workshops in groups, where detailed information, instructions and formats have been discriminated regarding Village Health Plan, Block Health Plan, Sub-Centre and District Health Action Plan.

The community participation has been ensured at Village, Block and District level with active participation of Panchayati Raj Institutions Integrated Child Development Scheme, Rural Development and other important stakeholders.

The capacity of development of Village Health Plan and Block Health Plan has definitely improved as far as local health functionaries are concerned. For the preparation of the District Action Plan detailed instructions have been issued along with the budget based on certain norms, so that the action plans at all levels are prepared logically and complied with in the form of District Action Plan.

District Action Plan data have been received by the State Programme Officers of Directorate of Medical and Health and Directorate of Family Welfare as well as by the concerned officers at State Programme Management Unit. The relevant data have incorporated in the State Programme Implementation Plan which has been submitted to the Government of India for appropriate discussion and approval.

Preparation of Programme Implementation data is collected from the Village and based on it Block/District plans are formulated. Thus, for these activities, various meetings are conducted. Finally based on district plans, state programme Implementation Plan has been compiled after several steps of reviews and discussions at divisional and State Health Quarters Level.

5.8. *Panchayati Raj Initiatives*

Panchayati Raj Institutions include orientation workshop and capacity building and establishing sub-centre level platform for effective Maternal and Child Health service delivery through front line workers.

5.8.1. *Orientation Workshop, Training and Capacity Building of Panchayati Raj Institutions at State/District Health Society, Community Health Centres, Primary Health Centres*

Village Health Sanitation and Nutrition Committee: National Rural Health Mission framework support decentralized planning monitoring up to grassroots level. It has been decided to entrust village level committee of the user groups community based organization for the planning, monitoring and implementation of National Rural Health Mission activities.

Village Health Sanitation and Nutrition Committee feed such purpose, it envisaged that the Village Health Sanitation and Nutrition Committee will be the key agency for developing village health plan and the entire planning of village panchayat for National Rurai Health Mission. This committee comprise of panchayat representative, Auxiliary Nurse Midwife, Anganwadi Workers, Teachers, Community Health Volunteers and Accredited Social Health Activists.

There are 52,374 Village panchayats where Village Health Sanitation and Nutrition Committee exists. It has been planned to orient committee on village health need identification and local action proposed and National Rural Health Mission.

It has been essential to build, capacity of Panchayati Raj Institutions Members, hence 50 per cent of the proposed amount is again being proposed for its approval.

The proposed activities are as follows:

- Letter to District Magistrate/Chief Medical Officer from Principal Secretary — Medical Health and Family Welfare regarding proposed Village Health Sanitation and Nutrition Committee.
- Chief Development Officers' orientation at the State Level in their routine monthly review meeting.
- District Panchayati Raj Officers' orientation at the State Level in their routine monthly review meeting.
- Orientation of District level Officers in the District Health Society with the proposed training programme.
- Master Training of Trainers for Additional Chief Medical Officers — Reproductive Child Health, District Panchayati Raj Officers — and state level Non-governmental organizations' members at the state level.
- District level Training of Trainers by Master Trainers (Additional Chief Medical Officers, Reproductive Child Health, District Panchayati Raj Officers and State level non-governmental organization's Members) for Health Education Offices, Panchayat and Non-Government Members (District Trainers).
- Training of Pradhans and Village Health Sanitation and Nutrition Committee members at the Nyaya Panchayat Levels in a cluster of 5 village Health Sanitation and Nutrition Committee to be Conducted by District Trainers.

- Monitoring of the training at different levels by —
  1. State level officers (Directorate, SPMU State Innovations in Family Planning Service Agency (SIFPSA) Staff.
  2. District level by DM, CMO and DPRO.
  3. Block and Panchayat level by Block Development Officer and Medical Officer Incharge.

5.8.2. *Establishing Sub-Centre Level Platform for Effective Maternity and Child Health Service Delivery through Front Line Workers*

Strengthening of capacity of field level workers to deliver quality health services and care at community level to improve coverage of critical intervention has been established globally and proven strategy. Proven approaches for strengthening capacity of field level workers includes equipping them with knowledge, skills, job aids, providing supportive supervision, ensuring work rationalization and improving motivation levels of field level workers.

(i) *Existing Block Level Platforms: Barriers and Challenges*

- Current block level meeting too large and inadequate for field level workers' level planning, review and supportive supervision.
- Inadequate Synergy between ICDS and NRHM.
- Inadequate skills and motivation among Field level workers.

(ii) *Sub-Centre Level Platform: The Proposed Model*

At sub-centre level monthly meeting of all the Anganwadi workers and Accredited Social Health Activists of the sub-centre area, overseen and facilitated by the Auxiliary Nurse Midwife and participation of block level officials have been proposed as a model for addressing the above barriers.

The sub-centre level meetings will be introduced in addition to the existing platform of Village Health Sanitation and Nutrition Developments and Block level meetings. The relatively small size of a sub-centre area will allow for the total number of participants at the sub-centre meetings to less than 20. A smaller group of the participants will provide a better opportunity and space to review and plan for each village, as represented by the corresponding Anganwadi Workers and Accredited Social Health Activists.

Auxiliary Nurse Midwifes are available as resource with better technical and some level of the supervisory skills that can be further enhanced with tailored capacity building inputs and hand holding until ANMs, learn to facilitate these meetings on their own, external facilitator will required to hand hold and support the meetings.

It has been planned that other facilitators from within the system would be drawn such as the Lady Supervisor, Block Community Mobilizers, Block Health Managers, etc.

It has been proposed that as an initial step for each Block, micro-plan with specific dates for each sub-centre meetings will be developed jointly by Block level Health and Integrated Child Development Scheme officials to ensure minimum overlap of meetings on a particular day.

The timing and scheduling of sub-centre meetings, can be flexible and largely locally determined, since it involves only a few, closely cluster villages and frontline workers at village level.

5.9. *Mainstreaming of AYUSH*

Ayurveda, Yoga and Naturopathy, Unani, Siddha and Homoeopathy (AYUSH) system of Medicine have been proven promotive, preventive and curative strengths, with a view to integrating AYUSH health care with mainstream health care services as per modified centrally sponsored scheme for development of AYUSH Hospitals and Dispensaries, operational guidelines, department of AYUSH, Ministry of Health and Family Welfare, Government of India for mainstreaming of AYUSH, under National Rural Health Mission with few Innovations and the State Government has proposed the following activities:

5.9.1. *Human Resource*

At the state level following human resource contractual/deputation posts have been proposed as per new structure, guidelines of the Government of India.

I. AYUSH — Programme Manager, Financial Manager, Accounts Manager and Data Assistant.
II. HMIS — HMIS Manager and Data Entry Operator.
III. Additional Proposal — General Manager, Dy. General Manager, Consultant and Programme Coordinator.

At the District Level, there are 1203 Male AYUSH Doctors, 841 Female AYUSH Doctors and 759 AYUSH Pharmacist are working in Uttar Pradesh at various health facilities at the District Level. Additional approval of Male AYUSH Doctors and Female AYUSH Doctors and Pharmacists have been ensured.

5.9.2. *Drugs and Consumables*

To purchase drugs and consumables at facility level under AYUSH, a provision of ₹ 1.25 lakh per unit has been made available. There are 2,044 units functional in Uttar Pradesh.

5.10. *Information, Education and Communication and Behaviour Change Communication*

It is well known fact that Uttar Pradesh is a very vast popular state. The rural community is mostly in difficult and unreached areas and the needs of the rural population is mostly unmet. To provide information regarding health services and to change in health seeking behaviour in our target audience, strong Behaviour Change Communication and Information, Education and Communication Campaigns are required.

5.10.1. *Strengthening of Information, Education and Communication/ Behaviour Change Communication Implementation Capacity*

The State of Uttar Pradesh realizes the need of establishing a fully Functional Information, Education and Communication Bureau under Family Welfare Directorate and IEC Cell at State Programme Management Unit level. All the Programme Managers will coordinate with IEC/BCC Cell under Family Welfare Directorate to implement programme related activities.

At the State Programme Management Unit level IEC/BCC Cell is established with one General Manager (on deputation from Provincial Medical and Health Services Cadre), One consultant, one Programme coordinator and one computer operator. However, Information, Education and Communication Bureau at Family Welfare Directorate level is not fully functional. There is only one Joint Director from PMHS Cadre along with supporting staff. The post of Director of IES Bureau is being vacant. The IEC cell wculd have the professional manpower recruited from the market or on deputation with expertise and requisite experience in IEC/BCC. The required logistic support for infrastructure including purchase of colour printers, photostat machines and computers have also been budgeted. Thus budget of ₹ 25.94 lakh has been proposed for the IEC Bureau.

5.10.2. *IEC/BCC Activities for Maternity Health*

The priority behaviour and target audience for BCC activities under the Maternal Health has been mentioned in Table 2.8.

Table 2.8: Maternal Health (JSY, JSS, MDR and Safe Abortion)

Priority Behaviour	*Target Audience*	
	Primary	*Secondary*
Complete ANC: 4 ANC Checkups 100 IFA 2 Injections T.T.	Married Women of Child Bearing age	Husband, Older Women in Household
Institutional deliveries and stay on hospital for 48 hours (focus on Janani Suraksha Yojana) and JSSK and introduce Post Partum Care	Pregnant Women and their husband	Decision Makers in household, Mother-in-laws
Essential New Born Care (Skin to Skin Care, Cord Care immediate exclusive BF) and 2 PNC	All married women on Child bearing age	ASHA, AWW older women in family
More emphasis on Registration and 48 hours stay in hospital after delivery	All unmarried and married women and adolescent	ASHA, AWW older women in family

Various activities are planned as per the State BCC strategy and included Household level, Community level and State level interventions of Inter-personal communication Mid Media and Community/Local Media and Mass media.

Inter Personal Community	*Mid Media*	*Mass Media State/ District Level*
Home visit by ASHA for need based counselling (IPC Total Flip Book)	Block level wall painting	Posters, audio, TV sports, Film shows
PNC Visit by ASHA	Facility level wall paintings, Hoardings, Nukkad Natak	Media workshop at State and District level and sensitization melas on Maternal Health, MDR, JSY, JSS and Safe Abortion at the occasion of Safe motherhood day
Village level activity VHND for ANC/PNC Service Provision	Safe Motherhood Booklets	

I. *Maternal Health Campaign "Chhar Gaanth"*

Maternal Health Campaign "*Chhar Gaanth*" has been launched by Bill Melinda Gates Foundation which includes Mid Media Campaign and Mass Media Campaign.

Maternal Health Campaign

Mid Campaign

- Street Play
- Inter Personal Communication
- Inter Personal Communication Maternal

Mass Media Campaign

- Audio Spots Airing
- Video spots telecast

II. *Maternal Health Campaign "Chance Kyon Lena Hai"*

Maternal Health Campaign has been launched through "Chance Kyon Lena Hai" which includes Mid Media and Mass Media Campaign.

- *Mid Media Campaign* — Wall writing, Governmnet sub-centre on ANC/NC and stay of the 48 hours in the hospital, hoardings, posters, etc.
- *Mass Media* — TV spots, Audio spots, two films produced by IEC Bureau (Surakshit Matritva) and by telecasted from Doordarshan Kendra Lucknow and local cable network. Safe Motherhood booklet, Sate level events and safe motherhood days, etc.

Memorandum of understanding has been signed between Government of Uttar Pradesh and Bill Mellinda Gates Foundation regarding promoting Health awareness in the State. Bill Mellinda Gates Foundation will develop IEC Campaign related health issues that will be used by the State Government. On the basis of this Memorandum of Understanding various Campaign have been included in the programme implementation plan.

- *Chhar Gaanth* — On Maternal Health.
- *Ek Tin Do* — On Family Planning.
- *Balgam Bhai* — On T.B. Control Programme.

5.10.3. *IEC/BCC Activities for Child Health*

An important area for communication interaction that have been identified under child health has been New Born Care. A set of three posters have been placed on labour room as IEC material, based on the Child Care after delivery. There are also posters related to maintenance of Child Health equipments. The language is easy Hindi and target audience is staff of labour room.

5.10.4. *IEC Activities for Family Planning*

Three IEC/BCC Campaigns have been proposed on Family Planning:

— Khushi Ka Mantra.
— Ek Teen Do.
— Chal Haat Ki or.

Thus IEC/BCC activities under Family Planning has been proposed in order to promote spacing and small family norm and other spacing method.

The priority behaviour and target audience of family planning has been mentioned in Table 2.9.

Table 2.9: Priority Behaviour and Target Audience Family Planning

Priority Behaviour	*Target Audience*	
	Primary	*General Public*
Intentions to adopt small family	Eligible Couples	General Public
Increase Birth Intervals	Couples with Spacing Needs	ASHA, AWW, ANMs, Mothers-in-law
Increasing men participation in contraception use of Limiting Method (Other Spacing Method)	Married Men Couples achieving desired family Size	VHSNC and Community influential ASHA, ANM. ASHA, AWW, Auxiliary Nurse Midwife, Eligible Couple

Various activities are planned as per the State Behaviour change communication strategy and include household level, community level and state level intervention of Inter-personal communication, Mid Media, Community/local media and mass media.

Inter-Personal Communication	*Mid Media*	*Mass Media State/ District Level*
1	*2*	*3*
Household Level ◆ Identification of Client for spacing ◆ IPC by ASHA (Tool Flip book)	*Sub-Centre Level* ◆ Hoarding Posters Fodder	◆ Workshop for correction of Developed Material ◆ Audio Video Spots
Block Level ◆ Job Aids for ANMs ◆ Group Meetings by ASHA	◆ Development of Flip ◆ Folk Media at Block Level ◆ Chal Haat Ki or ◆ Nukkad Natak	◆ Bus Panels
Village Level/Activity ◆ VHND Counselling of Pregnant Women by Auxiliary Nurse Midwife ◆ Liability of Pradhans	*Facility Level* ◆ Poster on Multiple Choice ◆ Folder ◆ Mobilization of Community	◆ Wide publicity of Small family norms through Mass Media ◆ Print Media ◆ Ads in Newspapers

5.10.5. *IEC/BCC Activities for Adolescent Reproductive and Sexual Health (ARSH)*

To promote Adolescent Reproductive and Sexual Health Clinics and its clinical services, posters have been proposed. The clinical posters are related to the services of ARSH and to promote the services among the adolescent and Menstrual Hygiene IEC/BCC activities related posters have been proposed.

5.10.6. *IEC/BCC Activities for School Health*

The IEC/BCC activities under the school health programme have been proposed in order to promote every child has right for good health to survive.

Iron is essential for every child, to reduce the anaemia De-worming Tablets are given on the six monthly basis. Wall paintings have been designed for the schools. Prabhat Pheri with school children once in a year on specific dates 15th August, 2nd October, and 26th January, has been organized at the District level. Banners, Bill Boards and Posters for the Prabhat Pheri has also been proposed.

5.10.7. *IEC/BCC Activities for Routine Immunization*

It has been noticed that there is very slow progress in the rate of fully immunized children from 30.03 to 40.9 per cent one of the barrier to complete and timely immunization schedule, prevailing myths and misconceptions, high dropout rate low parental motivation and lack of community ownership after immunization programme. To cover the above issues and create a healthy atmosphere on IEC/BCC activities under Routine Immunization has been proposed in order to promote the importance of Routine Immunization and reduce Infant Mortality Rate.

Primary Behaviour and Target Audience Routine Immunization

Priority Behaviour	*Target Audience*	
	Primary	*Secondary*
Importance to adopt routine immunization	Parents	General Public
To reduce disability and other deformities which increase without routine immunization	Parents	ASHAs, AWWs, ANMs, Mother-in-Law
To reduce Infant Mortality Rate	Parents	Community Influential ASHAs, ANMs

Behaviour Communication activities are as follows:

Behaviour Communication Activities on Routine Immunization

Inter-Personal Communication	*Mid Media*	*Mass Media State/ District Level*
Household Level ◆ Bandai Care for Parent with new born	*Sub-Centre Level* ◆ Routine Immunization booklets for frontline workers	◆ Posters and Audio-Video spots
Village Level ◆ Mobilization of Couples for importance of Routine Immunization	◆ Routine Immunization Sessions ◆ Posters and Banners ◆ Handouts	◆ Routine Immunization Secessions ◆ Posters/Banners
◆ Village Panchayat Level Celebration ◆ Liability of Pradhan	*Facility Level* ◆ Poster ◆ Handouts ◆ Banners	◆ Wide Publicity ◆ Mass Media

5.10.8. *IEC/BCC Activities for Emergency Medical Transport Services*

To provide Emergency Medical Transport Services to patients "108" Ambulance Services has been introduced. To promote services of "108" Ambulance Sewa, IEC Activities have been proposed which includes Mid Media, Posters and Mass media, Audio Spots.

5.10.9. *IEC/BCC Activity for Community Processes*

As most active worker at Village Level it is necessary to give recognition of ASHAs House, Name Plates of ASHA Houses as on Tin with Screen Printing has been proposed to provide early and quality health services for the villagers.

5.10.10. *IEC/BCC Activities for Tuberculosis*

With the view to reduce infections and deaths from Tuberculosis and to develop a healthy atmosphere it is necessary to develop IEC/BCC Campaign for the Tuberculosis.

A campaign "*Balgam Bhai*" has been developed by Bill Melinda Gates Foundation and soft copies are being provided for the utilization.

5.10.11. *IEC/BCC Activities for Pre-Conception and Pre-Natal Diagnosis Techniques*

National Rural Health Mission Uttar Pradesh has developed complete campaign on PCPNDT. The character of "*Shakti*" is introduced in the

Priority Behaviour Target Audience — Tuberculosis

Priority Behaviour	*Target Audience*	
	Primary	*Secondary*
"TB is a curable Disease" Importance to adopt TB Treatment	All Family Members	General Public
Intermediate Sputum if having cough more than 3 weeks	Parents	Family Members ASHAs
To stop death from TB	Parents	Community influential ASHAs, ANMs

BCC Activities on TB

Inter-Personal Communication	*Mid Media*	*Mass Media*
Group Meeting by ASHA (Tool Flip Book)	Nukkad Natak	Audio Video Spots

campaign. Two girls per Block will be selected and will be trained by ASHAs on PCPNDT issue. These girls will be given the name of the Shakti. The Shakti will collect the girls from schools and visit to nearly village in the form of Jattha raising their demand against sex ratio. IEC/ BCC activities under Sex ratio (PCPNDT) developed by NRHM UP has been proposed in order to reduce sex ratio related to female foeticide.

Priority Behaviour Target Audience Identified
Pre-Conception and Pre-Natal Diagnostic Test

Priority Behaviour	*Target Audience*	
	Primary	*Secondary*
To reduce pressure on women for reproduction leading to increase maternal mortality rate and maternal morbidity rate	Spouse	General Public
To create awareness regarding the affect of declining sex ratio of girls	Parents	ASHAs, AWW, ANMs, Mother-in-laws
To create awareness that girl can perform their duties towards their parents much better than son. To create awareness about the girl importance in the society	Elder Family Members	VHSNC and Community Influential ASHAs, ANMs, and Parents
To give proper information about the Act of 1994	Parents and Family Members Couples achieving desired family size	General Public

B.C.C. Activities on Sex Ratio PCPNDT

Block level/Village Level	*Mid Media*	*State Level and District Level Activities*
◆ *Group Meeting* by ASHA (Tool Flip Book)	◆ Folk Media Posters	◆ Posters, Audio-video spots
Block/Village Level ◆ Jattha Rally in the leadership of selected girl Shakti	◆ Jattha Folk Media poster, Banners	◆ Poster ◆ Audio-video spots.
Village Level (Community Sensitization (Tool Flip Book) ◆ Research Pretest (Block, Village and District Level) ◆ Monitoring ◆ District, Block and Village level ◆ Evaluation	ASHA Jattha Rally Banners ◆ All Print Maternal Rough cut of Audio video spots ◆ Guideline will be developed for campaign monitoring ◆ Mid-team and End line evaluation will be conducted by SIFPSA	◆ Phone in Programme from AIR ◆ By the selected agency NRHM and SIFPSA officials ◆ Monitoring by DPMU and time to time visit by NRHM, SIFPSA officers ◆ By the selected agency

Thus, all the audio-video spots will be aired and telecasted on State Hook-up rates and DAVP rates. The new activities introduced in IEC/BCC are as follows:

- Folk Media.
- Stage Play.
- Video and Radio Drama.
- Radio Phone in.
- Phone in Programme.
- Jattha and Prabhat Pheries.
- Pre-Test and Evaluation.

5.11. *Medical Mobile Unit*

The Millennium Development Goals aims at Access to the Health facilities and equitable distribution of health services among all inhabitants. To achieve this goal the Mobile Medical Units have been envisaged which will provide preventive, promotive and curative health care in the inaccessible areas, which are underserved or unserved areas, under usual circumstances. The factors that negatively influence the existing public health system and call for the exigency are:

1. Distance of the remote villages from the public health institutions.
2. Geographical Barriers to reach the pockets.

3. Lack of mobility support for field visit by the staff assigned to do the job.
4. Lack of Medicines/equipments/manpower.
5. Lack of awareness and health consciousness in the community particularly among disadvantaged people, who are socially and economically backward.

Mobile Medical Units are operative by the name of *National Mobile Medical Unit* along with Medical Officers, Pharmacists, lab-technician, nurse, a data entry operator/attendant and a driver, moves for at least 20 days a month to remote village in the Block area as per a schedule prepared jointly by the concerned District Programme Officer and Block Medical Officer.

Each Mobile Medical Unit is air-conditioned and equipped with a Generator Set (5.6 KVA) an air conditioner, a set of suction machine, a semi-auto Analyzer, refrigerator, a Binocular, Microscope, Eye Examination Kit, Centrifuge, 2 Numbers of Stethoscope, 2 set of B.P. apparatus, 2 set of clinical thermometer, 2 Nos. of weighing machine, 1 set of knee Hammer, 1 set of measuring tap, 1 set of ENT Diagnostic Kit, 1 set of First Aid Kit, 1 set of resuscitation Kits, 1 set of suture instruments and materials, 1 No. of needle cutter, 1 set of vaginal spechula, 1 set of 100 litre water storage device, 1 set of drinking water storage (with purifier), 1 set of 100 litre water storage device, 1 set of disposal globes, stationery, 2 packets of glass slides, 2 Nos. of dustbins with covers, 1 set of Bar light and siren, 3 Nos. of storage bins/Shelves for drugs, 1 No. of display Board on service offered by Mobile Medical Unit, 1 No. of folding structure, 2 Nos. of Fire Extinguisher of 2 kg weight, 1 No. of digital clock and 1000 Number of Patient card with National Rural Health Mission Logo. A computer set with DAV players and printer may be more beneficial. Examination Table with foot steps, Doctor's Chair and Patients' stool in sufficient number should also be there. As per the need more equipments, reagents, and medicine can be added or deleted. Sufficient quantity of medicine for the common ailments along with vaccine and syringes are being made available in Mobile Medical Unit.

Mobile Medical Unit will carry out the services like curative, care reproductive and child health services, Family Planning Services, Diagnostic Services, Emergency Services and care in times of disaster. They will also render Behaviour Change Communication activities to promote healthy lifestyle of the rural poor and counselling on Family Planning, RTI/STI or disease prevalent in that area. Information,

Education and Communication Material on Health Hygiene, proper nutrition are being displayed.

Priority Action: *Mobile Medical Units* are being operative by the name of *National Mobile Medical Unit* and are fitted with GPS for tracking the movements of vehicle. It will be integrated with the Primary Health Facilities and Anganwadi Centre will also be visited if nearby and will record the services rendered. Service data will be regularly put on public domain on National Rural Health Mission Website. Five Mobile Medical Units have been proposed for the Sultanpur District.

5.12. *The Referral Transport/Patient Transport System*

In view of the importance of access to ambulance services for reducing delays in access to care during acute emergency the ambulance services have been started in all the districts of Uttar Pradesh. These Services are basically depending upon the need and mode of operation.

1. "108" Emergency Medical Transport Services — Sewa.
2. U.P. Ambulance Sewa.
3. "102" Ambulance Sewa.

5.12.1. *Emergency Medical Transport Services*

An important objective is to provide immediate response during Emergency with basic First Aid to the patient and transport them to the nearest Government health facility. Initially 133 Ambulance operation has been achieved on 10 Feb., 2013. The operation of these Ambulances is being done by the service provider M/s. GVK, EMRI, U.P. It has a 100 seater centralized call centre branch in Lucknow. This service has gained wide popularity and 3,42,839 patients (including 1,84,440 Pregnancy cases) benefited till 31st March, 2013. This service has achieved the target of about four patients per ambulance per day as per agreement.

State Government has proposed to continue operation of these 988 Ambulances in the Programme Implementation Plan for which a sum of ₹ 1.287 lakh per Ambulance per month including 10 per cent increment has been proposed as per agreement between GVK, EMRI and Government of Uttar Pradesh.

5.12.2. *U.P. Ambulance Sewa*

Under State Basic Ambulance Services 972 Ambulances are already functional in all districts of Uttar Pradesh. The Ambulances are used for inter-facilities transport of Patient, Sick New Born Children and for the purpose of drop back under the Janani Shishu Suraksha Karyakram.

5.12.3. *"102" Sewa*

The 102 Sewa Ambulances are expected to serve transportation of pregnancy cases as well as neo-natal cases from home to the health facility. State Government has proposed to operate 1,000 such Ambulances.

5.13. ***Innovation***

The innovation include inter-sectoral convergence, District Specific, *Routine, Immunization, Management Information System, Effective Birth and Death Registration, Mobile Kunji, State Nutrition Mission and Mini Skills Lab and Mobile Nurses Trainers.*

5.13.1. *Inter-sectoral Convergence*

Inter-sectoral convergence includes the following programme:

A. *Proposed Establishing 151 Blood Storage Centres at First Referral Units*

National Blood Policy 2002 envisage universal availability of safe and quality blood and blood products with a view to reduce maternal and child mortality in the Uttar Pradesh. It has also been decided to make blood available at First Referral Units need licensing approval of FDA which is given only after the infrastructure for blood storage centre is set up.

The Blood Storage Centre has been established in the District Women Hospital, and Community Health Centres at Kadipur, Jagdishpur and Musafirkhana Community Health Centres in the District Sultanpur.

B. *Establishment of 4 Blood Banks in the Newly Created District*

As envisaged in the National Blood Policy-2002 and directives given by Hon'ble High Court, State Government is committed to establish Blood Bank in all districts of Uttar Pradesh. Presently 8 District Hospitals have no Blood Bank facility. In four District Hospitals Blood Bank infrastructure has been created and licensing procedure is underway, while the rest of the four newly created Districts namely — Amethi, Shamali, Hapur and Shambhal infrastructure along with equipment are required to initiate formalities of licensing for which budgetary provision of ₹ 71.88 lakh has been approved in the Programme Implementation for Plan of the National Rural Health Mission.

Table 2.10: Requirement for Establishment of New Blood Banks

Sl.No.	*Items*	*Quantity*	*Amount in ₹*
1.	Donor Couches	4	150000
2.	Blood Mixer and Shaker	4	65000
3.	Di Electric Tube Sealer	4	90000
4.	Blood Bank Refrigerator	4	145000
5.	Domestic Refrigerator	4	18000
6.	Laboratory Refrigerator	4	160000
7.	Bench top centrifuge	4	50000
8.	Serological Water Bath	4	10000
9.	Binocular Microscope	4	45000
10.	Elisa Reader and Washer	4	400000
11.	VDRL Shaker	4	5000
12.	Auto Clave	4	65000
13.	Air-Conditioner	4	35000
14.	Generator (15 KVA)	4	300000
15.	Computer with Printer and Internet	4	60000
16.	HC Calorimeter	4	10000
17.	Micro pipette (200 TTD 1000 MIC ROLT)	4	2500
18.	Micro pipette (STTPSO Microlt)	4	2500
19.	Haemoglobin meter	4	8000
20.	Recovery Beds	4	8000
21.	Syringe with Needle Destroyer	4	2000
22.	B.P. Apparatus	4	7200
23.	Hot Air Oven	4	3200
24.	Stop Watch/Timer	4	80000
25.	Storage Box for Transportation	4	60000
26.	Donor Weighing Balance	4	8000
27.	Oxygen Cylinder with Regulator	4	40000
28.	Rh View Box	8	40000
29.	Bed Side Stand	8	16000
30.	Stethoscope	4	3200
31.	Emesis Basin	8	4000
32.	Discard Containers	8	6400
33.	Sponge forceps	4	800
34.	Tube stripper	8	40000
35.	Big Lenin Box	4	4000
36.	Test Tube with racks	20	20000
37.	Test Tube with racks	20	4000
38.	Test Tube with racks	20	40000

Thus, a proposal of ₹ 41.888 lakh @ ₹ 17 per blood bank has been submitted for approval under National Rural Health Mission.

C. *Proposal for Establishing 20 Blood Component Separation Units*

As per directives of Hon'ble High Court, Allahabad in writ petition No. 10641/2010, the State Government has given an Affidavit to establish Blood Bank in each District of Uttar Pradesh in phased manner. Under first phase 27 Blood Component Separation Units were established by the State Government under second phase 20 more Blood component Separation Units are proposed to be established with the financial support of National Rural Health Mission.

D. *Strengthening of Blood Banks in Uttar Pradesh through National Rural Health Mission*

National Blood Policy-2002 envisaged universal availability of safe blood and Blood Products further to bring down Mother and Child morbidity and mortality in the safe. Blood storage centres have been proposed at First Referral Units in Uttar Pradesh to make blood availability at far flung areas. There is no separate staff cadre allotted to run Blood Banks in the State. At most of the Blood Banks the technical staff posted in the pathology are also working for Blood Bank.

It is pertinent to clarify that National Aids Control Organization provides only Blood Bank Technician and one counsellor at major blood Bank/Blood component separation Unit only. Thus staff is not enough to meet extra demand of Blood under Janani Suraksha Yojana.

E. *Proposal for STI/RTI Services at Sub-District Level*

(i) *District Level-STI/RTI Services* — STI/RTI Services at the District Level are provided through the Out Patient Department of Skin, Gynaecology and obstetrics departments of Medical College/District Hospital.

At District and select Sub-District Hospitals, if the concerned Departments/Specialists are not available, services are delivered through general duty medical officers in General OPD. These specific clinics are called designated STI/RTI clinics or "Suraksha Clinics". Such STI/RTI Services are being supported by National Aids Control Organization through State Aids Control Society. NACO has branded its sexual and Reproductive Health Services as "*Suraksha Clinic*".

Presently, 96 Designed STI/RTI Clinics have been established all-over the state with support from Uttar Pradesh AID Control Society (72 District Hospitals, 5 District Women Hospitals and

19 Medical Colleges). The support provided to these clinics are in terms of capacity building of Medical Offices, Counsellors and staff nurses, infrastructure strengthening, appointment of counsellor on contract, provision of colour coded drug kits for Syndrome case management, consumables and syphilis testing kits.

(ii) *Sub-District Level-STI/RTI Services* — As per the National STI/RTI guidelines — Health Worker, Auxiliary Nurse Midwife, Accredited Social Health Activists and link workers will conduct STI/RTI prevention and health promotion activities and refer individual with STI/RTI symptoms to Primary Health Centres, Block PHC, Community Health Centres for management of STI/RTI cases.

STI/RTI clinical services will be provided at sub-district level through existing health facilities with Syndromic Case Management approach.

Laboratory services wherever available will be used to corroborate syndromic diagnosis. This service delivery will be through health care delivery system under Reproductive and Child Health-II supported by National Rural Health Mission.

Proposal has been submitted to National Rural Health Mission for having provision of funds under Programme Implementation Plan:

- Training of Medical Officers and lab technician of sub-district heath facilities of 75 districts on STI/RTI and Syndromic Management through National Rural Health Mission.
- Provision of medicine for STI/RTI through NRHM.
- Provision of RPR/VDRL testing services including testing kits consumables and infrastructure) for Ante Natal Cases and STI/RTI Clinic Attendees at each sub-District Health Facility through NRHM.
- Provision of IEC Maternal for clinics through NRHM.

1. *Training*

Induction Training for Medical Officers and Lab-Technician at the Sub-District level are conducted — "*It has been experienced that training conducted in previous years were not organized within expected time period. Also technical inputs from UPSACS could not be arranged. Hence it is being proposed that funds for the training may be transported by NRHM to UPSACS and in turn UPSACS will coordinate with SIHFW/*

Training Institute for the conduction of training for Medical Officers and Lab-Technician as per National Guidelines".

Medical officers trained in the current and the previous financial years can be used as resource persons for the training in the respective districts.

It has been noted that there are 12 numbers of Community Health Centres/Block Primary Health Centres (2 Medical Officers per facility level will be trained) and 40 number of Additional Primary Health Centres/Primary Health Centres per 30,000 population (one Medical Officer per facility will be trained and 64 number of Medical Officers inducted for training and 12 number of Lab Technicians to be trained at CHC/BPHC (One Lab Technician per facility level) will be trained in the Sultanpur District.

2. *Colour Coded Medicine Kits/Loose Medicines*

The colour coded drug kits for syndromic case management have already been distributed to districts. These kits are supposed to be distributed to further districts level (CHC, FRU, PHC, etc.).

The Programme Implemented Plan of NRHM should include budget for the procurement of Medicines and RPR drug kits. RPR and Medicines are calculated only for 25 per cent of the Physical Target which will be procured at the State level and closely monitored by procurement officers and NRHM Programme Managers in State Programme Management Unit.

3. *Provision of Rapid Plasma Region (RPR) Venereal Disease Research Laboratory (VDRL) Testing Services*

It has been proposed that National Rural Health Mission should make necessary services for RPR/VDRL Testing available at all Sub-district Health Facilities. The provision of necessary infrastructure, availability of testing kits and consumables need to be ensured. The required kits and consumables need to be procured by National Rural Health Mission as per its procurement guidelines, coordinated and monitored by Reproductive and Child Health-II and Procurement Officer.

4. *Provision of IEC Material*

National AIDS Control Organization has already developed various IEC and training materials for STI/RTI services. It has been proposed that NRHM may have provision of funds for printing of these materials for its sub-District Health Facilities.

F. *Proposal for Free Transport Facility through UPSRTC to People Living with HIV/AIDS for their Treatment Related to ART/Link ART Centres*

There are 63,489 HIV Patients registered in different ART centres across Uttar Pradesh out of which about 25,500 HIV Patients are taking ARV from different ART centres on monthly basis and rest 37,989 HIV patients are enrolled as HIV care patients at ART centres who visit the ART Centre for their regular check up and opportunity Infections. Most of them belong to below poverty line category and have no means or resource to afford the regular travel. Hence, it has been proposed to provide them with the facility of free travel for visit to the ART Centre.

G. *Action Plan for NRHM-NACP Convergence for HIV Testing Services*

Strategic scale up of the PPTCT services in Uttar Pradesh has been ensured through establishment of FI-ICTC in high prevalence districts. It has been indicated that 21 high priority/high burden districts for HIV for facilities based ICTCs can be initiated. These districts have been identified based on the programme data showing high prevalence in general client or pregnant women or high vulnerability due to high migration. Among these 21 high priority/high prevalence districts CHCs have been selected on the basis of high migration blocks of the respective districts.

H. *Proposal for CPT Provision for ICTC/PPTCT Centres Located at the Districts/Sub-Districts Level*

Co-trimoxazole is a broad spectrum Antibiotic effective against a wide-variety of Bacterial Protozoal diseases, etc. Co-trimoxazole Phrophylaxis Therapy (CPT) is very effective against the common opportunistic infections frequently frequently encountered in People living with HIV/AIDS.

As per National Guidelines the co-trimoxazole Prophylaxis Therapy has to be provided to the babies exposed to the HIV infection, i.e. the babies born to HIV positive mother on breast led by HIV positive women.

Co-trimoxazole Prophylasix in HIV exposed babies has to be initiated at 6 weeks of age and continued till at least 18 months of age or till the time of HIV infection is reliably excluded in the baby.

I. *Establishment of Cold Storage Space*

Uttar Pradesh State Aids Control Society is working on HIV/AIDS project under National AIDS Control Organization, Department of AIDS, Ministry of Health and Family Welfare, Government of India.

Uttar Pradesh AIDS Control Society, Lucknow, is distributing HIV diagnostic kits to all ICTCI/PPTCT/Blood Bank/Community Health Centres of the state. Presently, Society does not have appropriate and sufficient facilities for the storage of kits under cold chain maintenance.

In order to maintain cold chain of HIV Diagnostic kits, it is proposed that one walk in cooler (size 2000 sq.ft. along with partition for cold space at 50 (L) × 30 (W) (Ext.) × 8'6" (Into. approx.) is established in the premises of a Government Hospital situated at Lucknow preferably nearby Gomti Nagar with the help of National Rural Health Mission.

J. *Proposal from Uttar Pradesh State AIDS Control Society for Better Utilization of Blood Mobile Van*

There are two blood mobile vans, provided from National AIDS Control Organization and allocated to Sanjay Gandhi Post Graduate Institute of Medical Sciences and Institute of Medical Sciences, Banaras Hindu University, Varanasi. To meet increasing demand of blood, more emphasis on collection to outreach blood donation camps is required and those Blood Mobile Vans are used for the same. Despite best efforts, then by both institutions and Uttar Pradesh State AIDS Control Society, the utilization of Blood Mobile van is much below the expectation of 20-35 days per month. To meet the challenge proposal for promotion has been made with the following objectives:

- To systemize and increase voluntary blood donation camps in licensed blood banks in Uttar Pradesh.
- To increase the level of awareness and motivation for voluntary Blood Donation in the State and Districts.

The proposal include more efficient utilization of two Blood Mobile Vans by implementing State and District level activities including organization of 40 voluntary Blood Donation Camps per month for initial 3 months followed by 56 camps per month through Blood Mobile Vans.

The key activities to be implemented includes technical support to Uttar Pradesh State AIDS Control Society in developing promotional communication material State Level advocacy, workshop with the partner agencies to increase voluntary Blood Donation including successful organization of Voluntary Blood Donation Camp.

5.14.2. *Innovations — District Specific*

Various local/district specific innovations are being proposed by districts. The Sanitation programme for Rural Child Health and Hygiene awareness programme "*Sanrachha*" has been launched for which a sum of ₹ 14.66 lakh has been approved.

5.14.3. *Innovation Routine Immunization*

Various innovation activities have been initiated to strengthen the routine immunization —

A. *Supportive Supervision for Strengthening of Routine Immunization*

The Universal Immunization Programme (UIP) also called "Routine Immunization" (RI) is primarily implemented by Government Health Services under National Rural Health Mission. Routine immunization is largest programme with respect to the human resources, number of beneficiaries, cold chain equipment, vaccines, etc. Routine immunization is provided at fixed sites in the District Hospital and Block Primary Health Centres and at outreach stations held by female health worker (Auxiliary Nurse Midwife) with the help of Anganwadi Workers and ASHAs in the village on Wednesdays and Saturdays.

❑ *Supportive Supervision as a Process*

The supportive supervision exercises comprise a participatory process that aims at supporting programme managers, health workers and other frontline functionaries to effectively perform their duties according to set programme benchmarks. The supportive supervision exercise consists of following activities:

1. District Sensitization Meeting.
2. Visit to all vaccine storage points and few randomly selected routine immunization session site.
3. Action Plan Meeting.
4. Concurrent Monitoring for follow-up of action plan activities.

❑ *District Sensitization Meetings*

One day district sensitization meeting is held for refreshing the knowledge about various components of routine immunization programme. The meeting is attended by district level health and ICDS officials, Block Medical Officer-in-charge of all the blocks, cold chain handlers and AROs (persons responsible for data management) and CDPOs of all the blocks of the District.

❑ *Visit to All Vaccine Storage Points*

Visits are made to all vaccine storage points of the district and few randomly selected Routine Immunization session sites during the next 2-3 days. During these, visits, specific programmatic information is collected by using standards.

❑ *Action Plan Meeting*

Once the field visits are completed, the data collected during the field visits are analyzed with the help of and Excel based compilation tool and a power point presentation is prepared showing various indicators. The presentation is shared with district and block officials. Based upon the findings of field visits an action plan is prepared.

❑ *Concurrent Monitoring for Follow-up of Action Plan Activities*

To facilitate the implementation of action plan concurrent monitoring is being done by field coordinators and Government officials. The feedback of the concurrent monitoring is shared with the district and state level officials on regular basis.

Based upon the results achieved, it has been decided to universalize the supportive supervision intervention and implementation of supportive supervision activity plan:

1. Training of Trainers.
2. Supportive Supervision Exercise.
3. Concurrent monitoring including joint field visits with district officials.
4. Data Management including feedback sharing.
5. Training of District Data Coordinator.
6. Regional District Data Coordinators.
7. Capacity building of other medical colleges.

1. *Training of Trainers for Supportive Supervision*

A pool of trainers for supportive supervision is being developed and 6 trainers (4 District level officials and 2 Block level officials) are being identified and trained in supportive supervision in each of the districts.

It has been planned to identify and train a total of 450 district/block health officials. These trainings are being organized at the division level.

2. *Supportive Supervision*

Two supportive supervision exercises are being conducted in each of the 75 districts. Technical support for carrying out these are being provided by UNICEF.

3. *Concurrent Monitoring including Joint Field Visits with District Officials*

To facilitate the implementation of action plan, concurrent monitoring is being done by the field coordinators from UNICEF representatives of medical college and the district health officials.

To provide hands on training to district health officials to perform concurrent monitoring, joint visits are being done by medical College/ Field Coordinators with district health officials. Subsequently, field visits are being planned and conducted by district health officials independently.

4. *Training of District Data Coordinators*

Generated data during supportive supervision exercise and concurrent monitoring will be collated by district data coordinator placed in the offices of the Chief Medical Officers of the respective districts with the support of UNICEF Office for the Uttar Pradesh one day training of data coordinator are being conducted.

5. *Data Management including Feedback Sharing*

The data generated during District Supportive supervision exercises and the concurrent monitoring visits will be compiled by the data coordinator at the District level. The compiled data will be shared at the State level UNICEF Office for Uttar Pradesh will support the analysis of data and generation of detailed reports. The reports will be shared by the Directorate of Family Welfare with the respective district for corrective actions one Deputy General Manager and one data coordinator at the state level will be made responsible for overseeing the activities related to supportive supervision activities.

A supportive supervision can be established with the support from UNICEF. A state supportive supervision coordinator has been placed in collaboration with SN Medical College, Agra. A state Data Manager will also be placed in supportive supervision cell for managing data generated during supportive supervision exercises.

6. *Regional Review Meetings*

To review the progress and also to identify bottlenecks/gaps, bi-annual review meetings will be conducted at regional level. Each meeting will be attended by the Government Official (Additional Directors, District Immunization Officers) of 3-5 divisions, representatives of respective Medical College and partners including UNICEF. The communication for these meetings will be done by the Directorate of Family Welfare in coordination with State Programme Management Unit.

7. *Capacity Development of Medical College*

In addition to the 5 Medical Colleges, *viz.* —

(1) MLB Medical College, Jhansi.
(2) BRD Medical College, Gorakhpur.
(3) LLRM Medical College, Meerut.
(4) MLN Medical College, Allahabad.
(5) S.N. Medical College, Agra.

The capacity building of other medical colleges will also be developed. UNICEF office for Uttar Pradesh will support a two-day sensitization workshop for the faculty Members of these Medical Colleges and they will be invited to attend the supportive supervision exercise for hands on training.

B. *Establishing Demonstration and Cross Learning Centres for Routine Immunization*

Universal Immunization Programme launched during 1985 in India is largest in the world in terms of quantities of vaccine used, number of beneficiaries and immunization sessions organized, geographical spread and diversity of areas covered. In broader perspective the Immunization delivery is also vehicles for health promotion and other health services addressing morbidity of public significance in all age groups.[1]

Annual Health Survey (2010-11) revealed proportion of fully immunized children in Uttar Pradesh as 45.3 per cent indicating the need to improve reach and quality of immunization services not only for reducing mortality and morbidity due to vaccine preventable disease but also for expansion of the public intervention including promotion of maternal and child health.

Multi-year Plan for Universal Immunization Programme (2005-10) highlights the major constraints underlying the programme at District and Health facility level includes:

- Available staff not technically sound who could practically plan and manage immunization services effectively.
- Lack of understanding about the importance of accurate recording and reporting of data for analysis and identification of necessary corrective actions.
- Poor planning and implementation of vaccine and logistics management leading of overstocking inadequate stocks and stock out immunization logistics.
- Poor management and monitoring of cold chain system and poor understanding of updated guidelines affecting potency and efficacy of different vaccines.
- Issues underlying immunization and injection of safety and appropriate disposal of waste.
- Low demand for an awareness of immunization services.

These "*Demonstration and Cross Learning Centres*" and identified Block Level Health Facilities (One Facilities per District) where immunization related processes and practices are implemented according to national and State Guidelines in a practical and integrated manner; and which serve as training and venue and provide an opportunity for building skills and capacity of staff members through demonstrations of correct techniques, hands and exercises interaction with peer group members and learning to utilize available resources in best possible manner.

Thus, practice related to different thematic areas including programme management (planning, review and supervision), vaccine-logistics and cold chain management, recording-reporting (Management Information System and use of data for action), immunization safety waste, disposal and community linkages can be demonstrated at the centres for capacity building of staff members.

❑ *Scale Up of Intervention*

Scale up of intervention as pilot has been implemented through encouraging and facilitating capacity building of not only supervisory staff and cold chain handlers rather also of programme managers and other functionaries. Scale up of this intervention with the financial and techno-managerial support from National Rural Health Mission can have significant impact on quality of immunization services and also quality coverage in the forthcoming years.

❑ *Process of Establishing Demonstration and Cross Learning Centres*

- *Orientation of District Immunization Officers:* One day orientation meeting is organized at various levels for sensitizing Programme Managers about the concept, objective and processes of developing demonstration sites. This meeting will also provide opportunity to orient the participants about standard operative procedures, timelines and readiness, assessment and monitoring check-lists. This meeting can also be merged with the quarterly District Immunization Officers review meetings where one day can be devoted for orientation on the demonstration sites.
- *Quarterly Review Meetings for District Immunization Officers:* The quarterly review of the activity is necessary to track progress and identify constraints for ensuring corrective actions. This can be merged with District Immunization Officers review meeting. Visits by State Official to selected poor performing districts to monitor and supervise demonstration site and facilitate cross learning visits.

❑ *District Level*

- *District Level Sensitization Meetings for Facilities Incharge:* This meeting is organized with an objective to sensitize all district level programme managers and facility incharge about the activity and process.
  This will also facilitate identification of underlying strengths of different health facilities including infrastructure, staff available locations for feasibility of cross learning visits, etc. Thus enabling identification of potential health facility to be developed as demonstration and cross learning centres.
- *Identification of Health Facility for Developing Demonstration Site:* In each district one health facility with adequate infrastructure and human resource availability is to be identified by District Officials in discussion with facility staff and other stakeholders (including development partners). Feasibility of organizing cross learning visits for staff Members from blocks health facilities of the District will be an important criterion for selecting health facility to develop as demonstration site. Standard check-list is to be used for selection of health facility in a subjective manner.
- *Review of Progress during the Monthly District Review Meeting:* During each monthly review meeting by Chief Medical Officer at

District Level the status and progress made and demonstration facility can be reviewed. Readiness assessment check-lists are to be used for assessing progress and readiness for organizing cross learning visits.

❑ *Block Level*

- *Orientation of Staff Members at the Identified Health Facilities:* The orientation meeting is to be organized at the health facility identified for developing demonstration and cross learning centre. During the meeting the staff members and other stakeholders are to be sensitized about the process and time lines of the activity for ensuring the involvement and support from all functionaries. During this meeting action plan including specific activities with time line is to be prepared for tracking progress and readiness for organizing cross learning visit.
- *Undertaking Specific Thematic Area-wise Activities for Strengthening the Processes and Practices over a Period of 2-3 Months:* Over a period of 2-3 months, the infrastructure and processes are to be developed in phased manner in line with the standard operative procedure under direct supervision of the District Immunization Officers facility incharge and cold chain handlers of the facility.

  The block level functionaries will work as a team to facilitate implementation of best practices for all thematic areas. The progress made at these sites will be measured on periodic basis on the basis of standard readiness assessment check-list which will enable programme managers to assess and monitor the intervention and plan cross learning visits for other staff members.
- *Cross Learning Visit:* Once the demonstration and cross learning centre is ready as per the readiness assessment checklist, cross learning visits are to be planned jointly by District Immunization Officers and facility Incharge for concerned staff members from other health facilities in batches. The different cadres of staff members that could be nominated for these visits include programme managers facility incharge of other health facilities, cold chain handlers, NRHM staff, supervisory staff and even health workers as part of formal two days training.

During these visits participants will be sensitized. Correct practices and guidelines and visits will be made to cold chain room, dry room, record room and waste management facility to demonstrate the implementation of guidelines. The visit will have a dedicated session interaction between participants and how the available resources can be utilized to implement guidelines at other health facilities.

The cross learning visits are to be organized at six monthly intervals and more visits can be planned for staff from poor performing health facility.

❑ *Specific Activities*

- Development of material for display at concerned areas including cold chain rooms, dry space rooms, management information system rooms, facility incharge room, Out Patient Department/ Immunization clinic and outside facility:
  - ◆ Flex banners for —
    - (a) ANM Roster.
    - (b) Immunization Schedule.
    - (c) Vaccine storage, contingency plan.
    - (d) Coverage monitoring chart.
  - ◆ Job aids on cold chain management injection safety waste disposal and inter-personal communication.
- Updated Micro Planning as per State guidelines and tools.
- Strengthening cold chain room including:
  - ◆ A correct placement of equipment appropriate clinical wiring connections and connection with voltage stabilizer, following correct practices related to vaccine storage and ice pack freezing storage of non-electrical cold chain equipment maintenance cold chain equipment room and dry space room.
  - ◆ Identifying assistant for assistant cold chain handler in cold chain maintenance vaccine and logistics management preventive maintenance of equipment and other immunization related works as specified by the facility in charge.
- Strengthening vaccine and logistic management as per guidelines.
- Using standing recording reporting formats as specified by state guidelines.
- Ensure correct immunization safety and waste disposal practices.

C. *Scale up of "My Village My Home" for Tracking of Immunization Beneficiaries*

Training of beneficiaries is an important aspect of immunization progress and is utmost necessary for achieving full immunization to beneficiaries. Preparation of due list before immunization sessions and mobilization of the beneficiaries in these due lists by ASHA workers and ICDS functionaries has come as an important activity and area of focus for monitoring appropriate implementation of immunization programme. It has been revealed that due to different and erroneous recording mechanisms and different in records of ANMs, ASHAs and Anganwadi workers the due lists prepared are many in times incomplete thus resulting into left out dropouts.

To address this issue of incomplete beneficiaries records with different frontline functionaries and resulting incomplete due listing of beneficiaries, a community level monitoring and tracking mechanism by name "*My Village My Home*" has been launched in the selected sub-centre area.

❑ *"My Village and My Home" Concept*

"My Village and My Home" is a mechanism not only for ensuring registration and tracking of all beneficiaries in a particular catchment area but also focuses on developing and strengthening channels of communication between the community and the service providers for approving routine immunization coverage.

It also serves as community monitoring tool where community members can monitor and assess the coverage of beneficiaries in their villages and take appropriate actions to improve coverage. This intervention, thus, emphasizes and addresses bottom up and a participatory approach and self-monitoring by community members, further helps in build confidence in the programme, creating demand thus, increasing the immunization coverage in respective area.

The objectives of 'My Village My Home' are as follows:

- To ensure coordination between health related department and other stakeholders for timely identification and tracking of eligible infants for full immunization.
- Strengthening channels of communication between the community and service providers and enable grassroots institution/community for self-monitoring of Routine Immunization service utilization.

My Village My Health intervention is to be implemented at all the immunization session sites (sub-centres/Anganwadi Centres/Outreach sites). The frontline functionaries information on the infant immunization status from their registers/records.

My Village My Health tool would be displayed at outreach session sites with names and immunization status of infants. This tool would serve the purpose of motivating and reminding the families for immunizing their children.

❑ *Activities for Roll Out of My Village My Health Interventions*

State Level Activities

- One day state level orientation of district officials and facilities incharge about their intervention.
- Discussion on progress made and status during quarterly District Immunization Officers review meeting.

District Level Activities

- One day orientation of District Officials and facilities incharge about the intervention.
- Printing of My Village My Health tool and required reporting format and distribution to blocks.
- Review during monthly review meeting at District Level.

Block Level Activities

- One day orientation of facilities staff, supervisors and health workers about the intervention.
- Orientating meeting with ICDS staff and orient them about the intervention.
- Development of supervision plan to review and provide supportive supervision to the frontline functionaries.

Session Site Activities

- Orientation of session functionaries (AWW, ASHA and other mobilizers) about the intervention by health worker and identifying suitable site for display of the tool at all session sites in respective sub-centre areas.
- Triangulation of beneficiaries data Maternal Child Health Register and records of ASHA and AWW and update information in the My Village My Health Tool.
- Ensuring mobilization of beneficiaries due for vaccinations as per the tool and update immunization information during the session day itself.

5.14.4. *Innovation-Management Information System: Leveraging Technology — New Innovation Programmes*

A. *Resource Mapping Management System for Health Facilities*

National Rural Health Mission, Uttar Pradesh is keen to take up e-governance initiative to adopt an information technology enabled operation across all key functions of Resource Management and Monitoring System. The specific objectives of this project are as follows:

- Collect geographic coordinates (spatial location) of health facilities/institutions.
- Collect baseline facility information of corresponding health institutions.
- Design and desire geo-data base on Google Earth.
- Incorporate data collected from baseline facility survey into geo-data base for visual mapping of service availability.
- Linkage of the desired system with the website of National Rural Health Mission, Uttar Pradesh.

B. *Video Telephony*

It has been proposed to connect all Chief Medical Officers, Additional Director of all divisions, Mission Director — NRHM, Principal Secretary, Medical Health and Family Welfare, all the three Directors General through Video telephony facility of BSNL.

At a time 19 users can interact with each other with video. This will enhance inter-office communication among all top health functionaries and will help in quick and timely decision making. In the first phase total 100 such connections are proposed to be taken. The estimated expenditure on each unit per annum is ₹ 3,500 which includes one time cost of equipment plus recurring expenditure of ₹ 2,750 per month and maintenance cost of entire network.

C. *Ring Tones/Caller Tunes*

The Jingles and spots are proposed to be played as caller tunes on existing and proposed CUG Network of National Rural Health Mission. Presently, there is existing network of 1,250 CUG connections and approximately 1.42 lakh CUG Phones are proposed to be given to ASHAs, ANMs and Medical Officer Incharge in all Districts. For this purpose monthly expenditure of ₹ 30 per CUG per month has to be paid to BSNL.

5.14.5. *Innovation-Effective Birth and Death Registration Increasing Citizen Registration System*

The strategy paper and road map for increasing birth and death registration, as per the conditionality of the Government of India, State Proposal along with detailed budget has been developed for approval in the financial year 2013-14.

1. *Training of the Registrars of Rural Areas:* The proposed training for the registrar of rural areas of total 52,029 registration units covering 9,000 Gram Panchayat Vikas Adhikaris and 20,737 ANMs working on sub-centre through 991 training workshops. The training venue is proposed Gram Panchayat Vikas Adhikari Registrars.

A. *Training Proposal for the Registrar of Rural Areas on the Processes of Citizen Registration System*

One day training of Gram Panchayat Vikas Adhikari:

1.	No. of Participants	30 (each batch)
2.	No. of Trainers	2
3.	Training Venue	Block Development Office
4.	TA/DA	32 × 100 = 3200
5.	Honorarium to Trainer	2 × 500 = 1000
6.	Working Lunch	32 × 50 = 1600
7.	Tea and snacks	32 × 10 = 320
8.	Workshop Material	30 × 50 = 1500
9.	Other Expenses overhead (Sound System and Generator)	1143
	Total Expenses	**8763**

B. *Printing of Formats for Birth and Death Scheme*

For the use of birth and death programme, the expected annual requirements of the formats have been calculated based on the mid-year population:

1. Birth Information Format - 1/7
2. Death Information Format - 2/8
3. Still Birth Information Format - 3/9
4. Medical Certificate of the Death Reasons - 4
5. Medical Certificate of the Death Seasons - 4 (a)
6. Birth Certificate Number - 5

7. Death Certificate Number - 6
8. Non-Availability Certificate No. 10
9. Summary of monthly Birth Information No. 11
10. Summary of monthly Death Information No. 12
11. Summary of monthly Still Birth Information No. 13

C. *Technical Human Resource for the Office of Chief Registrar (Birth and Death)*

The approved number of posts include Statistical Officer (Sankhya Adhikari), State Training Officer, Statistical Assistant, Analyst-cum-Data Assistant for Head Office and District, Panch/Verifier operator for head office. Thus, the approved post at head office level are 53 and due to lack of technical workforce the registration work are hurdled.

D. *Resources and Equipments for the Office of Chief Registrar (Birth and Death)*

Apart them the shortage of statistical staff at the office of the Chief Registrar (Birth and Death), Director General, Medical Health Services, Uttar Pradesh, there are some other sources which are required as the operationalization of Chief Registrar's related works are affecting.

5.14.6. *Innovation — Mobile Kunji*

Mobile Kunji is designed to be used by ASHAs during their home visits with families. The audio-visual job aid brings together an Interactive Voice Response based mobile service and a printed deck of Cards on a ring.

The virtually indestructible deck of 40 cards provides valuable information that can be shared with families. Unique toll free short mobile numbers printed of the bottom of each card enable Field Link workers to play related audio health messages to rural families using their mobile phones. The audio messages help to ensure standardized content delivery to beneficiaries without the need for reams of paper or expensive multimedia hardware.

❑ *Key Components*

- *A Deck of Illustration Cards:* Following the life cycle approach (nine months of pregnancy till the Child turns two) two cards containing key messages on pregnancy, birth, new born, health family planning, breast feeding, complementary feeding, immunization and hand washing. The cards are designed to be used by Field level link workers for effective inter-personal communication with families. The cards are durable, made from light weight credit card material which is convenient to carry and use.

- *Innovative Voice Response:* Mobile Kunji is a toll free service that can be accessed from any mobile phone. Media Action is in the final stage of negotiation with BSNL so the service will soon be available with BSNL tool.
- *Training:* The comprehensive three day training course orients field level link workers, in the use of Mobile Kunji as part of broader 'negotiated' communication skills. In addition to face to face training, a mobile based training course for ASHAs and Anganwadi Workers, called *Mobile Academy* will also be developed. The course contains technical contents on each behaviour tips and tricks for effective communication intended to provide supportive arguments to Field level link workers in their interactions with families.
- *Monitoring, Supervision and Handholding:* It is essential to simultaneous increase the number of home visits conducted by the Link workers at the appropriate time with appropriate and complete information.

5.14.7. *Innovation — State Nutrition Mission*

With a population of 200 million persons and 35 million children, Uttar Pradesh counts for India and for the world; Uttar Pradesh's population divided has an impact on India and the world —

- Every 5th Child Born in India is in Uttar Pradesh.
- Every 25th Child Born in the World is in Uttar Pradesh.

Any improvement in the situation of children in Uttar Pradesh will have an impact on the situation of children in India. Under nutrition accounts for one-third of under-five mortality.

The following figures reveal the poor nutritional situation of children in Uttar Pradesh:

- Only around 33 per cent of under 3 children (1 out of every 3) being breastfeeded for at least six months.

- Only around 18 per cent of 6-35 month children (one out of every 5) have been exclusively breastfeeded for at least 6 months.
- About 96,000 under 5 children lost every year.
- Uttar Pradesh has around 1.3 million served acute malnourished children. In Uttar Pradesh there are about 9,500 child death per year as a result of severe malnutrition.

It has been proposed that the Nutrition Mission be set up initially for a period of three years and subsequent decision be taken based on the results delivered by the Mission. UNICEF will be the lead technical partner in supporting the Nutrition Mission.

Nutrition Mission will be an autonomous flexible body which will liaise with Medical Health and Family Welfare Department and ICDS for strengthening select intervention.

5.14.8. *Innovation — Mini Skill Lab and Mobile Nurse Trainers: Concept of Mini Skill Lab and Mobile Nurse Training Team*

A. *Mini Skill Lab*

Each Mini Skill Lab will use equipment and instruments to provide simulation training to nursing staff. Some of the instrument will be available in the labour room and operation theatre of the Primary Health Centres, but in addition each mini-skill-lab will have the following mannequins, for training on skills, that are difficult to reach directly on patients:

- *Mama-Natalie* — To reach active management of third stage of labour.
- *Neo-Natalie* — To reach neo-natal resuscitation.
- *Zeo-Gynaecological Simulator* — To reach interval and post partum IUCD.

Therefore, mannequins will remain in the Primary Health Centres, housed in a mini-skill-lab demonstration counter, which is a table specially designed for demonstration training on specific clinical skills and for storing mannequins and other material when not in use.

B. *Mobile Nurse Trainer Teams*

- *Each district* will have two teams of mobile trainers. Each team will have two mobile nurse trainers. These mobile nurse trainers will be supervised and supported by master nurse trainers.

- *Mobile Nurse Training team* will provide on site on job training to nurses involved in the labour room and new born care duty in the identified facilities where Mini-Skill Labs will be established.
- *The entire training content* will be divided into two components — Basic and Advanced.
    - *Basic Component* includes skills related to infection control, waste management, normal delivery, care of the normal new born and basic standards of care in the operation theatre, for Family Planning Procedure.
    - *Advanced Component* includes the management of complication stabilization and referral.
- *Tentatively during* each month by ratio, mobile training team will visit each facility for one week duration.

5.15. *Planning Implementation and Monitoring*

Planning, Implementation and Monitoring includes the following activities:

5.15.1. *Quality Assurance*

The quality enhancement in health care has been recognized as an essential cornerstone for promoting equity and maximizing health gain. With the event of NRHM, a significant improvement has been made on multiple health indicators and promotional scheme for institutional deliveries have led to tremendous increase in the utilization of public health facilities. The State now strives to address the issue of enhancing the quality of health care services, rendered through establishment of quality assurance network at various levels.

In continuation to our quest for delivering high quality health services, quality assurance cell at State level has been established and state quality assurance working groups have been formed.

Quality Assurance Cell at State Level: Cell has been established under the Chairmanship of Mission Director and full time Deputy Director General Manger has been appointed.

- *State Nodal Officer:* Director, Medical Care, Medical Health and Family Welfare Department, U.P.
- *State Working Groups:* State Working Groups have been formed — RCH Service, NRHM Additionalities Routine Immunization and National Programme.

- *Monitoring and Evaluation Cell:* for quality assurance and improvement established through District Quality Assurance Cell.
- Appropriate actions have been initiated to award achieving Indian Pubic Health Standards.

Quality Assurance Cell — Divisional and District Level: To ensure the self-driven quality improvement at Primary Health Centres for improved quality of care objectives:

- Increasing participation of all stakeholders in a facility through development of quality teams.
- Increase engagement with District Quality Assurance Cell to ensure achievement of District Health Plan.
- Orient facility level staff to envision, plan and execute standard quality assurance paradigms like Indian Public Health Standard and Family Friendly Hospital Initiatives.
- Improve the quality of care provided to beneficiaries.

Essential Elements:

- *District Quality Assurance Workshop:* Orienting District Official on facility solution levels.
- *Block Level Workshops:* Orienting Block officials on facility solution levels.
- *Creation of Facility Quality Assurance Team:* Monthly Quality Assurance Team Meeting with recorded minutes.
- *Facility Assessment Tool Kit:* Standard tool kit (paper software based) for gap assessment and comprehensive facility assessment for readiness for IPHS.
- *Creation of Comprehensive Action Plan:* Gap assessment and achievement monitoring through monthly/quarterly Quality Assurance Team Meeting.
- *District Quality Assurance Cell Field Visits:* Periodic engagement of District Quality Assurance Cell with the facility to assess and monitor progress on comprehensive action plan.
- *Quality Management System:* Training to facility staff.
- *Following up Quality Management System Workshop:* Refresher and follow-up training on standard treatment protocols to facility staff.

Expected Outcomes:

- As a result of quality improvement, early identification of maternal and new born complication stabilization and timely referral to appropriate facility.
- Indian Public Health Standards accreditation by the State Government.

5.15.2. *Monitoring and Evaluation*

A. *Strengthening of Monitoring and Evaluation*

- Salaries of Monitoring and Evaluation, Management Information System and Data Entry Operators have been approved. The services of the same number of Health Management Information System operators are required at State Programme Management Unit as well as District Level.
- Strengthening of Management Information System has been made operational to look after the work of State and other on line portals for improvement of monitoring, evaluation and reporting and feedback mechanism.
- Training/Workshops are organized on monitoring and evaluation.

B. *Procurement of Hardware/Software and Other Equipments*

- *Hardware/Software Procurement:* Procurement of Hardware/ Software have been ensured.
- *Internet Connectivity:* Leased line internet connection at State Level and Broadband Connection at the District and Block level has been proposed.
- *Annual Maintenance:* For annual maintenance of Hardware and equipments has been proposed which were procured during first phase of NRHM programme. New Computers/Printers and UPS for State, Division has been proposed @ ₹ 50,000 computer system.
- *Contingency NRHM Website Development/Maintenance* and other online application including Web based reporting system has been procured, designed and developed.
- *CUG Mobiles for ASHA*, Auxiliary Nurse Midwife and Medical Officer Incharge has been planned but this may be dropped as already considered under committed expenditure of financial year 2012-13.

C. *Operationalization of Health Management Information System at Sub-District Level*

Operationalization of Health Management System at Sub-District level has been ensured.

- *Review of Existing Registers has been Ensured* to make them compatible with National Health Management Information System Portal.
- *Printing of New Registers/forms/formants* have been proposed.
- *Training of Staff* on HMIS, Tally, etc. will be required at all levels in order to enhance data quality of MIS. The persons included for training are computer operators, Assistant Research Officer, District Programme Manager/District Community Mobilizers Divisional Project Managers, Chief Medical Officer, Family Welfare, Additional CMOs, Dy. CMOs, Block Programme Managers, Routine Immunization Assistant, District Immunization Officer and Block Data Assistant.

D. *Operationalizing MCH Tracking*

Ongoing review of MCH tracking activities has been proposed and an appropriate budgetary provision has been made.

- *Monitoring Data Collection and Data Quality:* Work plan generation was proposed and honorarium for various officials has also been budgeted.

5.16. *Procurement*

Procurement of equipments, drugs and consumables have been analyzed.

5.16.1. *Procurement of Equipments*

Procurement of Equipments under various programmes including Maternal Health especially — MVA/EVA for safe abortion services and establishment of New Sub-Centre and Equipments for Child Health and Family Planning and equipments for Adolescent, Reproductive and Sexual Health and procurement of other diagnostic equipments have been proposed and requisite amount have been approved.

5.16.2. *Procurement of Drugs and Consumables*

The procurement of drugs and other consumables under various programmes has been proposed under Maternal Health, Child Health,

Bio-medical waste, Management, Cleaning/Washing, house keeping and laundry management at facility level, drugs and supplies for Health Facilities (Indoor and Outdoor Patient Department and drugs and supplies for AYUSH has been proposed for the procurement of drugs and consumables.

5.16.3. *Annual Maintenance Contract*

Annual Maintenance Contract for Valuable Medical Equipments including MRI, CT Scan machine, X-ray Machine, Ultrasound Machine and Pathological analyzer has been ensured. To make them continuously functional annual maintenance contract is greatly required. It is important to mention that at the time of Departmental procurement of these instruments through tender processes the rate of Annual Maintenance Contract is decided on open competition basis.

The budget proposed for Annual Maintenance Contract for the Programme Implementation Plan 2013-14 of National Rural Health Mission for the District Hospital Sultanpur for X-ray, Ultrasound Machine is proposed ₹ 96,396 and budget for Annual Maintenance Contract for X-ray Machine and Ultrasound Machine for District Women Hospital, Sultanpur has been proposed for ₹ 22,523 in the Programme Implementation of National Rural Health Mission.

5.17. *Drug Warehouses*

An appropriate logistic support is being ensured for the functioning of Drug warehouses.

5.17.1. *State Logistic Management Cell*

There is a State Logistic Management Cell to ensure operationalization of Drug warehouse at Naderganj, Lucknow. There is an ongoing activity which was also sanctioned in the previous year. State Logistic Management Cell will have the following contractual staff like Accountant-1, Computer Operator/Store Keeper-1, Fourth Class/Lift operator-cum-Mechanic-1, Store Keeper-1, Fourth Class Loader-1/ Generator-Operator-cum-Electrician/Mechanic-1 Armed Guard-1, General Guard-3, Gardener-1 and Sweeper-1.

5.17.2. *Operationalization of Regional Drug Warehouse*

There are 11 Regional Drug Warehouse in the State which is an ongoing activity sanctioned from previous years. Each regional drug warehouse has following contractual staff like accountant-1, computer operator/ store keeper-1/Fork lift operator-cum-Mechanic-1, Fourth Class Loader-1, Generator Operator-cum-Electrician/Mechanic-1, Armed Guards-1, General Guard-2, Gardener-1 and sweeper-1 will be deployed.

5.17.3. *Operationalization of District Drug Warehouses*

Government of India has sanctioned operationalization of District Drug Warehouses, which is an ongoing activity, the budget provision for contractual staff for District Drug Warehouses included — Computer operator-cum-store keeper, generator operator-cum-Mechanic/ Electrician, Loader, Chowkidar and Part-time sweeper, etc.

5.18. *Health Insurance Scheme*

Health Insurance Scheme has been proposed for all the ASHAs of the State by LIC of India. This scheme is called "*Jan Shree Bima Yojana*" desired by Central Government and LIC of India for the benefit of people below the poverty line.

Benefits — Various benefits of the *Jan Shree Bima Yojana* are as follows:

- *Natural Death:* In the event of death of the member under this scheme, a sum of assured amount of ₹ 30,000 will become payable to the nominee.
- *Accident Benefit:* In the event of death by accident or Partial/ Total Permanent Disability due to accident, the following benefit shall be payable to the Nominee —

I.	On Death or Total Permanent Disability due to accident	₹ 75,000
II.	On Partial Permanent Disability	₹ 37,000

- *Educational Benefit:* The benefit of children of the parents covered a scholarship of ₹ 600 per half year to be paid to students studying in standard XI to XII (including ITI courses). The benefit is restricted to two children of a family.
- *Premium:* ₹ 200 per member is to be shared as under 50 per cent of the premium is to be paid by the NRHM at the time of submission of proposal 50 per cent of the premium will be borne by social security fund of Government of India.

5.20. *Research/Studies/Analysis*

National Rural Health Mission seeks to provide accessible, affordable and quality health care to the rural people. For achieving goals and objectives of NRHM, U.P., the number of programme activities have been sanctioned in the Programme Implementation Plan for its implementation.

Programme evaluation is a valuable tool for strengthening the quality of programme and to improve outcomes. Programme evaluation answers basic questions about a programme's effectiveness and evaluation data can be used to improve programme services.

Programme evaluation is systematic method for collecting, analyzing and using information to answer basic questions about a programme. Process of evaluation assess whether an intervention or programme model was implemented as planned. Whether intended target population was reached and the major challenges and successful strategies associated with programme implementation. Outcome evaluation determine whether and to what extent, the expected changes occur and whether these changes can be attributed to the programme or programme activities.

5.21. *State Health Resource Centre/State Public Health Resource Centre*

State Health Resource Centre and State Public Health Resource Centre functioning are analyzed as under:

5.21.1. *State Health Resource Centre*

National Rural Health Mission mandates that each state set up a State level Health Resource Centre along with the State Programme Management Unit.

State Health Resource Centre envisions to serve as an apex body to provide Technical Assistance to facilitate State and District in Planning and Implementation of NRHM Programme as well as strengthening the Public health system in the State.

State Programme Management Unit was established in 2008. Most of the staff was hired on Contract, some on deputation and some staff was deputed from SIFPSA on loan basis. State Health Resource Centre was planned and set up in the year 2011-12 and a budget of ₹ 665.32 lakh was approved by Government of India but the Centre could not be established till date.

❑ *Institutional Requirements of State Health Resource Centre*

As per State Health Resource Centre models of different states following features can be adopted for Uttar Pradesh:

- State Health Resource Centre should be an autonomous body within its own governing body, executive committee and its rules/regulations. It should have sufficient Government representation in it to ensure transparency in all operations and to intervene as and when required.
- State Health Resource Centre should be a responsive organization with the flexibility to take subject experts on broad framework, from time to time for short or medium term.
- State Health Resource Centre should have collaboration with various National and International Technical Agencies/ Institutions for latest information and knowledge for application in the implementation process.
- While State Health Resource Centre should initiate activities to enable innovation, it should also take up tasks/assignments from Health Directorate and State Programme Management Unit to be delivered in a time bound manner. Its effectiveness will be desired from the quality of inputs, it will provide and its ability to internally champion process of change.

SIFPSA can be developed as State Health Resource Centre as various innovations have been done by SIFPSA. The SIFPSA also established partnership with public and private sector as in voucher project, social franchising, promotion of contraceptive social marketing, NGO Project capacity building of Panchayati Raj Institutions.

❑ *Plan for State Health Resource Centre*

For State Health Resource Centre organizational structure is being proposed. Since the State Health Resource Centre would require for providing very technical and specialized input, a provision is being made for hiring subject specialities experts and consultants intended for specific areas on short term basis.

5.21.2. *State Public Health Resource Institute*

In the National Rural Health Programme Implementation Plan, it was the mandate of First Phase of NRHM to establish State Health Resource Centre, at state level. But in the Second Phase of NRHM, the State has proposed to establish State Public Health Resource Institute through NRHM which will work in anchorship of State Institute of Health and Family Welfare and will coordinate Director General, Family Welfare and Director General, Health and SIHFW in the field of information/ data upgradation, Human Resource and Research Work in the field of the public health.

5.22. *Support Services*

Different support services have been initiated under National Rural Health Mission Programme which are as follows:

A. *Additionality for JE/AES and Malaria*

To support JE/AES and Malaria and National Vector-Borne Disease Control Programme has been proposed for additionality funds from National Rural Health Mission.

Name of Unit		*Unit Cost (₹ in lakh)*	*Total Amount (₹ in lakh)*
BRD Medical College Gorakhpur	Manpower (HR) for 54 bedded JE/ AES Ward	427.50	427.40
	Manpower (HR) for 100 bedded JE/ AES Ward	325.75	325.75
	Medicines	300.00	300.00
ICDS	Training for 1540 batches 40 participants per batch = 61600	0.4550 per batch	700.00
Department of Animal Husbandry for 20 Districts	Disinfection and Spray of Insecticides in PIG Shelters	20 Districts @ ₹ 9.364 lakh	187.28
Additionality for Malaria Rapid Diagnostic Kit @ ₹ 80.00 per Kit		5 lakh Kits	400.00
		Total	2473.59

B. *Additionality for Revised National Tuberculosis Control Programme*

To support Revised National Tuberculosis Control Programme, a sum of ₹ 1,166.46 lakh was proposed for the additionality funds from National Rural Health Mission.

C. *Additionality for National Leprosy Eradication Programme*

To support National Leprosy Eradication Programme, a sum of ₹ 129.96

lakh has been proposed for additionality funds from National Rural Health Mission.

D. *Additionality for National Programme for Control of Blindness*

To support National Programme for control of Blindness ₹ 137.50 lakh was proposed for additionality funds from National Rural Health Mission.

E. *Multi-Purpose Workers — Contractual*

Under National Vector-Borne Disease Control Programme an amount of ₹ 5,292.72 lakh was proposed for 7,351 Multi-Purpose workers (Contractual) @ ₹ 6,000 per month for 12 months. Services of multi-purpose workers are being utilized for Vector-Borne Disease Control Activities.

5.23. *Other Expenditures (Power Backup Convergence)*

Diesel for Generator at District Hospitals and Primary Health Centres/ Community Health Centres.

The availability of Electricity in the Uttar Pradesh is poor affecting the functionality of the health facilities. In some of the areas there is less than four hours of electricity available throughout the day. Further day-by-day increasing Janani Suraksha Yojana load and other services at facilities there is urgent need of regular power backup services.

As per proposal received from Director General, Medical Health, an amount of ₹ 3,359.10 lakh is required for 153 District level hospitals and Community Health Centres/Primary Health Centres of 75 districts.

6. Routine Immunization

The Immunization programme is the cornerstone of public health, world over, vaccination was practiced in India, since the early 1900s, especially against small pox, in the late 1940s. In 1962, BCG insulation was included in the National Tuberculosis Control Programme. A formal programme under the name of expanded programme of Immunization was launched in 1978. This gained momentum in 1985 under Universal Immunization Programme. Later on Universal Immunization Programme was merged in Child Survival and Safe Motherhood Programme in 1992-93. Since, 1997 immunization activities are an important component of Reproductive and Child Health (RCH) programme. A National Technical Advisory Group on immunization was set up in 2003 and a Mid-Term Strategic Plan developed in 2004. From April 2005, immunization is an important component of RCH-II under the National Rural Health Mission.

6.1. *Routine Immunization Strengthening Project*

A sum of ₹ 37.50 lakh has been proposed for morbidity support for supervision of district level officers under the programme Implementation Plan of Financial Year 2013-14. Appropriate budget has also been allocated for printing and dissemination of immunization card, tally sheet and monitoring formats, etc. and has been calculated @ ₹ 10 beneficiary (expected number of pregnant women).

6.2. *Review Meeting*

A sum of ₹ 17.06 lakh has been budgeted for district level quarterly review meetings. An amount of ₹ 413.88 lakh has been budgeted for Block level quarterly review meetings with ASHA as one of the participant and the amount has been calculated @ ₹ 75 per participant in Programme Implementation Plan of Financial Year 2013-14.

6.3. *Routine Immunization in Slum and Underserved Areas*

In the proposed Programme Implementation Plan of the Financial Year 2013-14, a total of ₹ 298.33 lakh was budgeted for focusing Routine Immunization in Slum and Underserved Areas.

6.4. *Mobilization of Beneficiaries through ASHA and Alternate Vaccine Delivery*

A sum of ₹ 3,147.33 lakh was proposed for mobilization of beneficiaries to session site through ASHA @ ₹ 150 per session. An amount of ₹ 310.47 lakh has been proposed @ ₹ 150 per session for Alternate Vaccine Delivery for hard to reach areas and ₹ 1,372.62 lakh was budgeted @ ₹ 75 per session for alternate vaccine delivery in other areas in Programme Implementation Plan.

6.5. *Consumables for Computers Including Internet and Bio-Medical Waste Management*

An amount of ₹ 3.58 lakh was proposed for consumables for computer including provision for internet access for Routine Immunization Management district. An amount of ₹ 142.07 lakh was proposed to the session site in the Financial Year 2013-14.

6.6. *State Specific Requirement*

A total of ₹ 261.33 lakh was proposed for State specific requirement which includes ₹ 14.40 lakh for annual maintenance at State and Divisional Level. ₹ 40.0 lakh for Electricity Bill and ₹ 38.0 lakh for generator and operational expenses at divisional vaccine stores, ₹ 2.0 lakh for mobility support for state level officers and ₹ 16.88 lakh for State level review meetings, ₹ 5.63 lakh for State level Training of Trainers for Medical officers, and ₹ 5.96 lakh for quarterly review meetings of Regional Managers and District cold chain store incharge at State level. ₹ 27.0 lakh for mobility fund for Regional Manager at District Level. ₹ 17.28 lakh for mobility for divisional RM at divisional level, ₹ 10.0 lakh for AEFI kit and ₹ 1.52 lakh for regional meetings for supportive supervision in Routine Immunization and ₹ 82.66 lakh for supportive supervision at Cold Chain points.

6.7. *Salary of Contractual Staff*

A total amount of ₹ 91.80 lakh has been proposed for salary of Contractual staff for computer assistant at State and District level and Salary of Cold Chain Staff was proposed ₹ 223.44 lakh out of which Government of India approved ₹ 98.01 lakh only.

6.8. *Training under Immunization*

A total amount of ₹ 601.90 lakh was proposed by the State in the financial year 2013-14 for training under immunization which includes a sum of ₹ 438.64 lakh which was budgeted for District Level Orientation training and ₹ 122.02 lakh for 3 days' training including Hepatitis-B, Measles and Japanese Encephalitis of Medical Officers, ₹ 34.58 lakh for 2 days' cold chain handlers, ₹ 2.92 lakh for Block level data handlers and ₹ 3.75 lakh for training of other categories.

6.9. *Training of Frontline Workers*

A budget of ₹ 80,000 per batch @ 30 frontline workers including Health workers, ASHAs and AWWs has been proposed for training of frontline workers planned to be conducted with the support from National Polio Surveillance Project.

6.10. *ASHA Incentive*

A sum of ₹ 6,531.61 lakh was budgeted for ASHA incentive for complete immunization of new born @ ₹ 150 for complete immunization of a child.

6.11. *Teeka Expenses*

A sum of ₹ 62.75 lakh had been approved in the budget for 2012-13 for Teeka Expenses, but the vehicle and guidelines were not available, hence, the budget remains unutilized.

6.12. *Innovation under Routine Immunization*

❑ *Supportive Supervision*

A group of experts including District Health Officers and officers from partner Agencies will be visiting all cold chain points in a planned manner and take "On the spot" corrective action to improve cold chain. Cold chain handlers and other working in the cold chain point will be trained simultaneously.

❑ *Demonstration and Cross Learning Centres*

Demonstration site will be developed in each district, exhibiting ideal practices, personnel from all cold chain points of the District will visit those sites twice in a year and will be expected to follow similar practices in their cold chain points.

❑ *My Village My Home*

Availability of due list at the Routine Immunization Session sites is essential, for ensuring successful immunization session. It has been a big challenge to make these due lists available and to ensure their completeness.

My Village My Home activity has been planned in each district. This will help to ensure coordination between health related departments — ICDS and other stakeholder for timely identification and tracking of eligible infant for full immunization. For this purpose an amount of ₹ 390.00 lakh only for high priority district for tracking of Immunization beneficiaries.

7. National Disease Control Programme

The National Disease Control Programme includes — National Iodine Deficiency Disorder Control Programme, Integrated Disease Surveillance Project, National Vector-Borne Disease Control Programme, National Leprosy Eradication Programme, National Programme for Control of Blindness, Revised National Tuberculosis Control Programme, National

Tobacco Control Programme and National Programme for Prevention and Control of Deafness, etc.

7.1. *National Iodine Deficiency Disorder Control Programme*

Iodine Deficiency Disorder has been recognized as a public health problem in India, since long ago. Iodine Deficiency Disorder was thought to be a problem in Uttar Pradesh. However, surveys carried out subsequently by the Ministry of Health and Family Welfare showed that no state in India was free from Iodine Deficiency Disorder.

The implication of Iodine deficiency for the unborn are of serious concern in India, where an estimated 11 million new borns are still unprotected against brain damage simply because their mothers did not consume Salt with adequate levels of iodine during their pregnancy.

Further loss of 10 to 15 Intelligence Quotient point attributable to iodine deficiency adversely impact on school performance of the 200 million primary school children in India and learning ability out of school children. This not only results in waste of social investment in education, but also compromised national development.

It has been indicated that almost half of the 17 districts assessed had level of urinary iodine below the WHO recommended level. In the districts with adequate urinary iodine execution level, the median was slightly above than 100 μg/lt indicating a precarious situation.

❑ *Iodine Deficiency Disorder Control Programme in Uttar Pradesh*

National Family Welfare Survey 1998 showed that only 50 per cent households consumed salt adequately iodized with iodine. Several initiatives were launched by the Government of Uttar Pradesh to accelerate the consumption of iodized salt by population. The achievement, however, suffered a setback when in the year 2000 Government of India lifted the ban on sale of non-iodized salt and increased the freight charges of rakes carrying iodized salt.

National Family Health Survey of 2005 showed a significant drop in the number of households consuming adequately iodized salt from 50 per cent in the National Family Health Survey-2. The consumption dropped to 38 per cent.

❑ *Overview of the Trade in Uttar Pradesh*

Uttar Pradesh is one of the States which continues to have the lowest consumption of iodized salt despite the fact there is a ban on sale of non-iodized salt for edible purposes.

Uttar Pradesh is a non-salt producing State and receives its quota of salt for industrial and edible purposes from the State of Gujarat and Rajasthan.

Reports from the Salt Commissioner's office indicate that the State receives a total 10,45,000 tonnes of salt annually of which 80 per cent (8,40,000 tonnes) is for edible purposes and the rest for industrial purpose (approximately 1,33,000 tonnes).

In a non-salt producing state like Uttar Pradesh, reaching the whole-sellers dealing in salt trade and linking them with State Iodine Deficiency Disorder lab will enable Public-Private Partnership critical for sustainability and programme evolvement. The salt whole-sellers procure salt by the rail or load, for supply for human and animal consumption as well as for industrial usage.

As this is a priority programme under National Rural Health Mission. The Social and Preventive Department of Medical College are already undertaking the task of titration support is expected from NRHM to strengthen monitoring of programme as well as improve the supply and availability of iodized salt in the market.

The Iodine Deficiency Orders Cell in Medical College will essentially comprise a titration unit set up within the existing laboratory of the community medicine department. The cell will be managed by a programme manager and a lab technician.

❑ *Objectives of Iodine Deficiency Disorder Cell in Medical College*

- Organize regular and frequent sensitization of wholesaler and retailers in the intervention distraction benefits of iodized salt and motivate them to procure and distribute good quality iodized salt for edible purposes.
- Organize Inter-sectoral advocacy/media meetings in the nodal district where Iodine Deficiency Disorder Cell is located with Government stakeholders (Education, Health, ICDS) under chairmanship of District Magistrate for generating demand for iodized salt using Government scheme.
- Encourage wholesalers/retailers to dispatch samples of procured salt received by rail or road for testing.

The reporting of these Iodine Deficiency Disorder Cells linked with 100 labs at State Health Institute, Lucknow and monthly analysis on samples tested for presence of Iodine will be shared with Iodine Deficiency Disorder Lab.

The analysis will be done free of cost and wholesalers and retailers who have volunteered to get the samples analyzed from Iodine Deficiency Disorder Cells will be provided prompt feedback using a feedback certificate.

7.2. *Integrated Diseased Surveillance Project*

Integrated Diseased Surveillance Project started in 2004 with support from World Bank to improve and Integrate Disease Surveillance in pursuance of recommendations by high powered committee, like Public Health System Committee of Secretaries of Environmental Sanitation. During 2007 with Avian Influence outbreak, human and animal components were added along with additional budget.

The following assumptions were made at the time of launch of project about infrastructure at the District and State Level —

- Units have adequate skills, resource and authority to respond.
- Communities and private sector have adequate incentive to participate.
- Good quality of lab information is available in timely manner and integrated into surveillance system.

It has been noted that these were not found to be fully correct, so the objectives could not be achieved as well as fund utilization was low. During 2009, after detailed analysis of the situation, World Bank agreed to restructure the project and extend it for 2 years focusing on what can be achieved by the end of two years. Keeping this in mind project development objectives was revised and a proposal for restructuring and extension of Integrated Disease Surveillance Project has been prepared.

❑ *Objectives of the Project Development*

- To improve the information available to the Government Health Service and Private Health Care providers on a set of high priority disease and risk factors so as to improve the responses towards them.
- To establish a decentralized State based system of surveillance for disease to ensure timely and effective health response towards health challenges at all level.
- To put greater emphasis on building the link between the collection and analysis of information and ground intervention by public or private sectors.

❑ *Activities to be Done under Different Components*

I. *Surveillance Preparedness*

- Training of Epidemiologist and Entomologist. It would be done regionally by drawing the faculty from the resource group.
- Training of Surveillance Team.
- Additional team for reporting and analysis for health supervisors, block health teams, pharmacists, etc.
- Ensuring fully functional I.T. System in place —
  - Mechanism to enhance data integration and flow from telephone, E-mail, and fax will be developed.
  - Revision of remuneration to bring these at par with other National Projects.
  - State Surveillance Unit and District Surveillance Unit will be authorized to have broad band connectivity through BSNL and also to distribute their broad band bills.
  - Training schedule and module for training.
  - Band with capacity of EDUSAT has been upgraded from 512 KG ps to 1 MG ps.
  - The issue of toll free numbers are being analyzed investigated and solved.
  - To promote the use of toll free services, the numbers will be publicized amongst the private and public sectors by advertisement, bulletins, etc.
  - The SMS Syndromic reporting model is being assessed to be incorporated in other priority areas.

II. *For Priority District Labs*

- Rigorous monitoring will be done for procurement of equipment.
- Development of specimen collection centre within the District.
- Placement of New Medical and non-medical micro-biologist at District and State's labs.
- Regular Monitoring of functioning of District Priority Labs.
- Implementation of guidelines for procurement of quality kits.
- To organize External Quality Assessment Scheme when District Priority Lab becomes functional for 3 months.

III. *For Entomological Surveillance*

(a) Training of Entomologist.

(b) Entomologist in consultation with National Vector-Borne Disease Control Programme Officer and Chief Medical Officer will do mapping, monitoring of entomological density and bionomics and sensitivity to insecticides.

(c) They will also do entomological investigations during vector-borne disease outbreak.

(d) Vaccine preventable disease diphtheria, pertussis and measles are going to be covered to Integrated Disease Surveillance Project. H1N1 has already been included in the programme.

❑ *Proposed Activities*

I. *Surveillance Activities*

- *Vaccine Preventable Diseases* — Measles, Pertussis, Diphtheria, and other diseases like Influenza A, H1N1 and other communicable diseases are being covered in the Integrated Disease Surveillance Project.
- All Medical Colleges of the State are going to be involved with proper guidelines of reporting from Areas of Prevalence in data collection disease surveillance.
- Strengthening the Surveillance of Epidemic Prone Disease especially AES/JE and Dengue.
- To ensure online data entry from all districts of U.P.
- To start video conferencing between State Surveillance unit and District Surveillance unit.

II. *Training*

(a) *Training of Hospital Doctors:* To help them in understanding the objectives and importance of surveillance. To train them for filling up various IDSP forms, so that complete and timely information from the hospitals is sent to the state unit. One day training will be given at District level under the guidance of District Surveillance officer. It will be given in 20 batches having 20 people per batch @ ₹ 50,000 per batch.

(b) *Medical College Doctors:* For their orientation of the Programme, so that exhaustive information of the health data may be provided. One day training will be given at state level in 5 batches having 20 people per batch @ ₹ 50,000 per batch.

(c) *Training of Hospital Pharmacist/Nurses:* For detecting and reporting early warming signals of outbreaks. One day training will be given at District level in 20 batches having 20 people per batch @ ₹ 38,000 per batch.

III. *Human Resources*

Recruitment for all the vacant position under the programme at state Head Quarter and District Surveillance Unit will be done during the 1st Quarter of the Financial Year 2013-14..Recruitment for the vacant posts will be done at state level by a committee chaired by Director General, Medical Health, Uttar Pradesh.

Under Integrated Disease Surveillance Project Programme to conduct various activities at State and District Levels an amount of ₹ 941.79 lakh was proposed out of which Government of India approved ₹ 888.62 lakh only.

7.3. *National Vector-Borne Disease Control Programme*

Important National Vector-Borne Diseases are Malaria, Dengue, Chikungunya, Filaria, Kala-Azar and AES/JE. Strategies for Prevention and Control of Vector-Borne Diseases are as follows:

- Integrated vector control (*Source:* Reduction, IRS, Fish, Chemical and Biolarivicide).
- Early Diagnosis and complete treatment.
- Vaccination against JE.
- Case Management as no specific drugs against Dengue, Chikungunya and JE are available.
- Annual Mass Drugs Administration for Lymphatic, Filariasis Elimination.
- Capacity Building.
- Behaviour Change Communication and Information, Education and Communication.

❑ *Goals*

- The elimination of lymphatic, filariasis and Kala-Azar.
- Control and Contain the outbreaks of Dengue, Chikungunya, and Japanese Encephalitis.
- Paving the way for pre-eliminating phase of Malaria.

❑ *Targets*

- Malaria:
  - — To increase ABER up to 10 per cent.

— To maintain API below 1 per cent.
— Spray of Insecticide (IRS) in Malaria Prone area.

- Dengue/Chikungunya:
  — All sentinel Surveillance, Hospital Labs to be made functional.
- Kala-Azar:
  — Focusing on Elimination of Kala-Azar.
- AES/JE:
  — To decrease Mortality and Morbidity.
  — Developing Paediatric ICU in 20AES/JE Prone area.

❑ *Priorities*

- Malaria:
  — To strengthening Human Resource.
  — Spray of Insecticide (IRS) in Malaria Prone Area.
- Dengue/Chikungunya:
  — Source reduction by putting more domestic breeding checkers.
  — Diagnosis and Case Management — Making Shelters in all District Hospitals.
- Kala Azar:
  — Focusing on Elimination of Kala-Azar and doing 2 rounds of DDT spray.
- AES/JE:
  — Initiate the activities as per recommendation of government.
  — To decrease morbidity and mortality.
  — Developing Paediatric ICU in 20 AES/JE Prone areas.

❑ *Challenges*

- Rurban slums are prominent Endemic site for malaria.
- Poor sanitation, water-logging, scarcity of drinking water for which people store drinking water for long time.
- Active surveillance is not been conducted effectively due to shortage of Multi-purpose workers.
- Population has increased relative to which infrastructure has not been strengthened.

- Presently ANMs and ASHAs are not able to fully contribute in vector-borne disease control programme because of other programmes.
- Current scenario of lab technician – Number of sanctioned posts = 2,224, working = 1,836 and vacant 338. Population and PHCs are increasing against the sanctioned post of Lab Technicians.
- Few Districts of Eastern Uttar Pradesh are affected by the Kala-Azar because of migration of labourers from Endemic State of Uttar Pradesh for livelihood.

7.3.1. *Malaria*

An important mission of the government is to bring down annual incidence of Malaria cases to less than one per 1,000 population at National level and its monitoring at District level.

❑ *Strategy and Innovation for Effective Disease Control and Treatment*

Epidemiological Surveillance and Disease Management

- *Microscopic Centres:* Strengthening the existing surveillance. All microscopic centres are to be made functional ANMs/ MPWs should make blood slides for malaria regularly.
- *Active Surveillance by MPWs and ASHAs:* Involvement of ASHAs for active surveillance. Honorarium @ ₹ 15 to ASHA amounts to ₹ 75.00 lakh. There are 1,38,200 ASHAs working and each expected to make 15 slides per annum. If they actively participate for giving radical treatment to the patient then per patient ₹ 75 will be paid.
- *Case Management:*
  - — All malaria Positive patients should get radical treatment earliest possible in the surveillance of Medical Officers and others.
  - — Epidemic preparedness and Rapid Response Team.
  - — Involvement of Private providers.
- *Integrated Vector Management:*
  - — Effective Entomological surveillance.
  - — Source reduction using Minor Engineering Method.
  - — Environment Control — Biological and Larvicidal Fish.
  - — Larvicides (Biolarvicides) and Larvicide (Chemical).

- Timely and good Quality and IRS is Important and implemented with sound technical skills.
- Operational Research.

• *Capacity Building:*

- Training of ASHAs in making blood smears.
- Training of ASHAs using Rapid Diagnostic Kit by Medical Officer Incharge in specified Primary Health Centres.
- Training of Health Workers and Supervisors in making solution of insecticides and in using spray pumps and fogging machine by District Malaria Officers and the Medical Officers should be well conversed with equipments and techniques.

• *IEC/BCC Activities:*

- IEC before straying and fogging operation about precautions to make it successful.
- Health Education Materials to be supplied to all health centres and to be distributed to public in the malaria month of June.

• *General Vector Control Strategy:*

- Main strategy for control of vector-borne disease in vector management.
- To control condition promoting mosquitoes breeding.
- One week day Saturday to be made dry day (emptying overhead tanks, coolers, defrost pans and plants' pots, etc.).
- Larvicide in open drains with stagnant water.
- Two round of IRS DDT — 50 per cent and three rounds of Malathian 25 per cent WDP in High Risk area.
- Spray wages from state resource for technical skilled labours.
- Fogging by Malathian Technical at dawn and dusk.
- To control outdoor mosquitoes density in village affected with JE/AES (Larvicidal Activity in morning).

7.3.2. *Lymphatic Filariasis*

An important goal of the programme is for elimination of Lymphatic Filariasis by 2015. To achieve elimination, the micro filarial rate in all the endemic areas should be less than 1 per cent to interrupt transmission.

Filaria is Endemic in 51 districts of Uttar Pradesh. One District, namely Sultanpur is bifurcated into two districts, *viz*. Amethi, so that the total number of endemic districts now become 52.

❑ *Specific Constraints for Implementation of Programme*

- Apart from disability, Management is great challenge to remove the social stigma for the population suffering from disease. Filaria is mainly urban disease and due to rapid urbanization the disease cases are increasing to manifold. No method for detecting parasite at early stage of infection. Resources are inadequate and insufficient due to 29 Filaria Units and 2 Filaria Clinics.
- MDA is expected to be successful. Interest in Health Education and Inter-sectoral cooperation is required.
- Under Filaria Control Programme MDA Programme is conducted every year on proposed date of 11th November.

❑ *Objectives*

- To progressively reduce and ultimately interrupt the transmission of Lymphatic Filariasis.
- To augment the disability alleviation programme to reduce the suffering of affected person through appropriate home based morbidity Management and Hydrocoelectomy.

❑ *Strategy for Lymphatic Filariasis*

- State Task Force and Technical Advisory Committee Meeting at State Headquarters.
- Coordination Committee Meeting at District Level.
- Line-listing of Filaria cases (Hydrocoele and Lymphodoema, etc.).
- Filariasis Survey at 4 sentinel and 4 random kits in each district.
- Training of Malaria Officers, Para-Medicals and Drug distribution.
- Identification of volunteers and Drug Distribution.
- Composition of Rapid Response Team.
- Preparation at Village and Sub-centre level involving Village Health and Sanitation Committee and Rogi Kalyan Samiti.
- Media Sensitization at District and Block level.
- IES activities at local level.
- Post MDA Assessment by Medical College/Institution.

7.3.3. *Dengue and Chikungunya*

Important objectives of the programme are as follows:

- To reduce the incidence of dengue and effective control on Chikungunya morbidity.
- Strengthening the state-wise surveillance mechanisms for Dengue and Chikungunya by increasing the number of Domestic Breeding Checkers.

❑ *Specific Constraints, New Strategy and Innovation Proposed for Implementation of the Programme*

- All municipalities and town areas should be involved in source reduction for vector breeding and logging of insecticides. The bylaws should be effective against those who create the situation favourable for mosquitoes breeding.
- Inter-sectoral coordination, involvement of the Village Health and Sanitation Committee, other community based organization, etc. should be ensured by all district level health officers.
- Emergency Hospitalization Plan in Case of epidemic/outbreak by reserving 5-10 beds in each District Hospital and ensuring availability of drugs, rapid response team.
- Monitoring and evaluation and constraints for analysis of entomological indices for early warning signals, time log in receiving reports from Sentinel Surveillance Hospitals and implementation of remedial measures, etc. should also be ensured.
- Availability of blood banks and blood component separation facility to District and State Level should be made functional.
- In high risk districts for dengue, domestic breeding checkers should be employed.

❑ *Strategy and Innovations Proposed for Implementation of Mid-Term Plan Strategy in Rural Areas*

- Identification of the entomological surveillance, vector control strategies including community involvement for elimination of vector breeding for transmission risk reduction and prevention of occurrence of outbreak.
- State of Uttar Pradesh has established 22 sentinel surveillance Hospitals with laboratory facilitating for enhancing the Dengue facility in the State. For back-up support these Institutes were

linked with SGPGI, Lucknow, which has been identified as one of the Apex laboratories in the State with advance diagnostic facility.

Vector control teams (volunteers required for breeding source reduction and social mobilization) selected and population targeted in High Risk Districts for Dengue.

❑ *Chikungunya*

Chikungunya fever is vital disease, caused by an arbovirus of the family TONGAVIRIDAE and transmitted by Aedes Mosquito. It is debilitating but non-fatal illness occurs principally during rainy season. The disease resembles dengue fever and is characterized by severe, sometimes persistent, joint pain (arthritis) as well as fever and rash.

It is rarely life threatening, Chikungunya is diagnosed by Blood tests (ELISA). Since the clinical appearance of both the Dengue and Chikungunya is similar. Laboratory confirmation is important.

7.3.4. *Kala-Azar*

An important goal of the Kala-Azar is targeted for elimination by 2015. The elimination is to bring down the number of Kala-Azar cases less than 1 per 10,000 population at Block level.

❑ *Situational Analysis of the Disease*

Kala-Azar is endemic in the six districts of Eastern Uttar Pradesh bonding Bihar State Kushi Nagar, Deoria, Ballia, Varanasi, Ghazipur and Sant Ravi Das Nagar. The principles of elimination are anti adult measures and complete treatment of patients.

❑ *Specific Constraints for Implementation of Programme*

- The disease has long incubation period of not detectable in early stage.
- The house of effected population are Kachha.
- Few District of Eastern Uttar Pradesh bordering Bihar, State are affected by Kala-Azar, because of migration of labourers from Endemic State to Uttar Pradesh for livelihood.

For Kala-Azar affected blocks, IRS of DDT 50 per cent (2 rounds) is being done. Spray Wages are given by Government of India. But during the year 2011 the spray wages were not released which created Pending Liabilities having adverse effect on the programme.

❑ *Proposed Strategy and Innovation*

- The Medical Officer Incharge/Superintendent of Primary Health Centres/Community Health Centres should be made responsive for conducting the case search. Case search activities are to be monitored by Chief Medical Officer/District Vector-Borne Disease Officer.
- Complete Treatment of Case.
- Behaviour change Communication/Information, Education, Communication/Advocacy for Kala Azar.
- Vector Control, Spray Pumps and accessories should be made functional and spray workers should be trained before starting the round of spray.

7.3.5. *Acute Encephalitis Syndrome (AES)/Japanese Encephalitis (JE)*

Acute Encephalitis Syndrome/Japanese Encephalitis are endemic mainly in Eastern part of Uttar Pradesh of which later is vector-born disease transmitted by Culex Vishunii gp mosquitoes. At intervals, the disease assumes epidemic form in the year 2005, the disease affected 34 districts of Uttar Pradesh. With concrete preventive and curative efforts, the departments have been able to contain the disease to only 18 districts in 2011 and 16 Districts in 2012. The districts of Saharanpur division were also involved up to 2010 to report AES/JE case but during 2011 and 2012, these districts did not report any case of AES and JE.

The department has been able not only to restrict the disease in Western part of Uttar Pradesh but has achieved drastic decline in morbidity and mortality due to Japanese Encephalitis in the State as decline by 37.95 per cent in morbidity and 14.81 per cent in mortality due to Japanese Encephalitis was observed during 2012 over 2011. Similarly, 0.17 per cent decline in morbidity and 4.46 per cent in mortality, due to AES was observed during 2012 over 2011.

However, the magnitude of the disease has declined but still it is a challenge to the department to contain the disease in Gorakhpur, Basti, Azamgarh and Devi Patan Division and Lakhimpur District and Lucknow Division.

Approximately 90 per cent of cases are reported from rural and peri-urban areas of these districts. The deaths due to the disease have been brought down to considerable level.

A. *Situation Analysis of the Disease*

Vaccination with SA-14-14-2 Vaccine to the children of 1-15 years age group was carried out in 34 districts in phases from 2006 to 2009 which had high response and acceptance in the community but keeping in view the independent assessment, the high level experts and officials decided to undertake another round of vaccination in highly Japanese Encephalitis sensitive districts of Basti and Gorakhpur Division in 2010, accordingly the good coverage of vaccination attribute decline in Japanese Encephalitis case considerably but the Number of AES cases still need attention for control.

B. *Proposed Strategy and Innovations*

I. *Disease Surveillance*

(i) The Surveillance staff for any disease at periphery level is inadequate leading to improved reporting of the AES/JE case. Presently ASHAs are working at every village, i.e. grassroots levels, who can notice the early patients of AES/JE in endemic area with symptoms of Encephalopathy.

The ASHA/AWW/Traditional Healers will convince the family members of the early patients to contact the nearly treatment centres for early treatment of the patient. They will be required to make a list of the early patients daily and will submit it to the respective Primary Health Centres of the area for this purpose they will be required to have exposure/training to identify disease so that they can recognize the patient at the earliest. The early reporting and treatment will lead to minimize the encephalopathy stage.

(ii) District Hospitals need to be strengthened for surveillance AES/JE ward already identified is required to be expanded and upgraded. There is a need to set up an ICU, in each district hospital out of which nine districts have been granted and released funds from Government of India and remaining districts will be provided funds for ICU set up.

Drugs and other medicines are requisite to be procured by the state. 14 District Hospitals of Gorakhpur, Basti, Azamgarh and Devi Patan Division and District Lakhimpur excluding district Gorakhpur will be equipped with the ventilators which will be made fully functional by training the Medical Officer.

There is need to strengthen CHCs/PHCs in the district. At present no admission is reported in the CHCs/PHCs and the mild and moderately sick patient for want of proper medical advice or reporting to BRD Medical College for Treatment. In order to provide early treatment at periphery by attaining confidence of the public, it is mandatory that moderately sick patients of AES get admitted in CHCs/PHCs which will take the patients load off from BRD Medical College.

In each CHC/PHC at least 5-10 beds to be assigned for treatment of ASE/JE patients. *Therefore provision of trained man-powers (clinicians, staff nurses and ward boys) is an important exercise which is required to be carried out besides provisions of adequate drugs and other medicines.*

II. *Prevention*

AES cases excluding JE cases make the major proportion of morbidity and mortality mainly in four divisions of eastern Uttar Pradesh. Community will be sensitized through different types of printed material to adopt various measures in order to prevent construction of the disease and the health education, material will be developed procured and supplied by the State Headquarters to the concerned districts.

III. *Diagnosis*

Early Diagnosis and prompt treatment will be ensured by strengthening the diagnostic facilities in 14 sentinel labs of highly sensitive districts and headquarter lab each, of which is equipped with one ELISA reader, deep freezers, and supplementary material.

However, pathologists and technicians will be reoriented for latest advancements in the techniques.

IV. *Treatment*

Treatment facilities including availability of adequate and ample stock of drugs and other medicines at different hospitals and treatment centres which will have proper legible and self-explanatory treatment schedule chart display to be followed by the medical and paramedical staff.

V. *Entomological Surveillance of Japanese Encephalitis*

(i) Vector Surveillance is an important component of AES/JE programme strategy. Though there is no direct relationship of Vector Density with impending outbreak of JE it is needless to mention that vector densities are required to be reduced significantly for avoiding outbreak situation.

(ii) Staff for Entomological Surveillance is meagre in the affected districts and districts are devoided of insect collector, which will be deployed in at least two contractual insect collector at each district. The collection made from all these districts will be recorded and some samples will be sent to NCDC Delhi and NIV Pune for detection of JE Virus antigen regularly at monthly intervals.

VI. *Vector Control for JE*

(a) Fortnightly fogging of Malaria by fogging Machine in the villages reporting JE cases for at last 2-3 years during the transmission period. Each district with vehicle mounted large thermal fogging machine and one small portable thermal fogging machine to each Primary Health Centre will be provided.

(b) Found stray/fogging of Malathion around 50 houses of a JE case to kill infective mosquitoes and prevent further transmission.

(c) The vector is of exophgic and expholic in nature, the high density built up population and house human dwelling Units inward movement of vector species may increase the risk of disease transmission during rainy season, hence Indoor Residual Spray with Malathion 25 per cent wdp or space spray with Pyrethrum 0.1 per cent solution will be done in the rural population assuming 50 houses coverage in each case.
The residual spray will be done in two round in 20 JE sensitive districts of 6 weeks each, i.e. first round starting from June 15th to July 31st and second round from August 1st to September 15th.

(d) Department of agriculture will be involved in vector control by enhancing its capacity building in the *Integrated Pest Management to the tune of Integrated Pest and Vector Management.*

(e) The fisheries department particularly in the JE affected districts will study and identify local indigenous mosquito Lavivorous fish and promote their hatcheries to cater among the aquatic based crop harvesting farmers and the health department will do their regular monitoring.

VII. *Training*

Appropriate training should be organized at various facility levels:

(i) *Training of Facility Level Workers:* Training of Medical Officers/ANMs/AWWs/Ward Boys/ASHAs from PHC/CHC/ District Hospitals of JE/AES affected districts, Health Education

Officers posted at Community Health Centres will be trained for dissemination of information to the Community for JE/AES prevention and control.

Auxiliary Nurse Midwife/ASHA/AWW will be educated for symptoms of disease personal perfection measures, proper sanitation, hygiene and early referrals of the patients to PHCs/ CHCs other para medical staff will be trained for providing immediate care life saving measures to the patient.

(ii) *Training of Traditional Healers:* Parents of sick children initially seek treatment from local traditional healers, resulting in late referrals, poor prognosis and leading to aggravating the disease. These traditional healers/fever treatment depot/drug distribution centres/holders will be trained so that their services can be utilized in early treatment of sick patient at their places Primary Health Centres/Community Health Centres/District Hospitals.

The Training material for various categories of trainees will be developed and supplied from State Headquarter to maintain the uniformity from State Headquarters to maintain the uniformity in the language of the Community in need.

VIII. *IEC/BCC*

Intensified IEC will be done in AES/JE affected districts to change the behaviour of the public in treatment seeking at nearly Government Hospital/Treatment Centres without delay.

Training of trainers modules for various Training of Trainers Groups, Health Education, booklets for children and health information books of adult will be made available from Headquarters to maintain uniformity.

Protection from mosquito bites through personal protection measures like use of mosquito's nets, wise gauging/screening of windows/ ventilators/doors, wearing clothing covering maximum body, isolation of pigs away from human habitation or wise gauging screening of piggeries.

Appropriate steps will be able to undertake towards prevention and control of waterborne diseases caused by Enter virus which also lead to AES. The message to be given to the community regarding proper sanitation, washing hands with soap after defecation and before meals, clipping of nails, use of water of India Mark-II Hand Pump only and not from shallow tube-wells/hand pumps, use of bleaching powder and chlorine tablets, etc. through different media also.

IX. *Supervision and Monitoring*

State Government has designated a separate programme officer for AES/JE in the State. State Cell comprises Director AES/JE and Jt. Director-AES/JE.

Weekly and fortnightly review meetings of JE/AES situation will be conducted ground zero. The activity and mobilization of District Malaria Officers and other paramedical programmes personnel at district level will be ensured.

Monthly review meetings of inter-sectoral department will be organized at District Level by the State Headquarters Regulars supervisory and analytical trips from state and divisional Headquarters.

X. *Vaccination*

Routine Immunization of all children at the age of nine months and 1.5 to 2 years to be carried out in all the districts which had vaccination of 1-15 years age group children as per revised strategy of Government of India and monitoring will be intensified to achieve 100 per cent coverage against the target proposed by the district.

XI. *Rehabilitation*

The children developing sequelae will be rehabilitated at rehabilitation centre functioning at BRD Medical College/District Hospital, Government and other autonomous bodies. Likewise other District Hospitals will have department of rehabilitation consisting of psychologist and various vocational therapist.

XII. *Nourishment*

High Level decision taken in the inter-sectoral coordination meeting chaired by Chief Secretary, Uttar Pradesh Government, the malnourished children of JE affected districts are to be provided with qualitative and adequate quantity of energy and protein rich food through AWW under the existing ongoing scheme of the integrated children development scheme. The monitoring and evaluation of the quality and quantity of the food will be borne by the Health Department Official at different level.

XIII. *Logistics*

Logistic arrangements pertaining to the treatment surveillance of the patients and vector, vector control diagnosis, IEC/BCC, drinking water disinfectants inadequate quality will be ensured at all levels from districts to periphery.

XIV. *Specific Constraints for Programme Implementation*

- Transmission cycle of JE is of complex nature.
- Disease affected districts mainly practice paddy cultivation as means of livelihood due to which expophilic and exophagic vector mosquito species of the disease JE get widespread breeding site and institution of anti vector control operations is very difficult. Larvivorous fish hatcheries and rearing not properly managed by the local people.
- The Ardeid birds, which are reservoir of JE virus are prevalent in the area.
- The pigs are also the means of livelihood of poor communities and these pigs act as amplifying host.
- Hon'ble High Court of Uttar Pradesh has instructed to remove piggeries from human habitations.
- Moreover veterinary based sero-surveillance of reservoir as well as amplifying host is lacking *which can be definite early warning signal for JE.*
- Inadequate human resources at different levels.
- Delayed treatment seeking approach of community at treatment centre, i.e. hospitals, CHCs and PHCs as they directly approach BRD Medical College, Gorakhpur on severity of the case.
- Shortage of Vehicles required for mobility of staff for undertaking intervention measures, surveillance, monitoring and supervision.
- Repeated training/reorientation training of the medical officer and the staff of Community Health Centres/Primary Health Centres as deployment of new staff after transfer.
- Lack of health consciousness pertaining to personal hygiene and sanitation in and around human habitation.

7.4. *National Leprosy Eradication Programme*

The main objectives of National Leprosy Eradication Programme are as follows:

- Elimination of leprosy, i.e. prevalent of less than 1 case per 10,000 population.

- Strengthen Disability prevention and Medical Rehabilitation of Persons affected by Leprosy.
- Reduction in the level of stigma associated with Leprosy.

❑ *Situational Analysis*

Uttar Pradesh has a prevalence rate of 0.79 per 10,000 population. Under the 12th Plan 45 high endemic districts were selected for special activity. Now in only 42 of these districts there are 378 Blocks with ANCDR more than 10 per lakh population (as per March 2010 report).

❑ *Result to be Achieved*

The following 8 results are to be achieved:

1. Improved early case detection.
2. Improved Case Management.
3. Stigma Reduced.
4. Development of Leprosy Expertise sustained.
5. Research supported evidence based programme practices.
6. Monitoring supervision and evaluation system improved.
7. Increased participation of persons affected by Leprosy in society.
8. Programme Management ensured.

❑ *Case Detection and Management*

Active case detection drive has been started in 147 high endemic blocks of high endemic districts.

(a) *Intensive Case Detection Drive:* Special activities in high endemic block of low endemic districts will be carried out in 31 Blocks with ANCDR > 10/10,000 population.

(b) *ASHA Involvement:* Performance based incentives to Accredited Social Health Activists and sensitization to new Accredited Social Health Activists.

(c) *Multi-Drug Therapy:* Multi-Drug Therapy should be supplied at the grassroots level.

❑ *Information, Education and Communication*

- To develop effective communication *vis-à-vis* the target audience and take on the task of effective delivery.
- To complement and support the detection and treatment services being provided through General Health Care System.
- To strive to remove stigma surrounding Leprosy and prevent discrimination against Leprosy affected person.

- To specifically cover client Health provider, influence in the masses.

One Para Medical worker's contractual basis for Leprosy supervision, monitoring and programme implementation in high endemic block of identified high endemic districts.

7.5. *National Programme for Control of Blindness*

National Programme for Control of Blindness was launched in 1976. The goal of the programme was to reduce the prevalence of blindness.

Out of the total estimated 45 million blind people (3/60) in the world, 7 million are in India and 1.85 million in Uttar Pradesh. This is due to the large population base and increased life expectancy. Every year 0.3 per cent of the population which means about 5.5 lakh blind persons are added to the total blind population. Out of 5.5 lakh total blind people 3.5 lakh become blind every year due to cataract.

As the number of cataract patient is reducing because the clearance of backlog blindness due to degenerative disease like diabetes and glaucoma and injuries related corneal opacities are increasing. The programme has to tackle emerging challenges.

An important goal of the programme is to reduce prevalence rate of blindness to 0.3 per cent by the end of year 2020.

❑ *Activities to Achieve the Goal*

- Cataract Surgery.
- School Eye Screening.
- Eye banking for Kerato plasty to treat corneal Blindness.
- Management for Disease other than cataracts (Diabetic, Retinopathy, Glaucoma management, Laser Technique, Corneal Transplantation, vitreorentinal surgery and treatment of child-hood blindness.

❑ *Activity-wise Situation of the Programme*

1. *Cataract Surgery*

As per the survey conducted by Government of India in 2004, 62 per cent of blindness is due to cataract. Estimated 3.5 cataract cases are added every year.

❑ *Strategies to Achieve the Target*

- Primary screening by ASHAs, MPW to identify high visual impediment.

- Case selection by Eye Surgeon at Screening camps, base and District Hospital.
- Transportation of Cataract Blind to have hospital for IOL Surgery free of all.
- Follow up of operated cases carrying out refraction and providing best corrected glasses.
- Promotion of NGOs those are good in technical skills.
- Extended IEC Programme by Electronic Media, Print Media and Local Agencies, AIB and National Channels to approach remote and rural areas.

2. *School Eye Screening*

It is estimated that 5-7 per cent of school going children aged 8-14 years have problems with their eyesight affecting their participation and learning at school which can be corrected by a pair of spectacles.

All schools having children in the age group of 8-14 years are expected to undertake eye screening activities. It is proposed that this activity will be undertaken by ASHA, MPW and primary school teachers trained for the purpose and optometrists under school health programme under NRHM. They will be trained for undertaking screening process and making referral for refraction to Block PHCs. District Health Society will supply the refractive glass to needy student.

❑ *Strategies to Achieve the Target*

- Training of ASHA, MPW and school teachers at primary level.
- Substracted refractive error children referred to Primary Health Centres/Community Health Centres Non-Government Organizations/Hospital/trained optometrist for proper refraction and will provide free spectacles to poor children.
- Involvement of NGOs in screening of children having low vision for non-school going children.
- Development of 75 vision centres at Primary Health Centres/ Community Health Centres level.
- School-wise report will be generated by ASHA depicting name of school, No. of children screened, No. of children with defective vision referred to PHC.
- Through the local IEC all schools will have wall painting/ writing in relation of ASHA for eye screening programme.
- The training of ASHA for eye screening is already included in regular ASHA training programme by NRHM.

3. *Corneal Blindness*

The prevalence of corneal blindness is about 1 per cent of total blindness. There are about 18,000 people in need of corneal transplant. The lack of corneal donation and functional institutions and major bottlenecks to address corneal blindness.

❑ *Strategies to Achieve the Target*

- Primary eye care medication will be available at PHC/CHC Level.
- 22 eye banks are already registered and 10 eye banks will be registered soon to achieve the target of 1,500 corneal transplanation and 1500 eye collection as well.

4. *Disease Other than cataract surgeries (Diabetic, Retinopathy, Glaucoma, Childhood Blindness, Vireo Vitreo Surgery, Laser Technique, Low vision aids, etc.*

About 16 per cent of total blindness is due to diabetes, glaucoma and of above mentioned disease. Currently, there is no mechanism to address this category of blindness which is gradually increasing.

It is proposed to set up screening clinic in every District Hospital and Treatment Centre. Equipments for diagnosis diabetes related problems by Government of Uttar Pradesh only indirect ophthalmoscopes are required to undertake screening process for both disease diabetic retinopathy and other posterior segment disorders.

❑ *Strategies to Achieve the Targets*

- All known diabetics to be examined by Eye Surgeon.
- Tonometry, furdoscopy and indirect ophthalmoscopy will be done at weekly clinic at all district hospitals.
- Medical management of diabetic retinopathy and surgical management of glaucoma at divisional level hospitals.
- For surgical intervention patients referred to Tertiary Centre. (Medical College, NGO Hospital) for diabetic retinopathy, Glaucoma and other eye diseases.)
- For operation of equipments optometrist should be trained at Medical College by State Government.
- Eye Surgeon to be trained in diabetic retinopathy and Glaucoma by Central Government.

Training of Paramedical Ophthalmic assistants/Optometrists to be conducted by State Refraction and instrumentation of 4 training centres.

Training of staff nurse in ophthalmic O.T. and Ward Management at recognized centre should be organized.

7.6. *Revised National Tuberculosis Control Programme*

An important objective of the revised National Tuberculosis Control Programme is to ensure universal access to T.B. Care and to ensure that All T.B. Patients are registered and treated under the programme.

- To achieve and maintain a cure rate of at least 85 per cent among newly detected infectious new sputum men positive case.
- To achieve and maintain detection of at least 70 per cent of such cases.

Priority areas at the State Level for Achieving the Planned Objectives have been illustrated in Table 2.11.

Table 2.11: Priority Areas for Achieving the Planned Objectives

Sl.No.	*Priority Areas*	*Activities Planned under Each Priority Area*
(1)	*(2)*	*(3)*
1.	Re-organization of RNTCP Services as per the National Strategic Plan (NSP) 2012-2017	Re-organization of TB Units as per community development blocks Recruitment of additional manpower as per sanctioned positions in NSP Advocacy with all stakeholders, arrangement of logistics
2.	Provision of Universal access to TB Diagnostic and Treatment Services to all	Ensuring that all DMCs function at the best of their capabilities Ensuring that all diagnosed TB patients are put on treatment Increasing No. of TB patients to know their HIV Status and TB-HIV Patients are linked to TB and HIV Services Strengthening of lab EQA Service Reaching out to the unreached population by contact investigation, screening of TB in population with co-morbidities, screening of vulnerable population, etc.
3.	Provision of Services for DR-TB Patients	Ensure all MDR-TB Patients to be put on treatment All diagnosed DR-TB Patients to be put on treatment

(Contd.)

Table 2.11 (*Contd.*)

(1)	*(2)*	*(3)*
4.	Building Partnership	Involvement of more and more NGOs undersigned schemes Seeking support from partners (Project Akshya, Professional Bodies, Faith Based Organizations)
5.	Promoting Research	Encourage Field based operational research Organize regular CMEs on current updates and new topics

7.7. *National Tobacco Control Programme*

Globally approximately 5.4 million people die each year as a result of disease resulting from Tobacco consumption. More than 80 per cent of these deaths occur in the developing countries.

Problems of Tobacco is more complex in India than probably and other country in the world. In the late 1980s, the number of tobacco contributable deaths in India was estimated at 6,30,000 conservative estimates reveal that the deaths attributable to tobacco currently range between eight to nine lakh people per year.

The overall prevalence of tobacco use in every form was 34.4 per cent in Uttar Pradesh. The observed prevalence was higher than the National Bidi was observed to be the commonest smoking material. The males are the predominant users and the prevalence was higher in rural areas. Persons with education in college has a lower prevalence of tobacco use.

Tobacco use prevalence crossed 50 per cent level among man in the age group of 25-29 years suggesting the early initiation of the habit.

Survey revealed that a very small proportion (3.5% males and 1.4% females) of tobacco users contemplated quitting their habit. A high percentage (90%) of tobacco users knew about at least one harmful effect of tobacco.

Considering that the public health implication of tobacco consumption and preventable nature of tobacco related morbidity and mortality the Government of Uttar Pradesh has issued notification To Enforce Cigarettes and Other Tobacco Products (Prohibition, Advertisement and Regulation of Trade and Commence, Production, Supply and Distribution) Act.

❑ *National Tobacco Control Programme in Uttar Pradesh*

1. National Tobacco Control Programme was launched in 2007-08 in U.P. District Tobacco Control Cells were established and activities pertaining to enforcement and prevention were implemented.
2. IEC/BCC Training of doctors, health and social workers, health melas and health activities carried out by NGO. Anti-tobacco awareness campaigns and training of health professionals were incorporated within the overall framework of the NRHM.
3. Training of DHOs, Doctors, Superintendent of Police, Dy Director of Public Health Institutions, Health and Social Workers and All concerned officer's Health camps activities are organized by the District Anti-Tobacco Control Cell.
4. Training and Capacity Building programme will target the school teachers, Health workers, Accredited Social Health Activists, Anganwadi workers, law enforcers women Self Help Groups and other civil society organizations, etc. for Tobacco control initiatives including implementation of the law.
5. Tobacco is risk factor for cancer, chronic pulmonary disease and T.B. Deaths, etc. IEC/BCC campaigns are helpful in changing the behaviour and lifestyle of the public. District level IEC/BCC campaigns must be include tobacco control and growing of alternate crops in tobacco farmers.
6. The school programme is aimed at creating awareness among the school children/teachers regarding the harmful effects of tobacco usage and passive smoke awareness.
7. World No Tobacco Day should be organized.
8. Anti Tobacco Cell and Medical Institutions are jointly planning various activities to raise awareness and advocate law enforcers and general public.

❑ *Interventions Proposed*

State Tobacco Control Cell should effectively coordinate the proposed initiative under the District Tobacco Control Programme.

- All the activities of the District Tobacco Control Programme should be carried out under the supervision and guidance of District Programme Manager, NRHM.
- Appropriate IEC Material and Campaign designs will be adopted to meet the needs of the local committee and in each district IEC

and mass media campaign be carried out in the implementing district.

- Awareness regarding ill effects of tobacco campaign will be an integral part of the states school health programme 50 of schools in each district and 250 school teachers will be trained to disseminate tobacco control message among the school children and the surrounding communities.
- 35 dedicated tobacco cessation centres will be established in the Internal Medicine Department of 35 hospitals. The centre will be managed by Psychologist who will be supported by the Medical Officer.

7.8. *National Programme for Prevention of Control of Deafness*

National Programme for Prevention and Control of Deafness is newly introduced Programme which has been launched to prevent hearing impairments found in children. The burden of deafness is relatively high in India with respect to world scenario.

The prevalence of severe to profound hearing loss is 291 per lakh population. 26.4 million of children in India are suffering from hearing loss which adversely affect their educational performance during their studies. Over 50 per cent causes of hearing impairment are preventable and 80 per cent of all deafnesses are avoidable by medical surgical method.

This programme is launched to prevent the avoidable hearing loss and no medically rehabilitate hearing impaired and action is in progress to sensitize the ENT Surgeon, Other Medical and Para-Medical personnel as well as Health workers.

Severe and profound loss of hearing adversely affects the physical and economic progress and productivity.

❑ *Objectives of the Programme*

- To prevent avoidable hearing loss on account of disease or injury.
- Early identification, diagnosis and treatment of ear problems responsible for hearing loss and deafness.
- To medically rehabilitate persons of all groups, suffering with deafness.
- To strengthen the existing inter-sectoral linkage for continuity of the rehabilitation programme for persons with deafness.

- To develop institutional capacity for ear care services by providing support for equipments, material and training personnel.

Long-term objective of the programme is to prevent and control major cause of hearing impairment and deafness so as to reduce the total disease burden 25 per cent of the existing by the end of Twelfth Five Year Plan.

❑ *Strategy*

- Capacity building of District Hospital, CHCs and PHCs.
- Identification of Potential District Hospital/Large Hospital to provide preventive/screening/curative services on daily basis —
  - — To provide above services there is need for.
  - — Strengthening of district hospital in terms of equipments/ instruments.
  - — Sound proof room for audiometry.
  - — Posting of manpower in adequate number (one ENT Specialist) and one Audiologist at least at District level.
  - — Skill development for service provider and paramedics.
  - — IEC for dissemination of information about availability of services, site, importance, etc.
- Sensitization of service providers and paramedics.
- Awareness generation in community through sensitization workshop with IEC support.
- Involvement of schools and ICDS for screening of children up to 14 years age.
- To utilize the existing health infrastructure for the project.
- District Hospital would be strengthened with the provision of equipment to enable diagnostic as well as therapeutic and rehabilitation exercise to be carried out.
- Doctors will be given training as well as the basic diagnostic equipment to enable them to disgnose, treat and refer the patients, with hearing and ear disease.
- School Teachers for the Primary section would be required to conduct a survey based questionnaire for Primary School Children.
- Screening camps one per month at District Hospital/CHC/PHC for early detection and control of deafness would be conducted by the District Nodal Officer and local ENT surgeon after

procurement of Audiological equipments and appointment of contractual staff including Audiologists.

- For audiometry and other proposed Activities, services of audiologist/audiologic assistant would be taken on the contractual basis.
- To develop institutional capacity for ear services and same programme will be extended in other districts where ENT surgeon is available.
- Monitoring, Evaluation and Auditing of the programme would be done periodically and review shall be done as well.

8. Conclusion

Significant progress has been noticed in improving the expectancy at birth, reducing mortality due to malaria as well as reducing infant and maternal mortality. HIV/AIDs, non-communicable diseases such as cardio-vascular, cancer, blindness, mental illness and tobacco related illness have imposed the chronic disease burden on the already over-stretched health care system.

Premature morbidity and mortality from chronic disease can be a major economic and human loss. The public spending on the preventive health services has a low priority over curative health.

Main objectives of the rural health programme has been reduction in child and maternal mortality, universal access to public health services, prevention and control of the communicable and non-communicable diseases and promotion of healthy lifestyle.

Under the Reproductive Child Health Flexible pool Maternal Health Programmes, specially Jnanai Suraksha Yojana and Janani Shishu Suraksha Yojana and operationalization of comprehensive abortion care services have been planned and strengthened. Maternal Health review — old activities and new activities, Training, Information, Education, Communication activities and procurement of equipments, drugs and supplies for maternal health programmes are being implemented at the facility level.

Navjat Shishu Suraksha Varsh is being celebrated to strengthen facilities, services and capacity building of health staff working at the delivery points to prevent the neonatal morbidity and subsequent reduction in the neonatal deaths.

Facility based interventions, i.e. Sick New Born Care Units, New Born Stabilization Units, New Born Care Corners, Nutrition, Rehabilitation

Centres have been established to fulfil the need of emergency care of the Neo-nate and to reduce neo-natal, pre-natal death.

Navjat Shishu Suraksha Karyakram, essential new born care equipments and Home Based New Born Care Community based intervention and drug kits and infant young child feeding and management of diarrhoea and Bal Swasthya Poshan Mah and Information, Education and Communication activities under Child Health Programme are being implemented at the facility level.

Population Policy looks at the issues related to population stabilization and improvement of the Health status of the people, particularly women and children in a holistic manner.

Family planning management activities and Terminal/Limiting Method (Providing sterilization services) Provision of fixed day for Non-scalpel Vasectomy (NSV) Services at each District Male Hospital (Combined Hospital and First Referral Units) should be continued. Accreditation of Private Centre/Non-Governmental Organization for sterilization services, plans for post part sterilization, spacing method and performance based reward to institutions and providers including incentives for ASHA and social marketing of Contraceptives, Training Information, Education and Communication, and Public Private Partnership activities under Family Planning activities have been strengthened and implemented at the facility level.

Adolescent, Reproductive and Sexual Health (ARHS) training, Major Hygiene and Rashtriya Bal Swasthya Karyakram, Pre-Conception and Pre-Natal Diagnostic Techniques, Information, Education and Communicable Training at various levels have been strengthened and implemented at the grassroots level.

To ensure effective management of activities, under National Rural Health Mission, of State Programme Management Unit, Divisional Programme Management Unit, District Programme Management Unit, Block Programme Management and Village Health Sanitation and Nutrition Committees have been formed to ensure need based delivery of health services.

Descriptive role of District Programme Manager, District Community Mobilizer, District Accounts Manager, District Data-cum-Accounts Assistant, District Programme Coordinator, District Data Assistant and responsibilities of Block Programme Manager, Block Data Cum Assistant, Block Coordinator, Data Assistants have been deployed, supportive supervision/mobility support/field visits, etc. have been ensured at the facility levels.

Rural Health Mission Flexible Pool includes Accredited Social Health Activists, Untied Funds, Annual Maintenance Grants, Hospital, strengthening, New construction, Renovation and setting up, mainstreaming of AYUSH, Information, Education and Communication, and Behaviour change, Communication, Medical Mobile Units, Referral Transport/Patient Transport System, Innovation, Planning, Implementation and Monitoring, Procurement, Drug, Drug warehouse, health insurance scheme, Research/studies/analysis, State Health Resource Centre/State Public Health Resource Institute, support services and other expenditures (power backup and convergence), etc.

Accredited Social Health Activists programme included the provision of ASHA Drug kits, incentives for ASHA and Annual ASHA Sammelan/ Diwas, ASHA Uniform, News letters for ASHA and ASHA award scheme and ASHA Mentoring Group and State Specific Innovation under ASHA Programme and ASHA support system have been strengthened and implemented at the facility level.

The untied funds especially maintenance grant, strengthening of hospital, including Trauma wings, spillover-maternity wings in District Women Hospital, Construction of 30 and 50 bedded Community Health Centres, Drug warehouse and construction of maternity wings and setting up of Emergency Caring Centre and strengthening of infrastructure have been implemented, Rogi Kalyan Samiti and involvement of community services and Panchayati Raj Institutions have been ensured at the facility level.

Orientation workshop, training and capacity building of Panchayati Raj Institutions at State District Health Societies, Community Health Centres/Primary Health Centres and village health sanitation and nutrition committees have been organized.

Establishment of Sub-centres platform for effective Maternity and Child Health service delivery through frontline workers has been ensured at the facility level.

Mainstreaming of AYUSH (Ayurveda, Yoga and Naturopathy, Unani, Siddha and Homoeopathy) system of medicines have proven, promotive, preventive and curative strengths. With a view to integrating AYUSH health care with mainstream health care services as per the modified centrally sponsored scheme for development of AYUSH Hospitals and Dispensaries, operational guidelines, Department of AYUSH, Ministry of Health and Family Welfare, Government of India have been ensured for its implementation at the facility level.

Strengthening of Information Education and Communication/ Behaviour Change, Communication and implementation capacity at the facility level has been ensured.

Maternity Health Campaign "*Chaar Ganth*" and "*Chance Kyon Lena Hai*" and "*Surakshit Matritva*" and "*Ab Aur Der Nahi*" campaigns have been launched at the grassroots level.

Mobile Medical Unit have been envisaged which will provide preventive, promotive and curative health care in the inaccessible areas which are underserved. Mobile Medical Units are operative by the name of National Mobile Medical Unit along with requisite logistics and technical staff and doctors.

Emergency Medical Transport Service "108" and U.P Ambulance Sewa and '102 Sewa' Ambulance services are made available to provide transportation of pregnancy cases as well as neo-natal cases from home to the health facility.

Sexual Transmitted Infection and Reproductive Tract Infection services at the district level are provided through the Out Patient Department of skin gynaecology and obstetrics department of medical colleges or district hospitals are provided.

National Aids Control Organization has branded its Sexual and Reproductive Health Services as "*Suraksha Clinic*".

Rapid Plasma Region Kits (RPR) and Venereal Disease Research Laboratory (VDRL) Testing Services has been made available at the Sub-District Health Facilities.

Proposal for free Transport facility through UPSRTC to people living with HIV/AIDS for their treatment related travel to Anti-Retroviral therapy centres has been proposed by the Government of Uttar Pradesh.

Sanitation Programme for Rural Child Health and Hygiene Awareness programme "*Sanrachha*" has been launched and innovation for strengthening routine immunization and concurrent monitoring for fallow-up action plan activities and regional review meetings and orientation of District Immunization Officers programme have been planned and implemented.

Scale up of "*My Village My Home*" programme have been launched for tracking of immunization beneficiaries.

My Village My Home is a mechanism not only for ensuring registration and tracking of all beneficiaries in a particular catchment area but also focuses on developing and strengthening channels of communication between community and service providers for improving routine immunization coverage.

"*Mobile Kunj*" is designed to be used by ASHAs during their home visits with families. The audio-visual jobs aid bring together an Interactive Voice Response based mobile service and a printed deck of cards on a ring.

Planning, Implementation and Monitoring have been ensured through quality assurance at the State Division-Block-Village or facility level.

Procurement of equipments, drugs and consumables have been ensured and Health Insurance Scheme known as "Jan Shree Bima Yojana" has been devised and launched by the Life Insurance Corporation of India for the benefit of the people living below poverty line.

State Health Resource Centre and State Public Health Resources Centre's establishment has been mandated under National Rural Health Mission.

Strengthening of routine immunization programme has been initiated through review meetings, and mobilization of beneficiaries through ASHA and alternate vaccine delivery.

Training of frontline workers and incentives for ASHA and TEEKA Express programme and various innovation under Routine Immunization has been launched and My Village My Home activity has been planned in each District.

Various Disease Control Programmes have been launched under the National Rural Health Mission programme. The National Disease Control Programme includes — National Iodine Deficiency Disorder Control Programme, Integrated Disease Surveillance Project, National Vector-Borne Disease Control Programme, National Leprosy Eradication Programme, National Programme for Control of Blindness, Revised National Tuberculosis Control Programme, National Tobacco Control Programme and National Programme for Prevention and Control of Deafness in which the surveillance, training, information, education and communication, specific constraints, strategies and innovations have been proposed for appropriate implementation of the various disease control programmes at the facility level.

Thus, the various programmes under National Rural Health Mission especially Maternal and Child Health, Adolescent, Reproductive and Sexual Health Routine Immunization and Rural Health Mission flexible pool and National Disease Control Programme should be launched equally, effectively, efficiently at the grossroots level. In the remote unserved rural areas and to provide promotive, curative and preventive health care to all at the facility level to save the human lives and reduce the economic loss and also to improve the socio-economic conditions of the resourceless, deprived rural poor multitudes surviving in the remote villages.

REFERENCE

1. *Multi Year Strategic Plan 2005-2010*, Universal Immunization Programme, Ministry of Health and Family Welfare, Government of India, 2005.

3

PUBLIC HEALTH PROGRESS

1. Introduction

In the last seven years after implementation of National Rural Health Mission, the public health delivery system has increased many folds which have affected the quality of services. In the next three years, it is necessary to increase and promote health delivery points so that the quality public health delivery services are provided to the needy interested people *equally, effectively* and *efficiently* at the facility level especially in the unserved, underserved and remote areas.

Under the National Rural Health Mission, Maternal Health, Child Health, innovations and initiatives, monitoring and review, Bal Swasthya Poshan Mah, Zindagi Ki Udaan, Golden Hour for New Born Tracking, Family Planning, Mainstreaming of AYUSH, etc. has been implemented at the facility levels.

A comprehensive study of Adherence and Cure rate of Tuberculosis using Technology enabled Monitoring and Supervision has also been implemented at various levels.

Immunization, Integrated Disease Surveillance Programme and National Disease Control Programme, National Vector-Borne Diseases including Acute Encephalitis Syndrome and Japanese Encephalitis Programme have also been implemented at the health facility level.

Various Non-Communicable Diseases including Injury and Trauma and National Mental Health Programme and National Programme for the Health Care of the Elderly and National Programme for Prevention and Control of Deafness, National Tobacco Programme, etc. under the National Rural Health Mission are being implemented at the health facility level.

An appropriate supervision, monitoring and review of the progress on National Rural Health Mission especially the 8th Common Review Mission of Uttar Pradesh was organized from 7th to 14th November, 2014 at State NRHM Headquarters, Lucknow.

Overview of the Important Health Indicators has been reviewed.

Table 3.1: Overview of the Health Indicators

Indicators	*Uttar Pradesh*	*Sultanpur District*
Maternal Mortality Ratio	258	362
Total Fertility Rate	3.3	5.6
Infant Mortality Rate	50 (SRS-2013)	95
Neo-Natal Mortality Rate	37 (SRS 2012)	66
Bacillus Calmette-Guerin Immunization (%)	86.3	51.9
Full Immunization (%)	40.9 (CES-2009)	25.7
Child Sex Ratio (0-4 Years)	919	903

It has been indicated in Table 3.1 that the Maternal Mortality Ratio is 258 in Uttar Pradesh and 362 MMR in Sultanpur District, while total Fertility Rate has been noted 3.3 in Uttar Pradesh and 4.6 total fertility rate has been recorded in Sultanpur District.

The Infant Mortality Rate has been noted 95 and Neo-Natal Mortality Rate has been recorded 66 in Sultanpur District. The BCG immunization has been found 51.9 per cent and Full Immunization has been recorded 24.9 per cent in Sultanpur District while Child Sex Ratio (0-4 years) has been found 903 in Sultanpur District and 919 in Uttar Pradesh.

There is District Male Hospital and District Women Hospital in Sultanpur District while there are one Primary Health Centre in Bhadainya Block. Sub-Health Centres are established mostly in all village panchayats of Bhadainya Block. The Sub-Health Centres are functional in Bhadainya, Babhangawna, Bokharepur, Purebaghrai, Palhanpur, Bikwajitpur, Bhapta, Pakhrauli, Kandhipur, Tewaripur, Teranye, Misirpur, Puraina, Bharathipur, Fatehpur and Mahanpur villages of Bhadainya Block. The Anganwadi Centres are also functional mostly in all the villages of Bhadainya Block. Auxiliary Nurse Midwife centres are also functional in most of the villages of Bhadainya Block.

The broad methodologies of the National Rural Health Mission Programme are as follows:

- Facility visits including visits to Anganwadi Centre.
- Record Scrutiny.
- Discussion Meeting with District Authorities and Health Care providers.
- Household interview with community members and beneficiaries.
- Interviews with Accredited Social Health Activists and Anganwadi Workers.
- Visits to school and interaction with school children.

The adequate infrastructure and physical facilities has been made available in the District hospital and the performance of facilities at the Primary Health Centre, Bhadainya has been found sub-optimal.

It has been noticed that the public health services are largely focused on immunization in Sultanpur District. The functional sub-centres are delivery points at the village panchayat level in Bhadainya Block. In Sultanpur District most of the delivery points/sub-centres have Auxiliary Nurse Midwife having clear division of work plans between post-2 Auxiliary Nurse Midwifes.

One Primary Health Centre in Bhadainya Block has 24 × 7 days and hours facility and provide only OPD Services and Lab Services not provided at Primary Health Centre Level in Bhadainya Block.

The progress of the various activities being implemented under the National Rural Health Mission Programme during the year 2013-14 as per the records/reports of the State Programme Management Unit of the National Rural Health Mission, Uttar Pradesh has been analyzed.

2. Maternal Health

Need based planning for operationalization of additional delivery points has been ensured under the National Rural Health Mission. In the last seven years after the implementation of the Janani Suraksha Yojana, case load at delivery points has increased manyfolds which have affected quality of the health care delivery services. Thus, in the next 3 years it is necessary to increase number of delivery points so that the quality health delivery services are provided to the women.

It is evident from the report of the Janani Suraksha Yojana that 19 per cent of the deliveries are being conducted at sub-centre and 18.7 per cent at the District level facilities. It clearly indicates that 62.3 per cent deliveries load is at L2 level Primary Health Centres, Caesarean percentage in the state is only 2.7 per cent and it has been planned to scale it up to at least 5 per cent in the next three years. The block level units are already overburdened and almost 90 per cent have been upgraded to Community Health Centre level and sub-Block Primary Health Centres are still underutilized.

It has also been planned to activate sub-block level Primary Health Centres (at 30-50 thousand population). The planning processes has focused on addressing inequities in terms of "Time to Care".

District Sultanpur have been planned for additional L-2 delivery points based on proposed increase in Institutional deliveries. Focus has been made to improve quality of care at L-1 sub-centre and planned to convert sub-Block Primary Health Centres into L-1 in year 2014-15 and convert them into L-2 in year 2015-16.

2.1. *Janani Suraksha Yojana*

District Sultanpur has been planned to increase in institutional deliveries taking into account their institutional deliveries in Public and Private Sector.

The Phenomenal success has been witnessed of the Janani Suraksha Yojana over the years. In the year 2011-12 there was nominal fall but in the year 2013-14 State has achieved 95 per cent target under Janani Suraksha Yojana which accounts to 44.92 per cent of the total expected deliveries in the year 2013-14.

It has been estimated that total 54,37,995 deliveries will take place in the State in the year 2014-15 out of which 48.86 per cent have been planned to be supported by Janani Suraksha Yojana with 4 per cent increase every year.

❑ *Home Deliveries*

State has planned 12,164 Home Deliveries of Below Poverty Line Women that will be attended by Skilled Birth Attendants for incentive under the Janani Suraksha Yojana. State has also removed the riders of age (> 19 years) and parity (up to 2 children) for availing this incentive in December 2013.

❑ *Institutional Deliveries*

Target of Institutional Deliveries have been rationaiized in the Sultanpur District. The ratio of the rural/urban deliveries is different and has been planned in the District Action Plan.

It has been noticed that the previous rate of ₹ 1,500 has been too meagre, therefore, the rate for C-Section in private accredited centre for BPL Women has been increased to ₹ 2,500 per case. State has proposed 3589 C-Section deliveries at private accredited centres for Below Poverty Line women this year.

Eighty five per cent of the rural deliveries are being proposed to be brought by Accredited Social Health Activists. Government orders have been issued for revisions, in ASHA incentives for entitlements for BPL home delivery and for ensuring account payee beneficiaries payments under *Janani Suraksha Yojana*.

State level administrative budget for 1 per cent of total budget has been allocated which is low due to lack of clarity and discontinuation of all accounts at the Directorate of Family Welfare level. During this year following activities have been proposed to be implemented with this fund:

- Maternal, Neo Natal Health Tool Kit for up to Block level.
- Skill Birth Attendant/Basic Emergency Obstetric Care/ Emergency obstetric care protocols for all delivery points.
- Standard Registers for the delivery points—
  - — ANC Registers.
  - — PNC Registers.
  - — Maternity Register.
  - — Referral in/Out register and slips.
- Printing of Information, Education and Communication Materials related to Maternal Health.
- Strengthening of Janani Suraksha Yojana Cell at Directorate of Family Welfare and Maternal Health Division at the State Programme Implementation Unit.
- State and Divisional Level Maternal Health reviews.
- Support for monthly/quarterly reporting system of maternal health programme and delivery points at District and State level.
- Support to obstetrics and Gynaecology Department of Medical College for reporting and Management Information System.

2.2. *Janani Shishu Suraksha Karyakram*

Janani Shishu Suraksha Karyakram has been rolled out in the Sultanpur District and 100 per cent coverage of pregnant women is being ensured.

The progress of the Janani Shishu Suraksha Karyakram over the year on free entitlements has been quite good comparing to the last year.

The details of the Janani Shishu Suraksha Karyakram and its progress over the years has been illustrated in Table 3.2 which is based on the available information from the National Rural Health Mission State Programme Management Unit.

(i) *Free Drugs and Consumables*

Requisite budget has been planned for drugs and consumables under Janani Shishu Suraksha Karyakram. This is proposed to benefit 47,89,990

Pregnant Women in Uttar Pradesh. This will cover Outdoor Patients Department and Indoor Patient Department in all delivery points as well as at least 80 per cent Ante Natal Cares by outreach services at facility level.

Table 3.2: Janani Shishu Suraksha Karyakram
(Progress Over the Year)

Janani Shishu Suraksha Karyakram	*Achievement March 2013*	*Target 2013-14*	*Achievement March 2014*	*Achievement March 2014 in %age*	*% Increase in One Year*
Free Treatment	15,33,199	40,00,000	27,67,754	69.19	80.52
Free Diagnosis	—	25,00,000	27,53,430	110.14	—
Free Diet	6,29,653	18,16,840	15,50,275	85.33	146.21
Free Drop back	3,38,008	13,48,112	9,02,861	66.97	167.11

The budget has been proposed @ ₹ 350 per case for Normal Deliveries and @ ₹ 1,600 per case for C-section but drugs and consumables required during the Ante-Natal period (outreach as well as institutional) will be covered with this budget pool only.

(ii) *Free Diagnostics*

It has been proposed to provide free basis investigations to 80 per cent of Pregnant women with quality Ante Natal Care through Village Health Nutrition Days and facility based surveys. The process for procurement of rapid diagnostic test kits has been initiated and permission has also been granted for local procurement at the District Level. It has also been proposed to cover a total of 47,89,990 beneficiaries in the year 2014-15.

(iii) *Free Diet*

A sum of ₹ 4,062.22 lakh is being proposed under the Free Diet Head. It has been observed that C-Section Patients start taking meals from 3rd day only and Normal Deliveries takes meals from 2nd day. The rate of approval of tenders is less than ₹ 100 per day at some of the Districts, therefore, the calculations have been made accordingly. Thus, a budget has been proposed @ ₹ 500 for 100 per cent of C-Section and @ ₹ 200 for Normal Deliveries, proposed for 80 per cent of Normal Deliveries at L2 and L3 only.

(iv) *Free Drop Back*

The 102 Call Centre is not fully functional yet and may take another

6-9 months, therefore, drop back of 11,25,620 beneficiaries has been planned for this year @ 250 per beneficiary with existing vehicle.

Important key points of the Maternal Health under National Rural Health Mission are as follows:

- Janani Shishu Suraksha Karyakram and Janani Suraksha Yojana Benefits has been properly implemented.
- Work on Maternal and Child Health Wing started at District hospital and Community Health Centres level.
- Labour rooms are well maintained and standard protocols displayed at facilities.
- Sanitary napkin being provided for post-delivery cases.
- Community aware of free ambulance services — 102/108 — Average 4/Case/Per day/vehicle.
- Lack of identification and line listing of high risk pregnancies Hb estimation, Urine, albumin not conducted for most of the mothers.
- First Ante Natal Care conducted in the fifth or sixth month.
- Limited knowledge about doses of key medicine such as Misoprostol.
- Maternal Death review has not been conducted as per guidelines.
- Lack of Gynaecologist/Obstetric Specialist at the District hospital and designated First Referral Units, knowledge and competencies also need improvement.

2.3. *Maternal Death Review*

Maternal Death Review has been analyzed for the old activities and new activities.

❑ *Old Activities*

1. It has been estimated that at least 60 per cent of the estimated deaths are reviewed at the Community by Block Team. An increased rate of ₹ 600 has been proposed for per Maternal Death Review and ₹ 300 will be for Medical Officer Incharge and ₹ 200 for Health Education Officer/Block Project Managers and ₹ 100 will be paid for the Auxiliary Nurse Midwife of the area.
2. Quarterly reviews at each division and address to media will be conducted at quarterly basis to spread messages for maternal

death reporting from all quarters. For this purpose ₹ 25,000 per review has been proposed.

3. District will conduct district level reviews of the programme on every alternate month. As per the guidelines of Government of India sample reviews will be put up before District Magistrate also and ₹ 200 each for 2 Family members of a family will also be paid from this fund.
4. Contingency support at Block level is proposed for printing of formats, etc. has been proposed @ ₹ 1,000 per block and ₹ 1,000 for urban areas.
5. Maternal Death Review teams in high focus Sultanpur District and high Maternal Mortality Rate in Faizabad Division ₹ 3,000 per review per team has been budgeted for each review visit.
6. *New Activities:* Training and orientation activities for Maternal Death Review programme. The District Officials have been oriented on Maternal Death Review programme three years back. Most of the officials have changed because of transfers and promotions. Revised guidelines of the Government of India have been incorporated since then. An innovative reporting mechanism for ASHAs, has been initiated. The programme is picking up in the State and the reporting has gone up from 1,337 (8.58%) to 3,274 (21.02%) in the last year.

2.4. *Incentives for ASHA under Maternal Health*

State Programme Management Unit of the National Rural Health Mission has proposed different incentives for the Accredited Social Health Activists under the Maternal Health Programme:

(i) *Incentive for Reporting Suspected Maternal Death by ASHA*

An incentive for primary informers for reporting a maternal death has been proposed under ASHA incentives @ ₹ 200 per case. District have estimated their expected Maternal Death and ASHA incentives for at least 33,812 suspected Maternal Deaths reporting (twice the expected number) have been proposed. A budget of ₹ 67.62 lakh is being allocated under the ASHA incentive programme.

(ii) *Incentive for Treatment of Service for the Anaemia*

The detection and line listing of severally anaemic pregnant women is an important activity and ASHA incentive @ ₹ 100 is being budgeted for preparing line listing and follow-up of severally anaemic pregnant women. The same is being proposed this year 2 per cent of the total expected Ante Natal Cares. A budget of ₹ 118.28 lakh has been proposed for this activity to ensure at least 1,18,280 anaemic women to be benefited by this intervention.

(iii) *Incentive to ASHA for Early Registration and Opening Beneficiaries Bank Account — New Activity*

The registration status of pregnant women in the first trimester in the State is unsatisfactory. During 2012-13, only 55 per cent of those registered for ANC got the registration done in the first trimester. As per Annual Health Survey 2011-12, only 46.5 per cent of the pregnant women got registered in the first trimester, complete check-up can be ensured and complications can be managed after early identification.

Timely identification of pregnant women and line listing of severally anaemic women, their timely referral in case danger signs, complete and quality ANC care, preparation of birth plans and safe institutional deliveries. Generation of work plans, proper immunization and vaccination of the targeted beneficiaries thus resulting in multiple gains.

The compliance of the new order of the Government of India regarding transfer of the beneficiaries incentive to their own account assistance of ASHAs can be taken in facilitating the opening of bank accounts.

Thus, it has been proposed that 37,98,282 of Rural ANCs will be covered by ASHAs to receive this incentive @ ₹ 100 per beneficiary.

2.5. *Orientation Training of ANMs at Block Level*

There are 20,576 sub-centres and only 1,928 are L-1 delivery points till date. It is very clear that majority of the sub-centres are performing outreach activities only but do not have skills to perform those with quality. It has also been observed that during monitoring visits that ANMs are not able to measure Blood Pressure, Haemoglobin, Urine testing for albumin and sugar. They are not able to fill MCP Cards properly, not able to prepare line list of severally anaemic women and not able to identify Human Resources and pregnancies.

Therefore, it has been proposed that an extensive training and capacity building programme is being taken up to cover all ANMs. The Training of Trainers for one batch of ANMs at Block has been proposed. This one day training of ANMs will be conducted at Block level facility on Tuesday which is a day designated for monthly meeting. Skill upgradation is being conducted by Medical Officer Incharge and Medical Superintendents will monitor after one month of training and certify that all the ANMs in their Block have the necessary skills to perform the outreach services.

2.6. *Procurement of Printing Plan*

It is planned to procure Maternal Neo Natal Health Tool Kits during this year, sufficient in numbers to distribute it till district and block level facilities. Standard format of ANC Register Referral Register/Slips and New Borne Registers are part of Maternal Neo Natal Health Tool Kit. A prototype of each will be developed and a set will be distributed up to block level. The cost of this activity will be met with Janani Suraksha Yojana State level Administrative Budget.

The Blood Pressure instrument with stethoscope, Haemoglobin rapid testing strips kits Uristix (Sugar Albumin) are necessary for effective ANC at Village Health and Nutrition Days.

The tests are very difficult to be carried out during outreach sessions and women are not able to come to Primary Health Centres for these tests. Therefore, it has been planned that these essentials will be procured and to be distributed to every Auxiliary Nurse Midwife before carrying out orientation of ANMs.

2.7. *Regional and State Level Maternal Health Reviews and Maternal Health Workshops*

It has been observed during the field visits that the information sharing is very poor in the Districts. The documents and the standard tools and guidelines that are shared with Chief Medical Officers/Additional Chief Medical Officer at the State Level are not shared with the Block officials and other District level officials.

Usually the tool kit like Maternal Neo Natal Health Took Kit, Maternal Death Review Booklet, Programme Implementation guidelines, standard prototypes of Registers, etc. are shared on State National Rural Health Mission Website but it has been noted that District/ Block officials are not very Information Technology Savvy.

It has been proposed to organize 5 one day regional workshops with all Additional Directors, Chief Medical Superintendents of L-3 delivery points, Additional Chief Medical officer, Chief Medical Officer, Medical Officer Incharge, Medical Superintendents, Division Programme Managers, and District Programme Managers of the region. Thus, at least, 1250 officials up to Block level are expected to participate in these workshops.

2.8. *Incentive for First Referral Unit Operationalization: Old Activities*

The incentive cover all facilities with the following criteria:

I. *Fixed Difficult Area Allowance*

It has been proposed to provide difficult area allowance to contractual specialists @ 20 per cent for District level facilities and 40 per cent for Sub-district Facilities. It has been proposed to provide ₹ 10,000 fixed monthly incentive to regular specialists posted at selected difficult areas to reach Community Health Centre's First Referral Units.

II. *Performance Based Incentives*

An incentive will be given where average number of C-sections is < 5 per month. If these facilities conducted 10 per cent more C-Sections in the same month last year, the incentive of ₹ 3,000 per C-Section will start after that for the team. It has been expected that at least 2,000 C-Sections will be increased in their units by starting this intervention.

An incentive will be given where average number of C-Sections is < 1 per month. If these facilities conduct 10 per cent more C-Sections conducted in the same month last year, the incentive of ₹ 3,000 per C-Section will start after that for the team. It is expected that at least 2,000 C-Section will be increased in these units by starting this intervention.

2.9. *Incentive for ANMs for Maternal Health*

The village having < 20 per cent institutional deliveries are being identified. The State is in the process of identifying ASHA areas where institutional deliveries are extremely low. In these areas if Auxiliary Nurse Midwife ensures institutional delivery, she will be given ₹ 500 per delivery. She will be prioritized for Skill Birth Attendant Training and if ANM is SBA trained and conducts home deliveries then also she will be given ₹ 250 per delivery. It is expected that at least *10 delivery per ASHA area will be added by this activity.*

2.10. *Human Resource at Delivery Points and Maternal Health*

Under the Maternal Health human resource are required at the delivery points level:

- Additional ANMs for L-1 sub-centre has been proposed. Additional ANM is necessary to look after women in labour, perform outreach services and delivery care services. Additional ANMs are required to be placed at all L-1 sub-centre delivery point on contract from NRHM to facilitate outreach as well as delivery care and sub-centre clinic services. The contractual ANMs are proposed to be placed at L-3 facilities @ 2 per facility to be placed Auxiliary Nurse Midwife record keeping and immunization of new born. Contractual ANMs are proposed to be hired on contract in the year 2013-15 @ ₹ 15,000 per month. The increment will be granted based in their outreach/ delivery performances.
- Contractual 1st ANMs against vaccines has been started. Directorate of Family Welfare has started regular recruitment of 3,300 ANMs in the State. Presently, the state has reported vacancy of 4,159 ANMs against regular sanctioned positions. Salary for 6 months is being proposed as the State Plans to fill the vacancies by regular appointment.
- Districts have been advised to calculate requirement of contractual Human Resources (Anesthetists)/Gynaecologist/ Staff Nurse) at delivery points based on the guidelines approved by the State government. The guidelines have been based on the standards illustrated in Maternal Neo Natal Health Took Kits.

3. Child Health

Reducing infant mortality is one of the key goals under National Rural Health Mission. Multi-pronged evidence based strategies have been adopted in the National Programme to prevent Neo Natal infant and child death. The infant and under five child mortality has shown a steady decline over the last three years. However, the progress is not uniform across states and even intrastate-inter-district-variations are quite evident from the recent surveys like the Annual Health Survey-2011. Moreover, the decline in Neo-Natal Mortality is slow and has not kept pace with the overall decline in child mortality.

It is well understood that for any further progress to be made the focus must shift to age groups, population and geographical area where mortality is higher/concentrated. Specific interventions are to be made the medical and systemic cause leading to mortality in new born and children < 5 years within a particular geographical area and population must be known. It is also essential that the annual planning process in District and State takes into account the local context and implementation of key child health strategies are prioritized and based on local morbidity and mortality patterns. This is possible only when a special effort is being made to investigate and record the sequence of events leading to child deaths and drawing inference from the data generated locally. Such analysis should guide the programme managers at all levels to recognize the key gap areas for service delivery and institute corrective measures.

3.1. *Childhood Diarrhoea Management*

Various surveys reveal the decline trend of Infant Mortality Rate in Uttar Pradesh but in comparison with India, the infant mortality rate of the State is unacceptably high. Diarrhoea is one of the major causes of child mortality in the State. India has a National Policy for management of Diarrhoea among children less than 5 years which recommends the use of Zinc tablets along with ORS in the treatment of Diarrhoea as the Ministry of Health and Family Welfare, Government of India, directive dated 2nd November, 2006.

Revised Diarrhoea Management Policy recommends administration of Zinc for every case of diarrhoea a dose of 20 mg/day for 14 days (even if diarrhoea Health and Sanitation stopped) for children aged 6 months to 5 years and 10 mg/day for 2-6 days.

❑ *Taken Initiative (2013-14)*

In confirmation to the recommended National Policy the Government of Uttar Pradesh, issued a detailed guideline of treatment protocol and implementation strategy of childhood diarrhoea during February 2013 and circulated with all Chief Medical Officers, Integrated Child Development Scheme and other partners. The Component of the capacity building of all functionaries — Medical Officer Incharge, Auxiliary Nurse Midwife Supervisors, ASHAs, AWWs of both departments treatment of diarrhoea by promoting the usage of Zinc and ORS and three level monitoring system from Auxiliary Nurse Midwife to CMO level has been included. The monitoring format have been developed with technical support of Micro-nutrient initiative.

The problems faced in the implementation of these guidelines in the State are as follows:

- To improve the situation, with the support of Government of Uttar Pradesh and National Rural Health Mission.

- Micro-nutrient initiative initiated interventions including Sultanpur District in Diarrhoea Alleviation through zinc therapy and achieved better results.
- Number of cases treated with ORS and Zinc increased 94 per cent and reporting of diarrhoea cases also improved.

❑ *Health Care Provides to Delivery Quality Care for Diarrhoea Management*

To ensure quality care for diarrhoea management, all different level functionaries of health and ICDS departments, i.e. Medical Officers CDPOs, HEOs, Staff Nurse, Paramedics, ANMs, ASHAs, ICDS supervisors and Anganwadi Workers in the intervention districts have been trained. To execute the training cascade model has been adopted and effectively implemented through concurrently supervised team.

Zinc and ORS supplies are available at all times and in the required volumes.

- Procurement and Distribution—
  - Around 10 lakh Combo Kit of Zinc and ORS procured.
  - Procurement and distribution mechanism has been strengthened.
- Zinc added in State Drug List.
- Technical support at all levels for preparing distribution plan as per requirement/supply.

❑ *Monitoring and Review*

- To strengthen monitoring mechanism by establishing 4-tier reporting system from grassroots to state level.
- Different level reporting and recording formats printed and distributed.
- Field coordinator involved in low performing block through local NGOs for supportive supervision.
- Provided support in monitoring through Divisional Coordinator, Field level workers directly supervised and care givers visited in the last 5 months.
- Reviews at District/Block and State Level.
- Facilitated to report Diarrhoea cases.
- Case load at facility level has been shifted to frontline workers.

Adherence for 14 days Zinc intake increase for visits Field Level Workers and follows-up with care givers:

- During the knowledge assessment 90 per cent ANMs are aware about the correct doses of Zinc followed by 67 per cent in ASHAs and 65 per cent in AWWs.
- Regarding the management of diarrhoea, 29 per cent ANMs were found able to treat some hydration level of Diarrhoea. More AWWs (35%) were able to manage dehydration level of Diarrhoea in comparison of ASHAs (29%).

❑ *Challenges*

- The number of treated cases declined due to non-availability of supply of zinc and ORS due to vendors through budget was timely transferred to districts.
- Treated cases reported only in intervention districts.
- Reported Data not integrated.
- No budget available to do district-wise activities.
- Low knowledge level of service providers about treatment plan, benefits of Zinc and ORS doses.
- Lack of clarity in distribution of supply to AWWs through health system.

❑ *Childhood Diarrhoea Intervention*

In view of the result of the above intervention, state proposed to scale up these activities in the entire state to increase the use of ORS and Zinc in the treatment of Childhood diarrhoea to at least 50 per cent in 2014-15.

- Orientation of Medical Officer, CDPOs, Supervisors and other ongoing meetings at different levels.
- Monthly monitoring and supervision by government officials and partners.
- Refresher training of All ANMs, AWWs, ASHAs on childhood diarrhoea management and recording and reporting through various exiting platforms (Auxiliary Nurse Midwife Weekly Meetings, ASHA Days and Anganwadi Monthly Meetings).
- Create awareness in the community about the importance of Zinc and ORS through various social mobilization activities.
- Observe ORS-Zinc day at the District and Block Level.
- Celebration of ORS day (29th July in Districts).

Presently along with micronutrient initiative other partners are also available for providing techno-managerial support through field team calling up activities will be executed with the support of these partners. The partners will provide support in District and Block level review meetings facilitating in developing distribution plan, supportive supervisions and other programme related activities.

3.2. *Bal Swasthya Poshan Mah*

Vitamin-A Supplementation Programme in Uttar Pradesh is in line with Government of India's policy of ensuring 9 doses of Vitamin-A supplementation for children between 9th month to 59th month age group. The strategy for administering Vitamin-A is to provide very first dose along with the measures in the age group between 9th month and 12th month. The second dose of Vitamin-A supplementation has to be done through a biannual exercise at a six months interval. In Uttar Pradesh these biannual rounds are held in the June and December.

❑ *Biannual Bal Swasthya Poshan Mah*

Uttar Pradesh is implementing biannual strategy in the form of biannual Bal Swasthya Poshan Mah Strategy. Two months, *viz.* June and December, six month apart have been identified as health and nutrition month, health sector is assigned with the task of providing immunization and other services to the beneficiaries while ICDS sector is responsible for mobilization of beneficiaries by organizing intensive social mobilization and information, education and communication activities. The biannual months have been linked to village-wise routine immunization sessions organized as per the immunization/outreach session's micro plan of ANMs.

The programme has been scaled up since December 2006 across the entire state and is implemented jointly by Directorate of Family Welfare and ICDS with support of development partners mainly UNICEF and Micronutrient Initiative. During the biannual rounds Vitamin-A is administered along with other high impact interventions, which are crucial for child survival and development. This package of services included immunization catch up, promoting optimal breast feeding and complementary feeding, screening and referral for severally malnourished children and education and demand generation for iodized salt.

The continuation and success of programme has been impacted by irregular and interrupted supplies. However, the supply during the year 2013-14 was able to be managed and appropriate funds were released to districts. During the year 2013-14 about ₹ 546.9 lakh has been given to districts to purchase about 9,36,974 Vitamin-A.

Infant Mortality Rate has been declining very slowly and State is committed to meet our goals, hence 2013-14 was celebrated as a year of *Navjaat Shishu Suraksha Varsh*. Emphasis was given to strengthen facilities, services and capacity building of health staffs working at the delivery points to prevent the Neo-Natal morbidity and subsequently reduction in neonatal deaths. At the Community level, trained ASHAs are being involved for home based new born care. The trained ASHAs are paying home visits 6/7 times to each of the month up to 42 days who delivered a baby to care the mother and neonates and accordingly action is being suggested by ASHA including referral services.

3.3. *Priorities to Reduce Neonatal Deaths*

Priorities to reduce Neonatal Deaths are as follows:

3.3.1. *Facility Based Intervention*

- *Sick New Born Care Units (SNBCUs):* Institutional deliveries are increasing at various facilities. There is a need of emergency care of Neonates. To reduce the Neo-Natal and Pre-Natal deaths, all facilities of Level-III type should have sick new born care unit.
- *New Born Stabilization Unit:* At level-3 health facilities, where there is no sick New Born Care Units, 4 Bedded New Born Stabilization Unit have been established to stabilize neonates of the facilities and work as referral unit for Level-2 and Level-1 facilities.
- *New Born Care Corners:* In each labour room at L-3 and L-2 facilities, new born care corners have been established to prevent, birth asphyxia, hypothermia and infections. A Government order to establish and making functional of New Born Care Corners has already been issued.

  The staff members working in the labour room have been trained Navjaat Shishu Suraksha Karyakram and equipment handling skills. This year onwards L-1 facilities (PHCs/ Accredited Sub-Centres) will be strengthened and New Born Care Corners will be established along with Navjaat Shishu Suraksha Karyakram and equipment handling training.
- *Nutrition Rehabilitation Centres:* To manage *Service Acute Malnutrition* (SAM) of Children, 26 Nutrition Rehabilitation Centres (including 5 medical colleges) have been established and made operational by March 2013, and additional 22

Nutrition Rehabilitation Centres are in the process of establishment in the District Male Hospitals. In the year 2014-15, 10 additional Nutrition Rehabilitation Centres are proposed for establishing in 10 District Male Hospitals of the State.

3.3.2. *Priorities for the Year 2014-15*

Priorities/target for the year 2014-15 to reduce Neo Natal Deaths are as follows:

❑ *Sick New Born Care Units*

Till 2013-14, 27 Sick New Born Care units have been established and are functional. In addition, 19 more sick New Born Care Units will be established in 2014-15 to have facility to treat severe sick New Born in all the High Priority Districts of Uttar Pradesh. Government of India has approved operational cost, renovation and repair and one time establishment cost for these 19 New Sick New Born Care Units in 2013-14, process of establishing has been initiated and are expected to be made functional in 2014-15. Therefore, State is proposing operational cost of old 27 functional Sick New Born Care Units including functional in Medical Colleges.

❑ *Development of Sick New Born Units in Medical Colleges*

Eight Medical Colleges of the State and one centrally aided Medical College in the State are providing support to various new born care and one centrally aided Medical College in the State are providing support to various new born care training, new born care scheme and care to very sick children in the community. Out of 27 functional sick New Born Care units in the State 8 are operationalized in Paediatric Department of the 8 Central/State run Medical University/College.

To strengthen sick new born units for providing specialized new born care to the children referred and admitted to these units, funds as approved by Government of India, for procurement of equipments as per demand and requirement was provided through respective District Health Societies.

However, these sick New Born Care Units established in the Medical University/College are being upgraded for providing super speciality services for the New Born of the respective area and also referral cases. Hence, the additional equipment with upgraded facility has been demanded by the Medical University/College and the same has been proposed in the year 2014-15.

These units will serve as centre of excellence/resource centres on new born care and also as potential training sites for all advanced training related to new born care.

Presently 27 Sick New Born Care Units in District Women Hospitals are fully functional and there is provision of 3 paediatricians (MD/DCH) and 8 staff nurses for each Hospital. At medical colleges there is provision of 8 staff nurses for each Medical College, further there is also a provision of 8 ward Ayas and 2 Safai Karmcharis at each of sick New Born Care unit.

❑ *New Born Stabilization Unit*

Up to March, 2014, 120 New Born Stabilization units have been made functional and for 2014-15, all the First Referral Units will have New Born Stabilization Units where there is no Sick New Born Care Units. Therefore, targets have been kept 205 Units, i.e. Additional 85 New Born Stabilization units are proposed for establishing in the year 2014-15. The doctors and staff nurses working in the Hospitals will manage the New Born Stabilization units. They are being trained for *Family Integrated Management of New Natal and Child Illness and Navjaat Shishu Suraksha Karyakram Training.*

❑ *New Born Care Corners*

Up to March 2014, 1473 New Born Care Corners have been established in all labour rooms of District Women Hospital, Community Health Centres and Primary Health Centres. During the year an additional 2,181 New Born Care Corners are proposed for establishing in L-1 facilities. But in the year 2014-15, a total of 1,000 New Born Care Corners would be established. The Doctor and the staff working in Hospital will manage the New Born Care Corners. They have been trained for *Navjaat Shishu Suraksha Karyakram and equipment handling training.*

❑ *Nutrition Rehabilitation Centres*

Up to March 2014, 26 Nutrition Rehabilitation Centres are to be established out of which 25 Nutrition Rehabilitation Centres are functional. In the year 2013-14, 22 Nutrition Rehabilitation Centres were approved by Government of India. Out of which 16 have been established and the rest 6 will be established very soon. In the year 2014-15, 10 New Nutrition Rehabilitation Centres are proposed. The

State has target to saturate with facility of Nutrition Rehabilitation Centres in all the 75 Districts by 2017.

3.4. *New Born Screening: A Preventive Child Health Care Initiative*

The preventive programme plays a major role in public health and are cost effective in terms of money, resources and quality of life. New Born Screening for treatable disorders in which early diagnosis and initiation of treatment before the onset of symptoms is an effective way of preventive disability and infant deaths for a number of disorders. With the improving health care in India and decrease in infections and nutritional disease establishment of New Born Screening programme as a part of child health care facilities is the need of the time.

As the infant mortality rate increases, decrease and approach towards 35 per 1,000, the contribution of birth defects and genetic disorders towards mortality and morbidity become significant and health care measures for these disorders are required.

New Born Screening for treatable disorder to prevent intellectual disability and early death is one such programme. The number of disorders included in New Born Screening programme worldwide has reached more than 40. It is only during last 5 years a few New Born Screening programmes were carried out in India with the support of Indian Council of Medical Research and Department of Bio-technology. The data available has given basic information about prevalence of the disorder tested and has proved the utility and feasibility of such a programme.

At Sanjay Gandhi Post Graduate Institute of Medical Science, Lucknow, Department of Genetic and Department of Endocrinology, recently completed a New Born Screening programme financially supported by Department of Biotechnology, Government of India.

Under this programme about 13,500 neonates have been screened for three disorders with easy, effective and cheap treatment. The disorders tested were congenital hypothyroidism, biotinidase deficiency and galactosemia.

In this project 11 Neonates were diagnosed with congenital hypothyroidism (2 with transient hypothyroidism) and were put on treatment within 2 to 3 weeks of life. Thus, preventing the life long disability due to untreated congenital hypothyroidism.

The crude cost effectiveness on the basis of calculators using minimum wages, shows that the new born screening programme is at least 10 to 50 times cost effective in addition to ensuring healthy baby to the family in this era of small family norms.

The experience indicates that the new born screening programme was accepted by all strata of the society with great enthusiasm and was considered as an important baby care measure. The media and medical community also welcomed the programme created much headed population awareness.

❑ *Methodology*

New born screening programme is a system involving peripheral hospitals providing obstetric care, providing information, counselling, sample collection, transport samples, laboratory testing, in timely manner, communication of results trickling cases with screen positive results, conformity tests, initiation of treatment, follow-up and audit. The disorders included in the screening programme are *congenital, hypothyroidism, biotinidase deficiency, glactosemia, congenital adrenal hyperplasia,* etc. Thus, all five disorders fulfil the criteria for inclusion in the new born screening most important of which is that early pesymptomatic diagnosis and appropriate treatment will help in preventing intellectual disability (mental retardation) and/or life threatening complications and early death.

The samples will be collected on a filter paper (five drops) along with the demographic information from all the new born delivered in the collaborating hospital after providing information about the utility of new born screening to the parents. Samples will be collected after 24 hours of life preferably within 48 to 72 hours after birth. Samples will be collected by heal prick using a very fine needle attached to lancet, making the process pain free.

The success of population based programme depends on the awareness amongst general population. Hence, the poster based and audio-visual based advertisement, awareness programme for general population and doctors. Training programme for medical social workers and paramedical staff will be organized at different levels.

3.5. *Girl or Boy: Healthy Baby is the Joy*

The new born screening programme for treatable disorders is a part of child health care. New born screening is not a test but a preventive programme and a system to be a part of established heath care system, with infant mortality approaching the target, it is the right time to start New Born screening initiative at the district level. This pilot programme will be role model which can be replicated with the aim of running a statewide New born screening programme as a part of Government supported Child Health Care and preventive programme over a period of next 5 to 10 years.

The burden of raising a handicapped child is immense and affects the financial, social and psychological aspects of all the family members. The *prevention is better* and *cheaper than Cure*.

New born screening programme is considered one of the major preventive programmes of modern medicine. It has been proved to be cost effective in the financial mode as well as an important way to ensure a healthy baby to a family, helping them to accept the small family norms.

Uttar Pradesh is one of the first states to provide new born screening to its population from all socio-economic strata. The initiative will lead to a statewide programme and to advocate and accept the moto of "A Girl or Boy: Healthy Baby is the Joy".

3.6. *First Passport to Life (Child Health Cards) 0-5 Years of Age (Zindagi Ki Uddan)*

India's Millennium Development Goals-4, target is to reduce Infant Mortality Rate by two-third between 1990 and 2015, i.e. from 80 infant deaths per 1,000 live births in 1990 to "28" by 2015, under Millennium Development Goals-4, another target is to improve the proportion of one-year old children immunization against measles from 42 per cent in 1992-93 to 100 per cent by 2015.

To a large extent, India shapes the global Millennium Development Goal's 4 and 5 targets, because of its share of the global burden of child (23%) and maternal mortality (19%). Moreover, during the past two decades, the 15 most populous states, which account for 95 per cent of India's population, have made variable progress on infant and/or maternal mortality reduction efforts.

Reaching the Millennium Development Goals on reducing child mortality will require universal coverage with key effective, affordable interventions, in order to achieve these Millennium Development Goals the 12th Five Year Plan (2012-2017) has defined the National Health outcomes of reducing Infant Mortality Rate to 25 per 1,000 live births by 2017.

❑ *Major Causes of Mortality in Children Less than 5 Yeas of Age*

The children who die before their fifth birthday almost one-third of them die of infectious causes, all of which are preventable. The causes of child mortality in the age group 0-5 years are as follows:

(a) Neo-Natal Cause (52%),
(b) Pneumonia (15%),
(c) Diarrhoea Disease (11%),
(d) Injuries (4%), and
(f) Others (15%).

❑ *Key Strategies to Address these Strategies*

- Early detection and management of illness in mother and new born.
- Immunization.
- First Level assessment and care for new born and childhood illness.
- Micro-Nutrient Supplementation.
- Danger sign recognition and care seeking for illness.
- Use of ORS and Zinc in Case of diarrhoea.

In order to follow-up on these strategies in a systematic way, "*Bal Swasthya Kunji (Passport to Life)*" has been proposed.

❑ *Bal Swasthya Kunji*

- A tool for community/families/individual learn, understand and follow practices for achieving good health of young infants and children.
- Card Helps them to know about various types of services which they need to access for the health and well-being of young infants and children.
- The card empowers them to make decisions for improved health and nutritional status of young children.
- The card tells us about the development milestones of the child.

❑ *Specific*

- Will be provided to each delivered Child (Live Birth/Still Birth).
- Bal Swasthya Card will have information about delivery and intermediate new born.
- Details about immunization.
- It helps in tracking and assessing the development milestones in children so that developmental delays if any can be identified and referred to appropriate level of care.
- It helps in knowing and identifying danger sign in young infant and children and what should be done.

- This card also works as on OPD booklet and helps to maintain continuing of treatment (if any given to the Child additionally helps us to track prescription practices and the appropriateness of the treatment-given to children in context of their birth record in the card.
- The card which will be issued to each delivered child will be linked with the check-list of case sheet (Mother and Essential New Born Care) where the child was born.

3.6. *Training*

Under Child Health Programme various trainings are being proposed at various levels for the year 2014-15. The status of training under Child Health Programme is as follows:

❑ *Navjaat Shishu Suraksha Karyakram Training*

All the staff posted at delivery points are to be trained for 2 days Navjaat Shishu Suraksha Karyakram. During 2013-14, 2 days training was organized for 2,174 Medical Officers, 2,035 staff nurses, 3,264 ANMs and the total achievement for the training has been 66.2 per cent to the total target of 10,807 personnel training.

❑ *Family Integrated Management of Neo-Natal and Child Illness*

The F-IMNCI training is being organized with the view to build capacity of Medical Officers and Staff Nurses posted at facilities to treat and manage sick new born babies. Presently, 9 medical colleges have been involved in various types of child health training. The achievements for the Medical Officers has been 46.1 per cent and for the staff nurse which is under progress has been 4.2 per cent during 2013-14.

❑ *Status of Integrated Management of Neo-Natal and Child Illness Plus for Medical Officers (Physicians Training)*

The IMCI Plus training is also being provided to Medical Officers posted at CHC/PHC to support to train ASHAs and ANMs. The achievement up to March 2014 has been 37.9 per cent. For coordinating with the District/State and other stakeholders; a post of training coordinator was created in the year 2008-09. State has included 4 additional Medical Colleges for F:IMNCI training of Medical Officer and other Child Health Training hence one training coordinators @ 40,000 p.m. for 12 months (9 × 12 × 40,000 pm. = ₹ 43.20 lakh) for each of 9 Medical colleges, total 9 posts have been proposed for the year 2014-15.

❑ *IMNCI Plus Training for ANMs*

To reduce Infant Mortality Rate, 10 days skill development training of Integrated Management of Neonatal and childhood Illness has been provided to ANMs/ASHAs. However, the training programme could not be undertaken due to unavailability of modules. During the year 2014-15, it is proposed to train 6,960 ANMs and local health volunteers with size of 24 in 290 batches. In addition 44 batches of training of trainees have been proposed. Site strengthening and priority of modules are proposed for the year 2014-15.

❑ *Home Based Born Care (Community Based Interventions)*

During the year 2013-14, the trained ASHAs in module 6 and 7 of 1st and 2nd Phase 36 IMICI + districts were taken up. ASHAs were given ₹ 250 per child as incentive after providing following services:

- Ensuring Birth Registration.
- Ensuring BCG and Zero dose polio.
- Ensuring recording of Birth Weight.
- Conducting 6/7 Post Natal Visits for Mother and ensuring Baby alive up to 42 days.

3.7. *Infant Young Child Feeding*

The rates of early initiation breast feeding in Uttar Pradesh is 36 per cent whereas exclusive breast feeding is about 19 per cent. There is an urgent need to improve the coverage of these indicators considering the impact of optimal breast feeding practices on child morbidity and mortality. In the subsequent years, the Infant and young child feeding components including promotion of complementary feeding and breast feeding will be taken up through community based actions and partnership.

The key features of Programme Implementation Plan 2014-15 on Infant Young Child Feeding will be as follows:

- Breast Feeding Week Celebration.
- Skill Based Training using existing Master Trainers available in the State.
- IEC and Communication activities during breast feeding week in communication and institutions.

(i) *Breast Feeding Week Celebration*

It has been proposed that the State will celebrate 'World Breast Feeding Week' jointly with ICDS. Technical support will be sought from UNICEF and other partners working in the State.

(ii) *Skill Based Training*

Skill Based Training will be undertaken for promoting optimal Infant and young child feeding practices. This training will be effective in building counselling, communication and problem solving skills among staff which will subsequently help in providing timely need based and quality counselling and practical support to mothers delivering in institutions or whenever the children are admitted to hospitals.

The Doctors will undergo 3 days training to become middle level trainers, while staff nurses will be trained for 7 days as counsellors. Training to these staff will be provided by pool of National Trainers with the technical support of UNICEF and support from other development partners will be taken for quality assurance of training and monitoring of the Infant Young Child Feeding practices for deliveries taking place in institutions.

Training will be imparted to staff of the District Male and Female Hospital. In addition, two staff nurses from each block will be trained on Infant Young Child Feeding. In this way all the staff nurses working close to children will be trained on Infant Young Child Feeding and 3 health staff from each block will be trained. Thus, on an average 30 Staff Nurses will be given 7 days training from each district.

(iii) *IEC/BCC Activities*

Under child health to carry out IEC/BCC activities celebration of breast feeding, new born care week, poster on New Born Care, IEC for All New Born Care Corners, requisite budget has been proposed for the year 2014-15.

3.8. *Facilities Based Management of Severely Acute Malnourisned: Nutrition Rehabilitation Centre*

Severely Acute Malnourished Children are at high risk of morbidity and mortality and such children need specific therapeutic care. Severe Acute Malnourished Children with complications need special therapeutic care at Nutrition Rehabilitation Care. There are already 25 such Nutrition Rehabilitation Centres functioning in 19 districts, 22 additional Nutrition

Rehabilitation Centres have been proposed and approved in 2013-14. Programme Implementation Plan shall be made functional till 2014.

For the Financial Year 2014-15, State shall be strengthening the Existing Nutrition Rehabilitation Centres by introducing some new innovations and improving quality of services through supportive supervision, quarterly reviews and reorientation/refresher workshops.

Management of severely Acute Malnourished — Nutrition Rehabilitation Centre are as follows:

- Revision of existing norms for Nutrition Rehabilitation Care is required.
- Cost of Medicine and Investigations is increased from ₹ 300 to ₹ 350 as it was reported by Nutrition Rehabilitation Centre that ₹ 300 is not sufficient in most of the cases as it also involves investigation, medicine and supplements which care sometimes not available from Government supply. Hence an increase of ₹ 50 has been proposed.

❑ *Daily Wage Compensation for Mother and Food for Mother during Stay*

Daily Wage Compensation is increased to ₹ 150 per day from a previous ₹ 100 also ₹ 50 per day is proposed as an additional fund to provide food to mother (Breakfast, Lunch, Evening Snacks and Dinner). After introduction of these two changes this will certainly motivate the mothers to stay back at Nutrition Rehabilitation Centres for longer duration thus increasing referrals, Bed Occupancy and Reduction of Number of Defaulters.

❑ *Transportation Cost to Family*

A sum of ₹ 200 for bringing child back home after discharge is introduced. Apart from these, an additional ₹ 200 per visit has been proposed for four follow-up visits of discharged children. These introductions shall definitely motivate the mothers to bring back their children to Nutrition Rehabilitation Centre for follow-ups.

❑ *Incentives for ASHAs for Follow-up Visits*

₹ 100 per follow visit within two months incentive is proposed for ASHAs for motivating and bringing the mothers and children to Nutrition Rehabilitation Centre for follow-up.

Contingencies — The contingencies per month is increased from ₹ 2,000 to ₹ 3,000 p.m.

❑ *Funds for Maintenance of Equipments and Purchase of Damaged Equipments*

A lump sum of ₹ 20,000 is proposed per Nutrition Rehabilitation Centre as Annual Maintenance Fund which is to be used for maintaining old equipment, painting or repairing of Nutrition Rehabilitation Centre.

Miscellaneous Items — like documentation, printing of documents, charts, discharge tickets, registers, etc. photographs, photocopying, display boards, etc. of ₹ 20,000 per Nutrition Rehabilitation Centre is proposed.

Internet Recharge — ₹ 250 p.m. is proposed for recharge of internet which is required for Nutrition Rehabilitation Centres Software.

Establishment Cost — The funds for purchase of mattresses is increased from ₹ 2,500 per set to ₹ 12,000 per set.

Deliverables — Operational funds shall make 26 old Nutrition Rehabilitation Centre operational. One should have capacity to treat and rehabilitate average 240. Severely Acute Malnourished Cases (10 Bed) and 120 SAM Cases (6 Bedded NRC) in the six CHC-NRC as these Units do not have sufficient place to expand existing Nutrition Rehabilitation Centre.

❑ *Child Death Review*

Child Death Review is a strategy to understand the geographical variation in the causes of child death and thereby initiating specific child health interventions. Analysis of Child Death provides information about the medical causes of death, helps to identify the gaps in health service delivery and social factors that contribute to Child Deaths. This information can be used to adopt corrective measures and fill the gaps in community and facility services delivery. With uniform Child Death Review process and formats across the states information can be compared over a period of time and common factors identified and addressed through national programme.

This contributes to overall improvement in quality of care and reducing child mortality. Data on the causes of Neo Natal and Child Deaths are also useful for health planners, administrators and medical professionals to evaluate trends in the causes of mortality over time and thus assess the impact of the ongoing health programmes and to make a decision on allocation of resources for different strategies to prevent and manage neonatal and childhood illness.

3.9. *"Golden Hour" New Born Tracking*

Introduction of Tablet computers as a tool for learning, training, counselling, documenting and reporting at high case load facilities has been initiated by the Government of Uttar Pradesh.

Government of Uttar Pradesh has made strides to reduce maternal mortality ratio and infant mortality rate, yet the State still lags behind Indian National averages. There are very critical periods in the life-cycle of both a mother and new born in which specific activities must be carried out within the first minute (Golden Minute) and hour (Golden Hour) following delivery in order to reduce morbidity and mortality.

Unfortunately, such *activities are not completely being carried out, and when they are, their quality is very poor.* State has identified poor implementation and poor monitoring during these golden minute and golden hours period as a contributing case of sustained Maternal Mortality Rate and Infant Mortality Rate in Uttar Pradesh. As a means to reduce these gaps, Uttar Pradesh wishes to initiate innovation solutions to improve service delivery implementation as well as improve monitoring of service activities at the facility level during the golden hour and golden minute.

3.10. *Zinc/ORS Social Marketing Programme*

The high mortality in Uttar Pradesh (68/1,000) of which 12-13 per cent results from Diarrhoea is due in part to the low reach of simple curative solutions, such as oral *dehydration* therapy. The awareness of ORS among mothers is high compared to that of zinc, usage is low due to preference for treatment perceived to provide immediate relief.

Due to the resulting low demand for these low-margin products, manufacturers do not see an attractive market for zinc and ORS and do not invest in the widespread distribution and product promotion activities that are required for building awareness and driving higher, uptake. This situation is the well-known 'market-trap' where limited supply constraint demand through unfamiliarity, which in turn, weakens the incentive to increase supply. Breaking this market trap, requires a non-profit intervention which is the basis of "Social Marketing".

The goal of social marketing scheme will be to create a market where Zinc and ORS are available in adequate quantities, informal providers prescribe its use and through repeated use mothers begin to recognize and demand it for their infants.

Important objectives of the programme are as follows —

- *To generate demand* and increase the perceived value of zinc and ORS as treatment for diarrhoea.
- *Expand access to Zinc and ORS products* at affordable prices, complement the free supply of zinc and ORS through the public health system and ensure the priority of quality health care products through good quality assurance system.

To implement the scheme following next steps are required:

(1) *To Set-up Social Marketing Unit*

Social Marketing Unit will be set-up for setting guidance, routing the subsidy, certifying the manufacturers and auding the social marketing unit will be jointly led by official from the Directorate of NRHM and headed by Director General Family Welfare will be supported by development partners.

(2) *Select Social Marketing Organization*

Social Marketing Organization will be a non-for profit organization with prior experience in social marketing and will invest in a procurement and distribution network of stockist and sales staff through which it will introduce the product to the Private Medical Practitioners. The demand generated by Social Marketing Organization will create a multiplier effect on the size of the market and attract a number of smaller players. The role of social Marketing Organization will be —

- Sale and distribution of products.
- Purchase of products from manufacturer.
- Branding.
- Trade Promotion.
- Design and implementation of marketing campaigns, targeting consumers and providers.

(3) *Provision of Subsidy*

The scheme will be supported by a trade subsidy from the government to be channeled through Social Marketing Unit. The amount of subsidy will be tied to the sales realized by the social marketing organization.

(4) *Allocate a Budget for Market Development Activities*

The scheme will require from Government to allocate an Information,

Education and Communication budget to generate and grow demand through Behavioural Change Communication initiative including a host of market development campaign targeted at both care given and the providers.

Social Marketing Organizations will be tasked with the role of implementing a behaviour change strategy aimed at getting rural practitioners to treat diarrhoea recommended and mothers to recognize and demand the appropriate products. The implementation plan for this strategy will be decided by each Social Marketing Organization but its broad components are expected to be as follows:

(a) Seek to influence demand at three levels — *Health Providers, Pharmacists and Care givers (mothers).*
(b) Establish Zinc, among health professionals through engagement of key opinion leaders.
(c) Improve recall through frequent sales visits and point of sale communication.

4. Family Planning

The Population Policy of Uttar Pradesh was launched on 11th July, 2000, to improve the quality of life, with unambiguous and explicit emphasis on sustainable development measures and actions. The population policy looks at the issues related to population stabilization and improvement of the health status of people, particularly women and children in holistic, open and transparent manner.

The Total Fertility Rate of Uttar Pradesh has declined from 4.1 to 3.8 per cent. However, compared to the National average of 2.7, the rates are still very high to enhance the performance of Family Planning, it is imperative to meet the desired unment needs. The unment need for spacing method has increased from 9 per cent in 1998-99 to 12 per cent in 2005-06 to 29.7 per cent in 2010-11.

❑ *Plan for Facilities Providing FEMALE Sterilization Services on Fixed days at Health Facilities*

The two days fixed for services "Under fixed day sterilization Service" (ligation/abdominal/tubectomy) will be continued at all District Women Hospital/PHC/CHCs having either a surgeon or gynaecologist.

Tuesday and Friday may be fixed as per suitability in consultation with the Chief Medical Officer wide publicity of the fixed days would be ensured through wall writing, leaflet, brochures, etc. A separate register would be maintained to record number of sterilizations conducted on fixed days including the details of clients and the surgeon conducting the sterilization.

❑ *Plan for Facilities Providing Non-Scalpel Vasectomy Services on Fixed Days at Health Facilities*

Provision of fixed days Non-Scalpel Vasectomy Services at each District Male Hospital/Combined Hospital and First Referral Units will continue. Any day may be fixed in consultation with Chief Medical Officer. Wide publicity of the fixed days would be ensured through wall writing, leaflet, brochures, etc. In case of non-availability of the service providers, efforts would be made to train them for non-scalpel vasectomy at the earliest.

❑ *Number of Female Sterilization Camps*

In order to achieve the target of sterilization, each district organizes sterilization camps at Block or Tehsils on regular basis. The expenditure on these camps relating to compensation money to clients and medicines is borne by the compensation head for female sterilization. In view of low performance (still shortage of service providers, so the fixed day/ daily services are not available at every facility) on sterilization, it is now proposed to provide funds for female sterilization camps.

❑ *Number of Non-Scalpel Vasectomy Camps*

Besides providing non-scalpel vasectomy services on regular basis, it is proposed that each district hospital will organize at least 2-12 NSV Camps per year depending on their performance and Client load. A total number of 667 NSV Camps are proposed for this year. For organizing NSV Camps @ ₹ 3,500 are admissible to districts.

❑ *Compensation for Sterilization (Female)*

Up to March 2014 around 3,19,917 sterilizations have been performed. Now with the availability of trained providers and accredited nursing homes, it is expected that in the year 2014-15 around 5,70,884 sterilizations would be performed. Out of this 5,44,884 cases are expected from public sector which will be compensated @ ₹ 1,000 and 26,000 cases are expected from private sector to be compensated @ ₹ 1,500.

❑ *Compensation for Sterilization Non-Scalpel Vasectomy (Male)*

Up to December 2014, a total of 7,046 male Sterilization have been performed. However, considering that this year all four centres of training for NSV are working more trained officers and work load is generated through them, therefore, it is now estimated that in this year 2014-15 around 15,262 sterilizations would be performed.

❑ *Accreditation of Private Centres/NGOs for Sterilization Services*

The purpose of this project is to evolve partnership with private nursing homes for offering Family Planning services and increase the acceptance of Family Planning Services through private sector. There are certain hindrances because of which private nursing homes and centres have not been accredited. For this purpose 6 regional workshops @ ₹ 50,000 to bring private hospitals and Government officers on one platform and to address issues in Accreditation of Private Centres/Nursing Homes to increase sterilization service. At the district level also one workshop @ ₹ 10,000 per district with private nursing homes for offering family planning service and increase the acceptance of family planning services through private sector should be organized.

❑ *Spacing Method*

After Sterilization, the newly introduced Cut 380-A is the most effective and reliable contraceptive. It is temporary method providing a long-term safety. Presently, 992 facilities are providing daily services. The accredited, sub-centres which have proper space and facilities with a minimum of 3 deliveries monthly average will be monitored for this activity.

❑ *Orientation/Review of ASHA/ANM/AWW Scheme for Home Delivery of the Contraceptives*

One day orientation meeting is planned for ASHA/AWW/ANM at the Block Level for 2 schemes promoted by ASHA: Social marketing of family planning methods and incentives for adoption of family planning method. They need hands on training on Collection of Data and record keeping.

❑ *Doorstep Delivery of Contraceptive by ASHA*

The contraceptives are supplied to the State by Government of India and distributed to the district as per their project requirements. In spite of trying various methodologies the distribution and usages of spacing methods, unmet need remains high. Identified reasons are many from timely availability of choice method to lack of privacy in distribution system. To overcome these constraints and promote usage of spacing methods in rural area, a new scheme has been launched in which packs of oral contraceptive pills, Emergency contraceptive pills and pack of 3 condoms have been supplied and distributed to ASHAs on an amount based on the eligible couple register data of Auxiliary Nurse Midwife to be distributed to the rural population on nominal prices.

❑ *Enhance Contribution of Panchayati Raj Institutions and Family Members*

To improve family planning programme, some activities are being proposed to improve outputs of programme activities to enhance contribution of Panchayati Raj Institutions and Family Members of eligible couples in family planning programme various incentives have been proposed:

(i) *Panch-Sarpanch Sammelan* — To create awareness in Panchayati Raj Institutions Organization of Panch-Sarpanch Sammelan at Block level has been proposed.

(ii) *Saas-Bahu Sammelan* — To emphasize the importance of small family and effect of more children on mother and child health it is important to create awareness in family so for that Saas Bahu Sammelan is proposed at Block Level.

(iii) *Non-Scalpel Vasectomy Satisfied Clients Meet* — For promoting Non-Scalpel vasectomy and male participation in family planning and to emanate methods from society, proposed NSV satisfied Clients meet at district level.

❑ *Plans for Partum Sterilization*

Deployment of Family Welfare Counsellor: Family Planning Counsellors are being developed in view of the opportunity of large number of institutional delivery under Janani Suraksha Yojana and they will have the opportunity to reach all the mothers and will counsel the women and address their concern for small family norms. Presently, there are 290 Counsellors who are counselling the ANC and PNC Members for adoption of post partum Family Planning methods. This year it is proposed today one family counsellor at all those facilities where more than average 200 deliveries are being conducted in a month and one additional family welfare counsellor for facility having average per month more than 600 deliveries.

❑ *Performance Activities to ASHA under Family Planning*

A sum of ₹ 150 may be paid to ASHAs for escorting the clients to the health facility for facilitating the insertion. For this activity expected number of clients escorting by ASHAs for institutional deliveries.

(1) *Pehel Sakhi Sammelan*

State is organizing a community event "*Pehel Sakhi Sammelan*". Nearly 250 people from the Block are expected to actively participate in the event. The target will be to have eminent Panchayati Raj Institutions, ASHAs, BPM and District Officials from CMO's Office like ACMO-FP, DPM, etc. to join this event. The importance of birth spacing in reducing maternal and child morbidity and mortality will be discussed. Doctors will clarify the myths and misconceptions regarding Intra Uterine Device and Post Partum Intra Uterine Contraceptive Device.

Pehel Sakhi Sammelan is way to bring satisfied users and eligible couples for spacing method on a common platform to promote the use of Intra Uterine Device and Post Partum Intra Uterine Contraceptive Device.

(2) *Male Group Meeting*

Male group meeting is being organized to increase awareness and correct knowledge of the spacing and limiting method among men. These meetings will enhance the acceptability of the IUD, PPIUCD and NSV among males. Nearly 250 people from block are expected to actively participate in the event. The satisfied couples or lady users of IUD, PPIUCD and NSV will share their experience and reveal how a log acting reversible contraceptive have made their family life healthy and happy. Token gift will be given to happy users.

Merry Gold Health Network—Merry Gold Health Network is being implemented by Hindustan Latex Planning Promotion Trust as the franchisor under guidance of *United States Agency for International Development and State Innovation in Family Planning Agency* (SIFPSA) since 2007, in order to engage the large and unregulated private sector through network and at the same time to standardize the prices of health services. Merry Gold Health Network is a proven and tested pilot of Social Franchising Mechanism under Public Private Partnership model, which has been the successful models of Public Private Partnership in health sector having quality Family Planning Services at affordable pre-fixed prices.

5. Rashtriya Kishor Swasthya Karyakram

National Adolescent Health Strategy, Rashtriya Kishor Swasthya Karyakram (RKSK) has been proposed in Uttar Pradesh as per the guidelines of Government of India. The target group is 10-19 years of age which will get with various components of Reproductive Maternal Neonatal Child Health and Adolescent (RMNCH+A).

Proposed key interventions are as follows:

- Selection, recruitment and training of peer educators.
- Organizing Biannual Adolescent Health Days at Block level.
- Weekly Iron Folic Acid Supplementation Programmes.
- Menstrual Hygiene Scheme.
- Rashtriya Kishor Swasthya Karyakram Training.
- Convergence within health and with other partner departments and scheme.
- Wide IEC/BCC pre-marital counselling.

❑ *Organization of Adolescent Health Days at Block Level*

It has been proposed to organize Adolescent Health Day at Block Level initially twice a year which may be expanded to quarterly as per experience/feedback in the next year. An estimated number of 250 participants (ASHAs, PEs, Adolescent Boys and Girls from various villages, selected school teachers, Panchayat Members, NGOs, ANMs and AWWs) will attend the function.

❑ *Weekly Iron Folic Acid Supplementation Programme*

Weekly Iron Folic Acid Supplementation Programme is being implemented from last two years. Weekly Iron Blue tablets are being provided to all the school going girls and boys in the age group of 10-19 years. The target in the year 2013-14 was about 60 lakh which has increased to 67 lakh in the year 2014-15.

Thus, a total number of about 116 lakh adolescent girls and boys (school going and out of school) are proposed to be covered under weekly Iron Folic Acid Supplementation Scheme. To create wide awareness among the communities, it is being proposed to organize workshop at various levels.

❑ *Menstrual Hygiene Scheme*

Menstrual Hygiene Scheme is being implemented in the State for the last three years. The utilization of sanitary napkins was as low as 11 per cent in March 2013 for which lots of efforts have been made with extensive monitoring, supervision and review meetings on a regular interval. The District Officers and Programme Managers have also tried hard and the utilization rate in March 2014 has increased to 45 per cent. As per scheme is highly subsidized, beneficial and empowering for girls, it has been decided by the Government of Uttar Pradesh to provide free sanitary napkins to school going girls in public sector from Class 6-12 from year 2014-15 the progress is under process.

To create awareness among communities it is being proposed to organize workshop at State level, District level, Block level and with SHG, Poster at Anganwadi Centre.

❑ *Convergence within Health and with Other Partner Departments*

To ensure positive results in various activities under Rashtriya Kishor Swasthya Karyakram Convergence within the Health Department with various section like Medical Health, Family Welfare Medical Education, State Institute of Health and Family Welfare and various units are most essential.

Convergence will be maintained by regular meetings and their involvements. Similarly, convergence with other departments like ICDS, Education, Mid Day Meal, Panchayati Raj Institutions, Rural Development and NGOs will be maintained by regular meeting at various levels under Rashtriya Kishor Swasthya Karyakram. Convergence with other schemes will also be ensured at various levels.

6. Rashtriya Bal Swasthya Karyakram

Rashtriya Bal Swasthya Karyakram is being implemented in the State from last three years which has been established by the 3rd quarter of the year 2013-14. Every Block of the State is supposed to have 2 Mobile Health Teams with 4 members in each team (2 Doctors, Para Medical and one Staff Nurse/Auxiliary Nurse Midwife), key components of the Karyakram are as follows:

- Programme Implementation under RBSK.
- Mobility support for mobile health team.
- RBSK Training.
- Procurement.

❑ *Mobility Support for Mobile Health Teams*

Provision of one vehicle per block (for 2 teams of 3 members each) in the year 2013-14 has been ensured. Presently, the number of members has been increased to 4 and it is not possible for vehicle to carry 8 members, logistics along with an additional driver. Hence, it is being proposed to provide one vehicle per mobile health team @ ₹ 30,000 per month in the year 2014-15.

❑ *Regular Management of Referral Cases*

About 5-6 per cent children are being referred to Community Health Centre or District Hospitals during 2013-14.

It has been made a practice to call all the referred children to nearest Community Health Centres on Saturday where team members are present to take personal care of the sick children and help in getting them investigated and managed at Community Health Centres by specialists. Those children who are referred to district hospitals are carried by the dedicated vehicles under Rashtriya Bal Suraksha Karyakram with one doctor of the team to district hospital for supervised investigation and treatment.

Mobility support is being proposed for transportation of referred children to neighbouring Medical College/Higher Centre which is about 0.14 per cent of the total screened children. An amount of ₹ 11 per km on an average from each district to the neighbouring medical college. It has been observed that there are many conditions which need specific investigations and are not free at medical college.

Therefore, an amount of ₹ 2,000 per case is being proposed for 0.1 per cent children to help them in sophisticated investigations done at Medical Colleges. Similarly, an amount of ₹ 5,000 per child on an average is being proposed for treatment of 0.1 per cent of Children supposed to be referred at Medical College. This amount will be kept at State level and a committee will be formed with Director General Family Welfare and Director General Medical Health, State Programme Management Unit, and K.G. Medical University to review the cost of such cases, verification of each case will be done through a committee at division level and funds will be reimbursed to concerned Medical College, through District Health Society. At local level District Nodal Officers, A.Ds. and nodal officers of the Medical College will be responsible for getting the Estimates and Bills, etc. In certain specific cases Mission Director may be authorized to advance some funds to the Medical Colleges as per requirement.

There are few conditions like congenital heart disease, retinoblastoma, plastic surgeries, etc. which need greater amount for treatment and a pool of ₹ 50.00 lakh (₹ 0.50 lakh × 100 such cases) is being proposed additionally for such peculiar conditions.

❑ *Human Resource under Rashtriya Bal Suraksha Karyakram*

There is a provision of two teams per block with 4 members in each team. There are two Doctors, One Staff Nurse/ANM and One Para Medical/Pharmacist. Some configuration will continue in the year 2014-15, with efforts to complete the teams as soon as possible in all the Districts.

7. Pre-Conception, Pre-Natal Diagnostic Techniques Act (PCPNDT)

Sex ratio is an important indicator to measure gender equity. The rapidly increasing sex ratio in the state is like to create severe gender imbalance that can destroy the social fabric. It should also viewed both as child right issues as girls are killed either through sex selective abortions or die prematurely due to violence and neglect. Figure below mentioned in Table 3.3 indicates the trend of violence and neglect. It also indicates the trend in sex ratio over the years in India and Uttar Pradesh.

Table 3.3: Sex Ratio Trends Over the Years

Year	*1901*	*1911*	*1921*	*1931*	*1941*	*1951*	*1961*	*1971*	*1981*	*1991*	*2001*	*2011*
India	972	964	955	950	945	946	941	930	934	927	933	940
Uttar Pradesh	942	916	908	903	907	908	907	876	882	876	898	909

But the results about the sex ratio among the children between age 0 to 6 years have decreased remarkably at National as well as State level.

Year	*India*	*Uttar Pradesh*
1991	945	927
2001	927	916
2011	914	902

The civil registration data clearly shows that sex ratio is declining in most of the commercially viable districts where Ultra sonography centres are in abundance indicating a direct correlation. Consequently, strategies will focus on these districts. Near about 4,430 centres have been registered under the Prevention and Control and PC and PNDT Act in the State. It is well known that it is difficult to regulate the private sector and therefore, initiatives to monitor the implementation of the PC and PNDT Act becomes even more essential. Given the above scenario, effective implementation of the PC and PNDT Act together with social reform efforts including enhancing of the value of a daughter is a significant step towards the prevention of female foeticide.

❑ *State PC and PNDT Cell*

A PC and PNDT Cell has been established at the Family Directorate, Presently one Programme Assistant and One Data Assistant is already working in this Cell. During the last one year there has been an increase in the number of court cases, formation of special Community to review the case Divisional and District Level Workshop for better implementation of PC and PNDT Act have also been done.

❑ *Zonal PC and PNDT Cell*

Uttar Pradesh is being a large State monitoring, follow-up of court cases, data collection, etc. is difficult from state level. For better implementation of PC and PNDT Cell Act it is proposed that the State is being divided into 6 Zones — Lucknow, Kanpur, Varanasi, Meerut, Gorakhpur, Agra, Each Zone will cover 3 divisions and 12 to 13 districts.

❑ *Divisional Level PC and PNDT Cell*

A separate divisional level PC and PNDT Cell is being established at Divisional Additional Director's Office.

❑ *District Level PC and PNDT Cell*

A separate district level PC and PNDT Cell will be established at Chief Medical Officers Office. This cell will work on line data reporting on web portal of PC and PNDT on regular basis.

❑ *State Inspection and Monitoring Committee*

State level Inspection and Monitoring Committee has been established, which will undertake inspection of Ultrasound centre in different districts.

❑ *Mobility for Zonal Programme Coordinator*

The follow-up of court cases, data collection, etc. is difficult from state. For better implementation of PC and PNDT Act State has been divided into 6 Zones — Lucknow, Kanpur, Agra, Meerut, Gorakhpur, Varanasi, each Zone will Cover 3 divisions and 12 to 13 districts. Coordination and monitoring with district team of different districts under the zone, the programme coordinator will travel to the districts.

8. Programme Implementation Plan for 2014-15

Various Programme Implementation Plans for the year 2014-15 have been formulated under the National Rural Health Mission Programme.

8.1. *Mainstreaming of AYUSHS*

World Health Organization has estimated that most of the people in developing as well as in developed countries received the bulk of their health care from traditional or indigenous health system.

Thus, the opportunity to increase the power and reach of the public health sector through integration of AYUSH systems in India cannot be ignored. Prevention of disease or illness is now being emphasized as more significant than treatment, whether we look at it from an angle of cost effectiveness or economic expenditure incurred by the State or by citizen.

AYUSH system highlights the preventive aspects rather than curative care. National Rural Health Mission has identified this significant aspect of AYUSH and thus mainstreaming of AYUSH at all levels in health care delivery system. Hence, the services of AYUSH Doctors and Paramedics are of the utmost importance in health care.

Ayurveda, Yoga and Naturopathy, Unani, Siddha and Homoeopathy (AYUSH) systems of medicines have proven promotive, preventive and curative strengths. The objective of mainstreaming of AYUSH is to provide AYUSH Health Care facilities at the PHCs, CHCs and District hospitals. The development of Health Care institutions scheme has been revised along with addition of some new components, in order to mainstreaming of AYUSH more effectively.

Most of the PHCs and CHCs are situated in rural areas, to promote basic health services by AYUSH system under one roof of PHCs and CHCs and District Hospitals in the light of Reproductive Maternal Neo-Natal Child Health and Adolescent to decrease Maternal Mortality Rate and Infant Mortality Rate. AYUSH Doctors and paramedics can be effectively and efficiently utilized in so many ongoing schemes/ programmes of National Rural Health Mission.

8.2. *Training*

There is a need for upgradation of in the professional competence and skills of AYUSH doctors. Emerging trends of health care and scientific outcomes necessitate time to time enhancement of professional knowledge of AYUSH Doctor. Good clinical practice are one major areas where AYUSH Doctors need to be regularly updated to keep up the standards of health care delivery in accordance with the emerging demands. Overall structure of the training and skill upgradation is aimed at encouraging AYUSH Doctors undergo need based professional training and bridge of knowledge gaps at various levels.

8.3. *Orientation Training of AYUSH Doctors*

The training programme for AYUSH Doctors aims to provide a comprehensive understanding of National Health Mission and the role and responsibility of AYUSH Doctor for various activities relating to National Health Mission in context to Reproductive Maternal and Child Health + Adolescent (RMNCH and A). Concept of AYUSH in the National Health Mission are as follows:

- Overview of National Health Mission.
- Maternal Health Programme.
- Adolescent, Reproductive and Sexual Health Programme.
- Family Planning Programme.
- Routine Immunization.
- Programme Monitoring and Evaluation and Review.

8.4. *Skill Upgradation Training of AYUSH Doctor*

Panch Karma/Ksharsutra/Illaz-ul-Tadaveer are helpful for management of certain lifestyle disorders and they are important and integral constituent of AYUSH treatment. In order to provide these specialized Devices of AYUSH System at newly constructed wings at District Hospitals, ₹ 19.2 lakh has been proposed in the year 2014-15. Programme Implementation Plan for skill upgradation focused on Panchkarma/ Ksharsutra/Illaz-ul-Tadaveer.

8.5. *Skill Birth Attendant Training for AYUSH Doctors*

As per the direction of the Government of India, under mainstreaming of AYUSH only those AYUSH Doctors who are posted at delivery points where ANC and PNC are conducted are proposed to be trained as Skill Birth Attendant Training, thus a total of 28 days training programme is scheduled for one batch. There are six medical colleges in the State which are selected for the purpose of the Skill Birth Attendant Training and each of them conducts 6 batches and 5 AYUSH doctors per batch thus a total of 180 AYUSH Doctors ($6 \times 6 \times 5 = 180$) are proposed for the Skill Birth Attendant Training.

8.6. *Intra Uterine Contraceptive Device Insertion Training for AYUSH Doctors*

In order to meet the unmet need of spacing there is an urgent need to train the AYUSH Doctors for Intra Uterine Contraceptive Device Insertion Services. Therefore, a six days training of AYUSH Doctors (except Yoga and Naturopathy providers) to perform Intra Uterine Contraceptive Device insertions as per the curriculum being planned.

9. Referral Transport/Patient Transport System

Various referral transport and patient transport systems have been made available to ensure proper delivery of health services at the facility level.

9.1. *"108" Emergency Medical Transport Services*

The objective of Emergency Medical Transport Services is to provide immediate response during emergency with basic first aid to the patient and transport them to nearest government health facility. Operations of 133 Emergency Medical Transport Services Ambulance started on 14 September, 2012 and fleet strength is increased in phased manner and all the 988 Ambulances were made operational on 10th February, 2013. These Ambulances are operated by Private Service Provider GVK-EMRI through toll free "108" centralized call centre. All ambulances are GPS fitted.

The service is very popular in community. The ambulances are performing much above the norms and doing about 6 trips per ambulance per day. The service has provided services to about 22 lakh patients of which more than 50 per cent were related to pregnancy.

Looking at the performance of the services the State has to continue operation of these 988 ambulances in future also.

9.2. *"102" National Ambulance Service*

In view of the importance of access to ambulance services for reducing delays in access to health care for Janani Suraksha Yojana and Janani Shishu Suraksha Karyakram beneficiaries, State Health and Sanitation started operation of "102" National Ambulance Service on 17th January, 2014. The service is operated through Private Service Provider M/s GVK, Janani Suraksha Yojana toll free "102" centralized Call Centre and adopting National Ambulance Service Guidelines of Government of India. These ambulances are used for transportation of beneficiaries of Janani Suraksha Yojana and Janani Shishu Suraksha Karyakram scheme from home to facility, inter-facility transport and for the purpose of drop back.

Target for Janani Suraksha Yojana for year 2014-15 in State is around 25,00,000. As per the JSY target total anticipatory trips required will be 62,50,000 @ ₹ 2.5 Trip per JSY beneficiaries as it includes bringing of JSY beneficiaries and neonates and their drop back as well as interfaculty referral. The trip cost as per agreement between GVK-EMRI Janani Shishu Suraksha Karyakram and state of U.P. is ₹ 360 per trip with annual increment of 10 per cent every year.

9.3. *Advanced Life Support Ambulance*

Government of Uttar Pradesh is operating 988 Ambulances under 108 EMTS (for Medical Emergencies). All the Ambulances are operational through Private Service Provider selected through transparent tender process and working as per the agreement signed with the State.

The patients are transported through these ambulances from site of emergency to the nearest health facility and in case of further requirement up to district level hospitals. In most of the district level hospitals only secondary level of health care is available. In case of need for tertiary level care the hospitals are in lack of Advance Life Support Ambulances Service. There are 14 Government Medical Colleges functional in the State where tertiary care facilities are available.

There is need of Advanced Life Support Ambulance for transportation of critically ill patients. Keeping norms of one Advanced Life Support Ambulance will be required in the State. The Ambulance will be equipped with equipments (cardiac monitor, defibrillator, etc.) and having trained manpower to handle critical patient.

9.4. *Paediatric Ambulance for Sick New Born Care Unit*

There are 25 Sick New Born Care Units functional in the State. The State has fleet of 108 ambulances as well as 102 Ambulances but both these services have basic life support Ambulance and do not have the capacity to provide care to critically ill infants and children. Advanced Life Support Ambulances are proposed in year 2014-15 but it will be more useful to have Paediatric Ambulance having equipments and trained manpower to handle critical paediatric emergencies, operation of 25 Paediatric Ambulance linked to Sick New Born Care Units is proposed to save lives of critically ill children and bringing down the Infant Mortality Rate.

9.5. *Monitoring Cell for Ambulance Services*

The fleet of 1972 Ambulance under "102" National Ambulance Service '988' Ambulance under Emergency Medical Transport Services is very large and covers all the 75 Districts of Uttar Pradesh. The service is operational through private service provider and rigorous monitoring and supervision is required to maintain quality of services Moreover, Department does not have the technical capacity to supervise and monitor it.

In order to provide quality care to the people of that establishment of monitoring and evaluation cell at the State Level has been proposed. The cell will be responsible to carry out data analysis. Verification of reports, suggestive measures for improvements of services, etc. on regular basis and will report the authorities of the concerned departments.

9.6. *Third Party Concurrent Evaluation of Ambulance Services*

Unbiased observations by third party is required for transparent assessment of any services. In accordance of above state is proposing concurrent third party evaluation of "102" National Ambulance Service and "108" Emergency Medical Transport Services for effective implementation of the scheme and corrective measures. The third party selection will be done either through transport open tender process or among firms empanelled with Government of India for such activities.

10. Bio-Medical Waste Management

Bio-Medical Waste must be properly managed and disposed of to protect the environment, general public and workers, especially health care and sanitation. Workers, who are at risk of exposure to bio-medical wastes and occupational hazards. Steps in the management of bio-medical waste include generation, accumulation, handling and storage, transportation, treatment and disposal.

Disposal occurs off-site at a location that is different from the site of generation. Treatment may occur off-site or on-site. Off-site treatment and disposal service (also called a truck service) whose employees are trained to collect and haul away bio-medical waste in special containers (usually Cardboard Boxes, or reusable plastic bins) for treatment at a facility designed to handle bio-medical waste.

❑ *Cleaning, Washing, House Keeping and Laundry*

Environment cleaning is very important part of infection prevention control in a health facility, more important of cleaning, washing, Housekeeping and Laundry in Hospital and Health Facility Units.

11. Adherence and Cure Rates of Tuberculosis using Technology Enabled Monitoring and Supervision

A critical challenge facing Tuberculosis control programme is to ensure that patient adhere to the full course of treatment. Non-adherence not only jeopardizes a patient's treatment outcome, but also leads to the emergence of drug resistant strains, which are increasing threat to global public health, while directly observed therapy, short course (DOTs) has greatly boosted adherence rates in Uttar Pradesh, there remains many challenges to measuring patient adherence and ensuring that it satisfies expectation.

In the public programme it is often difficult for every dose to be observed due to patients, travel transportation expenses missed work opportunities and other factors. In the private sector patients often default due to lack of awareness counselling and the financial burden of buying medication.

❑ *Reasons for Poor Adherence*

The existing mechanism of check patients 'adherence' to treatment is highly manual and relies on maintaining data on paper based files. The existing tracking for medication is supposed to be done through manual entering of information on scheduled chart in the treatment card maintained for each patient. The existing process also says that a new patient is to be registered on a TB Register file within a month of the initiation of the Treatment and Information from Treatment Card to be transferred to the Register monthly. The basic nature of data is non-electronic form leads to restrictions of delays in the information flow from DOTs providers. The delay in information flow is a major bottleneck to effective implementation of current supervision and monitor strategy. It is good to maintain records in electronic form for record keeping and later analysis but it is not at all useful for real time patient treatment adherence tracking.

❑ *Technology*

A low cost approach using the most widely used contemporary technology of cell phones is used for monitoring and improving T.B. Medication adherence. A research software system is developed to track and monitor the patients' adherence to treatment schedule. The patients dose intake information is entered into software based on the proposed SMS and missed Call mechanism.

As soon as new patient is registered an electronic software account of that patient adherence, research software system enables a wide range of reminders and follow ups to improve adherence behaviour. DOTs providers and other designated persons receive SMS notifications of missed doses, enabling timely counselling and follow-up. Programme Research Managers and their designated persons can also visualize the real time adherence records *via* a website.

12. Immunization

The immunization programme is the cornerstone of public health, world-over. Vaccination was practiced in India since early 1900s, especially against small pox, in late 1940s. In 1962 Bacillus Calmette-Guerin (BCG) inoculation was included in the National Tuberculosis Control Programme. A formal programme under the name of Expanded Programme of Immunization was launched in 1978. This gained momentum in 1985 under Universal Immunization Programme and it was merged in Child Survival and Safe Motherhood Programme in 1992-93. Since, 1997 immunization activities are an important component of Reproductive and Child Health (RCH) Programme. A National Technical Advisory Group on Immunization was set-up in 2003 and a Midterm Strategic Plan (MTSP) developed in 2004 from April 2005, immunization is an important component of Reproductive and Child Health-II under National Rural Health Mission Programme.

13. National Iodine Deficiency Disorder Control Programme

Iodine Deficiency Disorder is one of the major public health problems in India with around 200 million people estimated to be at risk. Uttar Pradesh with a population of 190 million is known to Iodine Deficiency Disorders endemic and no district in the State is reported to be free from Iodine Deficiency Disorders.

Iodine Deficiency can be prevented by using salt that has been forfeited with Iodine. Iodine Deficiency is particularly damaging during early pregnancy as it retards foetal brain development resulting in a range of intellectual motor and hearing deficits. Following disorders are associated with Iodine Deficiency:

- Goirte, Retarded Mental and Physical Development.
- Cretinism in Children.
- Repeated abortion and still birth.
- Poor School Performance.

❑ *Magnitude of the Problem in Uttar Pradesh*

As per the National Family Health Survey-3 in Uttar Pradesh while 77 per cent of households are using iodized salt, only 36 per cent households use adequately iodized salt. Furthermore 23 per cent of the population in the State is using non-iodized salt. The coverage Evaluation Survey of 2009 shows the coverage with adequately iodized salt 42.5 per cent.

National Iodized Deficiency Disorder Control Programme focuses on the following:

- Survey and Resurvey every 5 years to know prevalence rate.
- Supply of only Iodized Salt for human consumption (salt having 15 p.p.m. Iodine Salt at Consumer level).
- Creating demand for iodized salt especially in rural area.
- Information, Education, Communication and Health Education.

The goals on National Iodine Deficiency Disorders Control Programme are as follows:

- To bring down total goiter rate less than 10 per cent.
- To ensure 90 per cent households consume Iodized Salt (15 p.p.m. Iodine at Consumer level).
- Presently 77 per cent households are consuming Iodized Salt only 36 per cent households use adequately iodized salt.
- Supply of Iodized Salt through Public Distribution System.

In order to steer National Iodine Deficiency Disorder Control Programme (NIDDCP) in the State in forward direction and understand the progress made in NIDDCP in Uttar Pradesh there is a need to undertake following additional activities —

(i) Organizing regular activities under NIDDCP.
(ii) Organizing State Level review meeting.
(iii) Undertake Iodine Deficiency Disorder Survey across the State.
(iv) Celebration of Iodine Deficiency Disorder Day at District Level.

14. Integrated Disease Surveillance Programme

Integrated Disease Surveillance Programme started in 2004 with the support from World Bank to improve and integrate Disease Surveillance in pursuance of recommendation by high powered committee of secretaries on Environmental Sanitation.

During 2007 Avian Influenza Outbreak, human and animal components were added along with additional budget. Assumption of the programme is as follows:

- Units have adequate skills, resource and authority to respond.
- Communication and private sector have adequate incentive.
- Good quality of lab information is available in timely manner and integrated into surveillance system.

But these were not found to be fully correct so the objectives could not be achieved as well as found utilization was low. In January 2009 after detailed analysis of the situation, World Bank agreed to restructure the project and extend it for 2 years focusing on what can be achieved by the end of two years. Thus, after Project Development objectives were revised —

- To improve the information available to the Government Health Services and Private Health Care providers on a set of high priority diseases and risk factors, so as to improve the response towards them.
- To establish a decentralized State based system of surveillance for disease to ensure timely and effective health response towards health challenges at various levels.
- To put greater emphasis on building the links between the collection and analysis of information and ground intervention by public or private sectors.

❑ *Status of the Programme in the Year 2013-14*

I. ***Activities***

1. Integrated Disease Surveillance Programme Collectors receive information from all the districts and send weekly on IDSP portal on line to state headquarters.
2. Data Cell and Training Cell are present in all the Districts.
3. Micro-Biologists, Data Managers are working in the regional lab established in Health Directorate, Swasthya Bhawan, Lucknow.

4. Epidemiologists posted at District level are actively working whenever there is any kind of outbreak or are warning signal of epidemic in their respective area.
5. Data Managers appointed in the District are doing collection, collation, combination and dissemination of data.
6. IDSP has played a remarkable role in prevention and treatment of Swine Flu.
7. IDSP plays an important role in monitoring, testing and evaluating in case of an outbreak.
8. Monthly compiled report of communicable and non-communicable diseases from all the districts are regularly sent to the State Headquarters.
9. Online data reporting is being done from all districts.
10. Swine Flue vaccination complete in all the districts in two phases.

II. *Training*

(a) Training of Trainer of all District Surveillance Officers had been completed.

(b) Batches of District Surveillances officer have undergone Field Epidemiological Training Programme.

(c) Micro-biologist posted at regional lab, Headquarters has been given induction training at J-Medical College, Pune.

(d) Data Manager posted at State Surveillance Unit has undergone TOT Training at NCDC, New Delhi.

(e) Training of District Rapid Response Team Members have been done by Government of India.

(f) All currently posted Epidemiologists have undergone Training of Trainers by Government of India.

III. *Laboratory Components*

State Priority Laboratory (Regional Lab at State Headquarters and District Hospital Lab Ghaziabad):

(i) No procurement has been done for priority labs under IDSP as the existing infrastructure is well furnished.

(ii) Tests done stool culture for Cholera, ELISA for Dengue, Chikungunya, J.E., Malaria, Measles, Hepatitis A&E and Water Bacteriology.

15. National Vector-Borne Disease Control Programme

Vector-borne diseases are prevalent in Sultanpur District and prioritized as high risk district. District has also been Categorised as priority district for AES/JE, Malaria, Kala Azar and Dengue diseases. The AES/JE are the major public health problem in Sultanpur District and Uttar Pradesh.

The disease situation of the National Vector-Borne Disease of the Uttar Pradesh has been illustrated in Table 3.4.

It has been noted that Malaria, Dengue, Chikungunya, Filaria, Kala-Azar, AES/JE and vector-borne diseases are prevalent in Sultanpur District.

15.1. *Malaria*

ABER > 10 per cent per thousand population (during 12th FY Plan) the objective is to bring down annual incidence of Malaria cases to less than 1 per 1,000 population at National Level by 2017 and its monitoring at District Level. The detailed informations related to Malaria Vector-Borne Disease over the year has been mentioned in Table 3.5.

❑ *General Vector Control Strategy*

- Main strategy for control of vector-borne disease is vector management.
- To control condition promoting mosquito breeding.
- One week day — Saturday to be made dry day (emptying overhead tanks, cooler, defrost pans and plant pots, etc.).
- Larvicide in open drains with stagnant water.
- Two rounds of IRS NDT — 50 per cent and three rounds of Malathion 25 per cent wdp in High Risk Districts.
- Spray wages from state resource for technical skilled labours.
- Forging by malathion technical at dawn and dusk.
- To control outdoor mosquitoes density in village affected with JE/AES (Larvicidal activity in morning).

15.2. *Lymphatic Filariasis*

Elimination of Lymphatic Filariasis by 2015. To achieve elimination, the micro-filaria rate in all the endemic districts should be less than 1 per cent to interrupt the transmission. The details of the Lymphatic Filariasis has been mentioned in Table 3.6.

Table 3.4: Disease Situation in Uttar Pradesh

Year	*Malaria*			*Filaria*		*J.E./A.E.S.*		*Dengue*		*Kala Azar*		*Chikun Gunia*
	Positive	*P.F.*	*Death*	*Diseased*	*M.F.*	*Cases*	*Death*	*Cases*	*Death*	*Cases*	*Death*	*Suspected*
2006	105302	3149	0	7613	619	5581	1593	121	4	68	2	0
2007	91566	3875	0	5738	725	2073	476	617	14	83	0	0
2008	81580	1989	0	5791	437	2675	577	130	2	69	1	4
2009	93383	2310	0	5134	477	2730	468	51	2	26	0	0
2010	54488	660	0	2815	452	3073	556	161	2	17	1	0
2011	64468	1389	0	2291	412	3548	498	960	8	14	0	5
2012	56829	1857	0	2109	364	3490	579	155	5	11	1	0
2013	47400	740	0	1969	322	3484	557	369	4	5	0	13
2014	48112	581	0	2006	327	3096	609	1414	5	11	1	1

Table 3.5: Malaria

Year	*Population (lakhs)*	*BSC*	*BSE*	*Total Malaria Positive*	*P.F. Cases*	*P.F. %*	*ABER*	*SPR*	*API*	*SFR*	*Death*
2005	1671.2	4229061	4223366	105302	3149	2.99	2.53	2.49	0.63	0.07	0
2006	1671.2	3882984	3872475	91566	1875	2.04	2.33	2.35	0.54	0.05	0
2007	1744.2	3527918	3524829	81580	1989	2.56	2.02	2.35	0.47	0.06	0
2008	1744.2	4158441	4150306	93383	2310	2.47	2.38	2.25	0.54	0.06	0
2009	1744.2	4171162	4171162	54488	660	1.21	2.38	1.31	0.31	0.02	0
2010	1880.1	4040902	4040902	67468	1389	2.06	2.32	1.67	0.39	0.03	0
2011	1998.8	4142930	4142930	56829	1857	3.27	2.37	1.37	0.33	0.04	0
2012	2039.7	3904034	3904034	47400	740	1.53	2.24	1.19	0.27	0.02	0
2013	2039.7	4211429	4211429	48112	581	1.12	2.06	1.14	0.27	0.01	0

Notes: BSE — Blood Slides Examined. API — Annual Parasite Index (Malaria Case per thousand population).
ANER — Annual Blood Slides Examination Rate %. PF — Plasmodium Falciparum Positive Case per cent of Total Malaria Cases.
SPR — Slides Positivity Rate %. SFR — Slides Falciparum Rate.

Table 3.6: Lymphatic Filariasis

Sl.No.	*Year*	*Cases*	*Mf Positive*
1.	2007	5791	637
2.	2008	5134	477
3.	2009	2815	452
4.	2010	2291	412
5.	2011	2109	364
6.	2012	1969	322
7.	2013	2006	327

❑ *Specific Constrains for Implementation of Programme*

- Apart from disability, management is great challenge to remove the social stigma from the population suffering from disease. No method for detecting parasite at early stage of infection. Resources are inadequate and insufficient due to 29 Filaria Units and 2 Filaria clinics.
- MDA is expected to be successful — Interest in Health Education and Inter-sectoral Cooperation is needed.
- Under Filaria Control Programme MDA Programme is conducted every year on proposed tentative date of 11th November. In the year 2011-12 because of the partial release of funds against the total allocation, the MDA Programme was conducted in only 14 Districts and in 2012-13 due to delay in supply of DEC 100 mg, MDA was observed in February/ March 2013 in four rounds. This year in 2013-14 MDA in observed in three rounds (January, February and March 2014).

❑ *Objective*

- To progressively reduce and ultimately interrupt the transmission of Lymphatic Filariasis.
- To augment the disability alleviation programme to reduce the suffering of affected person through appropriate home based Morbidity Management and Hydrocoelectomy.

15.3. *Dengue and Chikungunya*

Important objectives of the programme are as follows:

- To ensure the incidence of Dengue and effective control on Chikangunya morbidity.
- Strengthening the state-wise surveillance mechanism for Dengue and Chikungunya.

Status of Dengue and Chikungunya deaths over the years have been depicted in Table 3.7.

Table 3.7: Dengue and Chikungunya

Year	*Dengue Cases*	*Deaths*	*Chikungunya*	*Deaths*
2008	51	2	0	0
2009	161	2	0	0
2010	960	8	5	0
2011	155	5	0	0
2012	369	4	13	0
2013	1414	5	1	0

❑ *Situational Analysis*

Districts which are highly affected by the Dengue are the urban areas and the activities to be performed and logistics with respective cost or as below should be reflected.

❑ *Effective Disease Control and Treatment*

Strategies and innovations for effective disease control and treatment, epidemiological surveillance and disease management activities have been initiated at the facilities level.

❑ *Microscopic Centre*

Strengthening the existing surveillance, all microscopic centres are to be made functioninal.

❑ *Active Surveillance*

Auxiliary Nurse Midwife/Multi-Purpose Workers should make blood slides for malaria regularly.

❑ *ASHAs*

Involvement of ASHAs for active surveillance collection of ₹ 15 to ASHA for each blood slide. If the ASHAs actively participate for giving radical treatment to the patient, per patient ₹ 75 will be paid in remote areas, ASHAs and ANMs/ MPWs to be provided RDT kits.

❑ *Case Management*

- All malaria positive patients should get radical treatment as earliest as possible.
- Epidemic preparedness and rapid response team.
- Involvement of Private Providers.

❑ *Integrated Vector Management*

- Effective Entomological Surveillance.
- Source reduction using minor engineering method.
- Environment Control Biological and Larvivorous Fish.
- Larvicides (Bio-Larvicides) and Larvicide (Chemical).
- Timely and good quality of IRS is important and implemented with sound technical skill.
- Operational Research.

❑ *Inter-Sectoral Coordination*

Optimal utilization of local Panchayati Raj Institutions especially village Health Nutrition and Sanitation Committee, to play a crucial role in National Vector-Borne Disease Control Programme.

High risk areas for Vector-Borne Disease are mainly rural area and urban slums — close coordination as well as supervision and monitoring of village Health Nutrition and Sanitation Committee/ local institutions will improve Community ownership especially in the area of sanitation and reduction of vector breeding site.

❑ *Capacity Building*

Training of health workers and supervisors in making solution of insecticides and in using spray pumps and fogging machines by District Malaria Officer and the Medical Officer should be well conversed with the equipments and techniques.

Intensification of the entomological surveillance, vector control strategies including community involvement and school education for elimination vector breeding for transmission risk reduction and prevention of occurrence outbreak.

As per guidelines of Government of India, State of Uttar Pradesh has established 25 sentinel surveillance Hospitals with laboratory Facilities, for enhancing the Dengue facility in the State. For back up support these institutes were linked with SGPGI, Lucknow which has been identified as one of the Apex Referral Laboratories in the State and Advanced diagnostic facility.

❑ *Chikungunya*

Chikungunya fever is a viral disease caused by an arbovirus of the Family TONG AVIRIDAE and transmitted by Aedes Aegypti mosquito.

It is debilitating, but, non-fatal illness occurs principally during rainy season.

The disease resembles dengue fever and is characterized by severe sometimes persistent, joint pain (arthritis) as well as fever and rash. It is rarely life threatening, Chikungunya is diagnosed by Blood Test (ELISA). Since, the clinical appearance of both the Dengue and Chikungunya is similar. Laboratory confirmation is important.

15.4. *Kala-Azar*

The Kala-Azar is targeted for elimination by 2015. The Elimination is to bring down the number of Kala-Azar cases less than 1 per 10,000 population at Block level.

❑ *Situational Analysis*

Kala-Azar is endemic in the six districts of Eastern Uttar Pradesh bordering Bihar State, namely Kushi Nagar, Deoria, Ballia, Varanasi, Ghazipur and Sant Ravi Das Nagar (Bhadohi). The principles of elimination are anti-adult measures and complete treatment of patient.

The situational analysis of Kala-Azar yearwise has been illustrated in Table 3.8.

Table 3.8: Situation of Kala-Azar (Year-wise)

Year	*Cases*	*Deaths*
2007	69	1
2008	26	0
2009	17	1
2010	14	0
2011	11	1
2012	5	0
2013	11	1

15.5. *Acute Encephalitis Syndrome/Japanese Encephalitis*

Acute Encephalitis Syndrome and Japanese Encephalitis are endemic and mainly observed in Uttar Pradesh of which later is Vector-Borne Disease transmitted by culex vishunil gp mosquitoes. At intervals the disease assumed epidemic form in the year 2005, the disease affected 34 districts of Uttar Pradesh. With concrete preventive and curative efforts, the Department has been able to contain the disease to only 18 Districts in 2011 and 16 Districts in 2012. In the year 2013, 28 Districts of Uttar Pradesh have been affected by this disease.

The situational analysis of Kala-Azar in the affected districts of Eastern Uttar Pradesh has been mentioned in Table 3.9.

Table 3.9: Situation of Kala-Azar in the Affected Districts

Sl. No.	*District*	*Total PHC*	*Kala-Azar Affected*		
			PHCs/ Block	*Village*	*Name of PHCs*
1.	Deoria	15	1	1	Bankata
2.	Kushi Nagar	14	3	3	Kasya, Khawan and Nagwa Angina
3.	Ballia	17	2	2	Murli Chhapara and Dubhar
4.	Varanasi	8	4	4	Cholapur, Chiraigaon, Horruhua Kashi Vidya Peeth
5.	Ghazipur	16	1	1	Goru
6.	St. Ravi Das Nagar	5	1	1	Bhadohi
	Total	75	12	12	

The details of Kala-Azar affected districts during the year 2012 has been illustrated in Table 3.10.

Table 3.10: Details of Kala-Azar Affected Districts (2012)

Sl. No.	*District*	*Total PHC*	*Kala-Azar Affected*		
			PHCs/ Block	*Village*	*Name of PHCs*
1.	Deoria	15	1	1	Bankata
2.	Ghazipur	16	1	1	Barathaur
	Total	31	2	2	

During 2013 the geographical area Health and Sanitation increased to 28 Districts which includes Sultanpur. However, the magnitude of the disease has declined but still it is a challenge to the Department to contain the disease in Basti, Gorakhpur and Azamgarh Divisions and District of Lakhimpur in Lucknow Division. Approximately, 90 per cent of cases are reported from rural and periurban areas of the Districts. The disease incidence has been brought down to considerable level as it is evident from Table 3.11.

For Prevention and Control of disease Government has identified 20 Districts of Uttar Pradesh for intensified intervention measures, but during 2013 the disease spread to larger geographical area and as such 10 more districts including Sultanpur has also been reported disease

cases which also require intervention measures, accordingly steps required area also incorporated in the programme implementation Plan.

Table 3.11: Acute Encephalitis Syndrome/Japanese Encephalitis

Year	*No. of Affected Districts*	*RES*		*JE*	
		Cases	*Deaths*	*Cases*	*Deaths*
2005	34	5581	1593	1042	304
2006	22	2075	476	170	49
2007	24	2575	577	235	29
2008	23	2730	483	168	36
2009	26	3061	555	328	50
2010	20	3548	498	344	59
2011	18	3490	583	224	27
2012	16	3484	557	139	53
2013	28	3069	281	281	47

Source: State Programme Management Unit, National Rural Health Mission, Lucknow.

❑ *Specific Constraints for Programme Implementation*

The transmission cycle of Japanese Encephalitis is of complex nature.

Disease affected districts mainly practice paddy cultivation as means of livelihood due to which exophilic and exophagic vector mosquito species of the disease of Anti vector control operations are very difficult. Larviorous fish hatcheries and rearing not properly managed by local people.

- The Ardied birds, which are reservoir of JE virus, are also prevalent in the area.
- The pigs are also means of livelihood of poor communities and these pigs act as amplifying host. Hon'ble High Court of Uttar Pradesh has instructed to remove piggeries from human habitation. Concerned department is trying to comply with the orders of the Hon'ble High Court.
- Moreover, veterinary based sero-surveillance of reservoir as well as amplifying host is lacking which can be definite early warning signal for JE.
- Inadequate human resource at different levels.
- Delayed treatment seeking approach of community at treatment centres, i.e. hospitals, CHCs and PHCs as they directly approach BRD Medical College, Gorakhpur on severity of the cases.
- Shortage of vehicles required for mobility of staff for undertaking

intervention measures, surveillance, monitoring, supervision, etc.

- Repeated training/reorientation training of the medical officer and the staff of CHC/PHC as deployment of new staff after transfer.
- Lack of health consciousness pertaining to personal hygiene and sanitation in and around human habitation.

15.6. *Strategies and Innovations*

❑ *Disease Surveillance*

The surveillance staff for any disease at periphery level is inadequate leading to improper reporting of the AES/JE cases. At present ASHAs are working at every village (grassroots level) who can early track the patients of AES/JE in endemic areas with symptoms of fever, headache and altered sensorium (Encephalopathy). The ASHA/AWW will convince the family members of the tracked patients to contact the nearby treatment centres for early treatment of the patient. They will be required to make a list of the early patients daily and will submit it to the respective PHC of the area. If the case motivated/assisted case declared to be of JE/AES, then the concerned ASHA shall be entitled for honorarium worth ₹ 300 per case (Fever tracking of AES/JE cases).

District hospitals needs to be strengthened for surveillance. AES/JE ward already identified have been expanded and upgraded. There is a need to set-up an ICU, in each district hospital out of which 12 districts have been granted and released funds from Government of India and remaining 8 districts (Balrampur, Shrawasti, Ballia, Mau, Hardoi, Sitapur, Kanpur Dehat and Saharanpur) will be provided funds for ICU set-up. In the year 2014-15, 3 ICUs establishment has been proposed in the PIP at current price index. Drugs and other medicines are required to be procured by the State. For running of already established ICUs, 10 Medical Officers and 10 Staff Nurses from each district have been proposed for training in operation and critical care management.

❑ *Diagnosis*

Early Diagnosis and prompt treatment will be ensured by strengthening the diagnostic facilities in 20 Sentinel labs of highly sensitive districts and HQ Lab., each of which is equipped with one ELISA reader, deep freezers, and supplementary material. However, Pathologists and

Technicians will be reoriented for latest advancements in the techniques, which will be trained at State APEX Lab, Lucknow. Recurring funds need to be made available to these Labs and capacity building of the technicians/pathologists is reflected in the present PIP.

❑ *Treatment/Case Management*

Treatment/Case management facilities including availability of adequate and ample stock of drugs and other medicines at different hospitals and treatment centres which will have proper legible and self-explanatory treatment/Case management schedule of AES/JE cases to be displayed inwards and clinician chambers and accordingly followed.

❑ *Entomological Surveillance of Japanese Encephalitis*

Vector Surveillance is an important component of AES/JE programme strategy. Though there is no direct relationship of vector density with impending outbreak of JE, it is needless to mention that vector densities are required to be reduced significantly for avoiding outbreak situations. To monitor the entomological parameters, one Consultant/Entomologist with sufficient background of knowledge and experience will be engaged/ utilized for collecting and analyzing different related parameters.

❑ *Vector Control for Japanese Encephalitis*

Fortnightly fogging of Malathion by fogging machine in the villages reporting JE cases for last 2-3 years during transmission period. Each district with vehicle mounted large thermal fogging machine and one small portable thermal fogging machine to each PHC have been provided but 11 districts identified still require vehicle mounted fogging machine for which the proposal has been included in the present PIP. In the PIP guideline it is stated to procure 3 MT Malathion Technical which in turn will require 15,200 litre diesel for 1 MT quantity. Accordingly, the recurring expenditure to be incurred on fogging machine procurement/ arrangement and operational expenses are proposed in the PIP in relevant FMR code.

The agriculture department will be involved in Vector control by enhancing its capacity building in *Integrated Pest Management* (IPM) to the tune of Integrated Pest and Vector Management (IPVM),

The fisheries department particularly in the JE affected districts will study and identify local indigenous mosquito Larvivorous fishes and promote their hatcheries to cater among the aquatic based crop-harvesting farmers and the health department will do their regular monitoring. The impact of already released Gumbushia fish in Gorakhpur and Basti Divisions shall be monitored in regular intervals. The recurring expenditure towards this is proposed in the PIP in relevant FMR code.

❑ *Training of Medical Officers*

Medical Officers of JE/AAES affected districts, Health Education Officer posted at CHC will be trained for dissemination of information to the community for AES/JE Prevention and Control.

❑ *Information, Education and Communication/Behaviour Change Communication*

AES cases excluding JE cases make the major proportion of morbidity and mortality mainly in four divisions of the Eastern UP.

Community will be sensitized through different types of BCC activities such as electronic (Radio, TV, FM, etc.) and Print media as well as Railway and Bus tickets bearing key messages for prevention of the disease. Printed material to be made available through group meeting and inter-personal communication in order to prevent contraction of the disease and the prototype health education material will be developed and communicated to the affected districts.

❑ *Operational Research*

Impact assessment of IEC/BCC activities on the community *vis-à-vis* change in treatment seeking behaviour, trend of disease incidence and mortality by medical institutions/independent agencies/IMGOs in 11 highly affected districts @ ₹ 2,00,000 per District (for HR, mobility and contingent expenditures, etc.).

❑ *Supervision and Monitoring*

For effective monitoring and the supervision of the prevention and control activities at least one vehicle for transmission period of 6 months is proposed in the PIP more over computer with accessories, State and district consultants have also been proposed. Weekly and fortnightly review meeting of JE/AES situation will be conducted at ground zero. The activity and mobilization of District Malaria/VBD Officer and other paramedical personnel at district level will be ensured.

Regular supervisory and analytical trips from State and Divisional Headquarters should be ensured.

❑ *Vaccination*

Vaccination with SA-14-14-2 vaccine to the children of 1-15 years age group was carried out in all 34 districts in phases from 2006 to 2009 which had high response and acceptance in the community but keeping in view the independent assessment, the high level experts and officials decided to undertake another round of vaccination in highly JE sensitive districts of Gorakhpur and Basti division in 2010, accordingly the good coverage of vaccination attributed decline in JE cases considerably. Further, it is stated that JE vaccination has been included in UIP since 2011 and two doses of JE vaccine at the age of 9 month and 16-20 month are being administered, but the occurrence of AES cases still needs attention for its containment.

16. National Leprosy Eradication Programme

Important objectives of the National Leprosy Eradication Programme are as follows:

- Elimination of Leprosy, i.e. prevalence of less than 1 case per 10,000 population in all the Districts.
- Strengthen Disability Prevention and Medical Rehabilitation of persons affected by Leprosy.
- Reduction in the level of stigma associated with Leprosy.

The performance under National Leprosy Eradication Programme has been illustrated in Table 3.12.

Table 3.12: Performance under National Leprosy Eradication Programme

Sl.No.	*Indicators*	*2009-10*	*2010-11*	*2011-12*	*2012-13*	*2013-14*
1.	No. of New Cases Detected (ANCDR/100,000)	27473 (13.4)	25509 (12.52)	24530 (12.3)	24222 (11.0)	22565 (10.90)
2.	No. of Cases on Record at Year End (PR/10,000)	16484 (0.81)	15719 (0.77)	13939 (0.68)	14865 (0.72)	14308 (0.69)
3.	No. of Grade II Disability Among New Cases (%)	594 (2.16)	645 (2.53)	671 (2.74)	703 (2.90)	722 (3.20)
4.	Treatment Completion Rate	92.81	93.1	94.78	93.17	U. Comp
5.	Reconstructive Surgery Conducted	405	190	295	311	268

The following eight results are proposed to be achieved at the end of the 12th Plan Period, i.e. by March 2017:

1. Improved early case detection.
2. Improved case management.
3. Stigma reduced.
4. Development of leprosy expertise sustained.
5. Research supported evidence based programme practice.
6. Monitoring, supervision and evaluation system improved.
7. Increased participation of persons affected by leprosy in society.
8. Programme management ensured.

17. Non-Communicable Disease including Injury and Trauma

The Non-Communicable diseases include National Programme for Control of Blindness, National Mental Health Programme, National Programme for the Health Care of the Elderly, National Programme for Control of Deafness, National Tobacco Control Programme, National Programme for Control of Cancer, Diabetes, the National Disease Control Programme have been launched under National Rural Health Mission at the facility level.

17.1. *National Programme for Control of Blindness*

India was the first country to launch the National Programme for Control of Blindness in 1976. An important goal of the programme was to reduce the Prevention of Blindness. Out of the total estimate 45 million blind people (3/60) in the world, 7 million are in India and 1.85 million in Uttar Pradesh. This is due to the large population base and increased life expectancy.

Every year 0.3 per cent of the population, which means about 5.5 lakh blind persons are added to the total blind population. Out of 5.5 lakh total blind 3.5 lakh become blind every year due to cataract.

As the number of cataract patients is reducing because of clearance of backlog, blindness due to degenerative diseases like diabetes and glaucoma and injuries related corneal opacities are increasing. The programme has to tackle emerging challenges.

It has been recorded that the prevalence rate of blindness in Uttar Pradesh is 1.0 per cent. The goal of the programme is to reduce prevalent rate of blindness to 0.3 per cent by the end of year 2020.

❑ *Activities to Achieve the Goal*

- Cataract surgery.
- School Eye Screening.

- Eye banking for keratoplasty to treat corneal blindness.
- Management of disease other than cataracts (diabetic Retinopathy, Glaucoma management Laser Techniques, Corneal Transplantation Vitreo relinal Surgery) and treatment of child blindness.

1. *Cataract Operation*

The target for cataract operation in the year 2014-15 is 11.36 lakh out of which 50 per cent will be operated in Hospital owned by Government/ NGO Sector (5.68 lakh) and 50 per cent will be operated in private sector hospitals (5.68 lakh). As Government of India provides ₹ 450 for an operation in Government and ₹ 1,000 for operation in NGO owned hospital, to total requirement is (450 × 284000 Cataract operations = ₹ 1,278.00 lakh in Government Sector) and ₹ 1,000 × 2,84,000 cataract operations = ₹ 2,840.0 lakh in NGO Sector. The component-wise progress of the programme is illustrated in Table 3.13.

Table 3.13: Component-wise Progress of the Programme

Sl. No.	*Intervention*	*Targets*	*Achieve-ments Till February 14*	*Expected Achievement by March 14*	*Remarks*
1.	Cataract Operation	11,36,000	6,12,546	8,75,000 lakh	◆ Delayed procedural exercise for purchase of IDL ◆ The targets will be achieved till March as most of the cases are operated in winters
2.	School Eye Screening	50,00,000	24,16,602	30,00,000	◆ Expecting better results than targeted as the activity has been linked up with School Health Scheme (Ashirvad)
3.	Free Spectacles for poor Children	1,50,000	75,797	1,00,000	◆ Less availability of manpower for screening of school children
4.	Corneal Collection	1,500	719	1,500	◆ Due to lack of public awareness
5.	Vision Centre Eye	100	0	0	◆ Grant could not be recorded from GoI
6.	Eye donation Centre	5	0	0	◆ After full functioning of eye banks it will take off gradually ◆ Lack of response from the field

The Government of Uttar Pradesh is also proposing to increase this amount to ₹ 1,000 for an operation in Government sector too, so that the quality eye services like lenses, proper medicines and better transportation on services can be provided.

2. *School Eye Screening*

It is estimated that 5.7 per cent of School going children aged 8-14 years have problems with their eyesight affecting their participation and learning at school. This can be corrected by a pair of spectacles.

All school going children in the age group of 8-14 years are expected to undertake eye screening activities. It is proposed that this activity will be undertaken by ASHAs, MPW Male and primary school teachers trained by the purpose and optometrists under school health programme under NRHM. These workers will be trained for undertaking screening process and making referral for refraction to Block PHCs. District Health Society will supply the refractive glass to needy students.

❑ *Targets for 2014-15*

- Screening of 50 lakh children of aged 9-14 years.
- Free distribution of 2 lakh spectacles to poor children (one lakh and SES programme under National Programme for Control of Blindness and One lakh in School Health Programme under NRHM @ ₹ 200 each in year 2014-15.

❑ *Strategies to Achieve the Target of 2014-15*

- Training of ASHAs, MPWs and school teachers at Primary level.
- Suspected refractive error children also screened by contractual PMOAs under school health programme of NRHM and referred to PHC/CHC/NGO Hospitals/trained Optometrist for proper refraction and will provide free spectacles to poor children.
- Suspected refractive error children referred to PHC/CHC/NGO Hospitals/trained Optometrist for proper refraction and will provide free spectacles to poor children.
- Involvement of NGOs in Screening of Children having low Vision for non-school going children.
- Development of 75 vision centres at PHC/CHC level each in every 75 districts and in NGO/PVT sector with the equipment and furniture and fixture in the year 2014-15 so that in next 3 years all block health facilities will have a vision centre. The

concept of vision centre arises from fact that one time provision of equipments and supportive material hardly ever gets replaced resulting into non-functional facility.

- The training will be completed by June and screening programme by September 2014. School-wise report will be generated by ASHA depicting name of school, number of children screened, number of children with defective vision referred to PHC.
- Through local IEC all schools will have wall painting/writing in relation to eye screening programme.
- The training of ASHA for eye screening is already included in regular ASHA training programme by NRHM.

3. *Corneal Blindness*

The prevalence of corneal blindness is about 1 per cent of total blindness. There are 18,000 people in need of the corneal transplant. The lack of corneal donation and the functional institutions are major bottleneck to address corneal blindness.

❑ *Target for 2014-15*

- Target of 1,500 eye collection and 1,500 corneal transplantation in the year 2014-15 is targeted.
- Collection of donated eye providing Keratoplasty Services in all Medical Colleges, and registered eye banks. The total Number of Eye Banks available in U.P. are 23 and approximately 5 more will be added in 2014-15.

❑ *Strategies to Achieve the Targets*

- Primary Eye Care medicine will be available at Primary Health Centre/CHC level.
- 23 Eye Banks are already registered till 2014-15 and 5 eye banks will be registered in 2014-15.

4. *Disease Other than Cataract Surgeries*

The disease other than cataract surgeries included Diabetic Retinopathy, Glaucoma, Childhood Blindness, Vitreo Retinal Surgery, Laser Technique, Low visions Aids.

About 16 per cent of total blindness is due to diabetic glaucoma and other above mentioned diseases. Currently there is no mechanism to address this category of blind persons which is gradually increasing.

It is proposed to set-up screening clinic in every District Hospital and Medical Colleges. Equipment for diagnosis diabetes related problems by Government of Uttar Pradesh. Only indirect Ophthalmoscopes are required to undertake screening process for both disease — diabetic retinopathy and other posterior segment disorders.

❑ *Strategies to Achieve Target*

- All known diabetics to be examined by eye surgeon/ophthalmic assistant.
- Tonometry, fundoscopy and indirect ophthalmoscope will be done at weekly clinic at all district hospitals.
- Medical Management of diabetic retinopathy and surgical management of glaucoma at divisional level hospital.
- For surgical intervention patients referred to Tertiary centres (medical colleges and NGO hospitals) for diabetic retinopathy, glaucoma and other eye diseases.
- For operation of equipments optometrist should be trained at medical colleges by State Government.
- Eye surgeons to be trained in diabetic retinopathy and glaucoma by Central Government.

17.2. *National Mental Health Programme*

It is estimated that 6-7 per cent of general population suffers from mental disorders. Together these disorders account for 12 per cent of the global burden of disease (GBD) and an analysis of trends indicate this will increase to 15 per cent by 2020 (World Health Report, 2001). Most of them (> 90%) remain untreated. Poor awareness about symptoms of mental illness, myths and stigma related to it, lack of knowledge on the treatment availability and potential benefits of seeking treatment are important causes for the high treatment gap.

Apart from a large population suffering from mental illnesses, the well-being of rest of the population also needs to be ensured by increasing their resilience through mental health promotive components like life skills training and counselling services in schools, college counselling services, workplace stress management and suicide prevention services.

The Government of India has launched the National Mental Health Programme (NMHP) in 1982, keeping in view the heavy burden of mental illness in the community, and the absolute inadequacy of mental health care infrastructure in the country to deal with it.

❑ *Objectives*

1. To ensure availability and accessibility of minimum mental health care for all in the foreseeable future, particularly to the most vulnerable sections of the population.
2. To encourage mental health knowledge and skills in general health care and social development.
3. To promote community participation in mental health service development and to stimulate self-help in the community.
4. To increase awareness about mental illness through change of attitude and public education.

❑ *Strategies*

1. Integration of mental health with primary health care through the NMHP.
2. Provision of tertiary care institutions for treatment of mental disorders.
3. Eradicating stigmatization of mentally ill patients and protecting their rights through regulatory institutions like the Central Mental Health Authority, and State Mental Health Authority.

❑ *Mental Health Care*

1. The mental morbidity requires priority in mental health treatment.
2. Primary health care at village and sub-centre level.
3. At Primary Health Centre level.
4. At the District Hospital level.
5. Mental Hospital and Teaching Psychiatric Units.

As envisaged in National Health Policy 2002 and following globally accepted trend of community care of mentally ill, it is proposed to extend DMHP to 565 more districts. Under the scheme, support will be provided to districts to implement DMHP to provide basic mental health services at the community level. Scheme consists of support for staff, medicines, IEC activities, training, and contingency for running DMHP. Scheme is being revised to include Life Skills Education and Counselling in schools, Counselling services in colleges, Work Place stress management, District Counselling centre and Crisis Helpline with an enhanced outlay.

❑ *Components*

1. Training programmes of all workers in the mental health team at the identified Nodal Institute in the State.

2. Public education in the mental health to increase awareness and reduce stigma.
3. For early detection and treatment, the OPD and indoor services are provided.
4. Providing valuable data and experience at the level of community to the State and Centre for future planning, improvement in service and research.

17.3. *National Programme for Health Care of the Elderly*

The National Programme for the Health Care for the Elderly (NPHCE) is an articulation of the International and national commitments of the Government as envisaged under the UN Convention on the Rights of Persons with Disabilities (UNCRPD), National Policy on Older Persons (NPOP) adopted by the Government of India in 1999 and Section 20 of "*The Maintenance and Welfare of Parents and Senior Citizens Act, 2007" dealing with provisions for medical care of Senior Citizen.*

❑ *Objectives*

To provide an easy access to promotional, preventive, curative and rehabilitative services to the elderly through community based primary health care approach.

To identify health problems in the elderly and provide appropriate health intervention in the community with a strong referral backup support.

To build capacity of the medical and paramedical professionals as well as the care-takers within the family for providing health care to the elderly.

❑ *Strategies*

- Community based primary health care approach including domiciliary visits by trained health care workers.
- Dedicated services at PHC/CHC level including provision of machinery, equipment, training, additional human resources (CHCJ, IEC, etc.).
- Dedicated facilities at District Hospital with 10 bedded wards, additional human resources, machinery and equipment, consumables and drugs, training and IEC.
- Strengthening of 8 Regional Medical Institutes to provide dedicated tertiary level medical facilities for the Elderly, introducing PG courses in Geriatric Medicine, and in-service training of health personnel at all levels.

- Information, Education and Communication (IEC) using mass media, folk media and others.
- Communication channels to reach out to the target community.
- Continuous monitoring and independent evaluation of the Programme and research in Geriatrics and implementation of IMPHCE.

❑ *Expected Outcomes*

- Regional Geriatric Centre (RGC) in one Medical Institution by setting up Regional Geriatric Centre with a dedicated Geriatric OPD and 30-bedded Geriatric ward for management of specific diseases of the elderly, training of health personnel in geriatric health care and conducting research.
- Post-graduates in Geriatric Medicine (2) from the 1 regional medical institution.
- Video Conferencing Units in the Regional Medical Institutions to be utilized for capacity building and monitoring.
- District Geriatric Units with dedicated Geriatric OPD and 10-bedded Geriatric ward in District Hospitals.
- Geriatric Clinics/Rehabilitation units set-up for domiciliary visits in Community/Primary Health Centres in the selected districts.
- Sub-centres provided with equipment for community outreach services.
- Training of Human Resources in the Public Health Care System in Geriatric Care.
- Coverage of District.
- In Uttar Pradesh, 9 existing districts and 19 new districts are being proposed for the successful implementation of the programme.

17.4. *National Programme for Prevention and Control of Deafness*

National Programme for Prevention and Control of Deafness has been launched and Non-Communicable Disease Components of the National Rural Health Mission programme.

The burden of deafness is relatively high in India with respect to world scenario. The prevalence of severe to profound hearing loss is 291 per lakh population in India. Thus, 5.8 lakh people are estimated to be suffering from profound to severe deafness among 19.96 crore population (Census-2011) of Uttar Pradesh, adversely affecting their educational and social performance, over 50 per cent cases of hearing impairment are preventable and 80 per cent of all deafness is avoidable by medical or surgical method.

Presently National Programme for Prevention and Control of Deafness is being implemented in Barabanki and Gorakhpur (2006-07) and in 2008-09 three districts Varanasi, Banda, Lucknow and in 2009-10 three more districts, namely Agra, Saharanpur and Moradabad have been taken under National Programme for Prevention and Control of Deafness in Uttar Pradesh. Additional 5 new districts, i.e. Allahabad, Aligarh, Bahraich, Jhansi and Shahjahanpur have been proposed under the programme in 2014-15.

❑ *Information by State under National Programme for Prevention and Control of Deafness*

- *Prevalence of Hearing Impairment:* Estimated 5.8 lakh having severe to profound Hearing Impairment.
- *District Covered under NPPCD:* Agra, Banda, Barabanki, Gorakhpur, Lucknow, Moradabad, Saharanpur and Varanasi.
- *New Districts proposed to be covered under NPPCD:* In the year 2013-14 additional 5 districts, *viz.* Aligarh, Allahabad, Bahraich, Jhansi and Shahjahanpur have been proposed.
- *Number and Name of Districts where ENT Surgeon is posted in the District Hospital:* Seven existing and four new proposed districts (Existing — Agra, Banda, Barabanki, Lucknow, Moradabad, Saharanpur and Varanasi and new proposed districts are Allahabad, Bahraich, Jhansi and Shahjahanpur.
- *Number and Name of Districts where Audiologist/Audiological Assistant/Instructor for the Young Hearing Impaired Children is Posted in the District Hospital:* None for efficient and smooth running of National Programme for Prevention and Control of Deafness, maintenance of records and monitoring it is required to establish suitable infrastructure at Medical and Health Directorate.

National Programme for Prevention and Control of Deafness is being run in Agra, Banda, Barabanki, Gorakhpur, Lucknow, Moradabad, Saharanpur and Varanasi. Five new districts are being proposed to be included under this programme in 2014-15, *viz.* Allahabad, Aligarh, Bahraich, Jhansi and Shahjahanpur.

As per NSSO-2001, prevalence of severe to proposed hearing loss is 291 per lakh population in India. Thus 1.41 lakh people are estimated to be suffering from profound to severe deafness in these 13 districts of

Uttar Pradesh, adversely affecting their educational and social performance. Over 50 per cent causes of hearing impairment are preventable and 80 per cent of all deafness is avoidable by medical or surgical method.

It has been proposed to rehabilitate cases of deafness by providing them medical and surgical treatment of PHC/CHC/District Hospital/ Medical College level and by providing them hearing aid after proper evaluation to bring them in the mainstream of society.

17.5. *National Tobacco Control Programme*

Tobacco is the foremost preventable cause of death and disease in the world today. Killing half of the people who use it. Globally it kils nearly 6 million people, of these 0.6 million premature deaths can be attributed to exposure to second hand smoke.

As per World Health Organization, if current trends continue by 2030 tobacco use will kill more than 8 million people worldwide each year. It is estimated that 80 per cent of these premature deaths will occur among people living in low and middle income group.

As per report of the Tobacco Control of India 2004 more than 0.9 million people die due to tobacco consumption every year. There are studies to indicate that approximately 40 per cent of the diseased burden on the country is associated with some form of tobacco or others. Approximately 50 per cent of all cancers in males and 20 per cent cancers in females can be attributed to tobacco use. The burden of the disease for treating just 3 major diseases (Cancer, Cardio-Vascular disease and lung disorder) attributable to tobacco use was more than ₹ 30,800 crore. Tobacco is a risk factor for six of the eight leading causes of death.

The overall prevalence of tobacco use in any form was 34.4 per cent in Uttar Pradesh. Males were the predominant users and the prevalence was higher in rural areas as compared to the urban area. Persons with education in collegè had a lower prevalence of tobacco use. Although the prevalence of tobacco was less in the secondary school education children also as compared to illiterate and less educates, the differences were not sharp.

Prevalence of tobacco use increases with age. Tobacco use prevalence crossed 50 per cent level among men in the age group of 25-29 years suggesting the early institutions of the habit. A very small proportion of 3.5 per cent males and 1.4 per cent females of tobacco uses contemplated quitting their habit. A high percentage (90%) of tobacco users knew about at least one harmful effect of tobacco.

Considering that the public health implications of tobacco consumption and the preventable nature of job related morbidity and mortality, Government of Uttar Pradesh has issued notification to enforce the "Cigarettes and other tobacco products" (Prohibition of Advertisement and Reduction of Trade and Commerce, Production, Supply and Distribution, 2003). The state proposes the strategy to reduce the demand as well as supply of tobacco so as to decrease the disease/disability and deaths associated with tobacco use.

It has been noted that 21 per cent of students currently use any form of tobacco, 8 per cent currently smoke cigarettes, 14 per cent currently use some other form of tobacco.

Environment exposure indicates over 4 in 10 students live in homes where other smokes in their presence, over 5 in 10 are exposed for smoke in public places, over 4 and 10 have parents who smoke. Over half of the students think smoke from others is harmful to them.

Over 6 in 10 students think smoking in public places should be banned. Over 8 in 10 students think smoking in public places should not be banned. Over 8 in 10 students saw anti-smoking media message in the past 30 days; roughly 7 in 10 students saw pro-cigarette advertisements in the past 30 days.

The current tobacco use in any form 33.9 per cent of Adult (Male 48.8% and Female 16.9%) and the current Cigarette smokes 2.3 per cent of Adults (Male 4.1% and Female 0.2%) and current Bidi smokers 12.4 per cent of Adults (Male 20.1% and Female 3.5%) and current users of smokeless tobacco 24.5 per cent of adult (Male 35.4% and Female 13.7%) has been recorded.

17.6. *National Programme for Prevention and Control of Cancer, Diabetes, Cardio-Vascular Disease and Strokes*

India is experiencing a rapid health transition with a rising burden of *Non-Communicable Disease* (NCDs). Overall, NCDs are emerging as the leading cause of deaths in India accounting for over 42 per cent of all deaths (Registrar General of India). NCDs causes significant morbidity and mortality both among urban and rural population with considerable loss in potentially productive years (aged 35-64 years) of life.

It is estimated that overall prevalence of diabetes, hypertension, Ischemic Heart Diseases (IHD) and Stroke is 62.47, 159.46, 37.00 and 1.54 respectively per 1,000 population of India.

Nine Districts of Uttar Pradesh are being supported by the Central Government to supplement their efforts by providing technical and financial support through National Programme for Prevention and Control of Cancer, Diabetes, CVD and Stroke (NPCDCS). The NPCDCS programme has two components, *viz.* (i) Cancer and (ii) Diabetes, CVDs and Stroke. These two components have been integrated at different levels as far as possible for optimal utilization of the resources. The activities at State, Districts, CHC and Sub-Centre level have been planned under the programme and will closely be monitored at different levels.

❑ *Objectives*

1. Prevent and control common NCDs through behaviour and life-style changes;
2. Provide early diagnosis and management of common NCDs;
3. Build capacity at various levels of health care for prevention, diagnosis and treatment of common NCDs;
4. Train human resource within the public health setup, *viz.* doctors, paramedics and nursing staff to cope with the increasing burden of NCDs; and
5. Establish and develop capacity for palliative and rehabilitative care.

❑ *Prevention and Control of Non-Communicable Diseases: "Prevention through Behaviour Change"*

- Prevention of identified risk factors for NCDs by creating general awareness about the Non-Communicable Diseases (NCD).

❑ *Screening/Early Diagnosis*

- Opportunistic screening of persons above the age of 30 years for diabetes and hypertension, at the point of primary contact with any health care facility.
- Providing support for strengthening screening services at sub-centre, PHC, CHC and District Hospitals.

❑ *Treatment of NCDs*

Appropriate treatment and management of various NCDs will be provided at PHC/CHC and district hospital level. The uncomplicated diabetes and hypertension can be treated up to district level. The cancer cases may require referral to higher facilities, i.e. medical colleges and Regional cancer centres. The follow-up chemotherapy can be given in the district hospitals with advice from higher centres.

Implementation of National Programme for Prevention and Control of Cancer, Diabetes, Cardio Vascular Disease and Strokes

The following packages of services is to be provided at various levels of health care delivery at the facility level.

I. Sub-Centre (SC)

- Health Promotion for behaviour change and counselling.
- 'Opportunistic' Screening using B.P. measurement and blood glucose by glucostrip method.
- Identification of early warning signals of common cancer.
- Referral of suspected cases to CHC/nearby health facility with referral card.
- Designate one day for NCD clinic.
- Screening of common cancers (oral, breast and cervical), if possible.

II. Primary Health Centre (PHC)

- Health promotion for behaviour change and counselling.
- 'Opportunistic' Screening using B.P measurement and blood by glucostrip.
- Clinical diagnosis and treatment of simple cases of Hypertension and Diabetes.
- Identification of early warning signals of common cancer.
- Referral of suspected cases of NCDs to CHC.
- Designate one day for NCD clinic.

III. Community Health Centre (CHC/FRU)

- Prevention and health promotion including counselling.
- Early diagnosis through clinical and laboratory investigations (Common lab investigations: Blood Sugar, lipid profile, ECG, ultrasound, X-ray, etc. if not available, may be outsourced).
- Management of common CVD, diabetes and stroke cases.
- 'Opportunistic' Screening of common cancers (Oral, Breast, Cervix and prostate).
- Referral of difficult cases to District Hospital/higher level of health care facility.

IV. District Hospital

- Early diagnosis of diabetes, CVDs and Cancer.
- Investigations: Blood Sugar, lipid profile, Kidney Function

Tests (KFT), Liver Function Tests (LFT), ECG, Ultrasound, X-ray, mammography, etc.

- Outsource investigations for poor and needy, if not available.
- Medical management of cases (outpatient, inpatient and intensive care).
- 'Opportunistic' Screening of common cancers.
- Referral of difficult cases to higher level of health care facility.
- Health promotion for behaviour change and counselling.
- Follow-up chemotherapy for cancer patients.
- Rehabilitation and physiotherapy services.

❑ *Screening, Diagnosis and Treatment*

- The screening of target population (age 30 years and above, and pregnant women) shall be conducted either through opportunistic and/or camp approach at different levels of health facilities and also in urban slums of large cities.
- Screening of pregnant women would be integrated and through Ante-Natal Clinic (ANC) under RCH programme of NRHM. This is expected to be done for all pregnant women.
- The screening of school children shall be carried out during the routine school health check-up activity under the school health programme.
- The suspected cases of diabetes and high blood pressure shall be referred to higher health facilities for further diagnosis and treatment/management.
- The ANMs shall be trained for conducting screening for NCDs at sub-centre level.
- Each district shall be linked to nearby Tertiary Cancer Care (TCC) facilities to provide referral and outreach services.
- The suspected cases of various cancers shall be referred to District Hospital and Tertiary Cancer Care (TCC) facilities.
- For screening of diabetes, support for Glucometers, Glucostrips and lancets are provided to the State under NRHM.

❑ *Strengthening of Health Infrastructure*

Community Health Centre (CHC)

- Support is provided to the CHC/FRU to establish a '*NCD Clinic*' (NCD here refers to Cancer, Diabetes, Hypertension, Cardiovascular diseases, and Stroke) where comprehensive examination of patients referred by the Health Workers as well as reporting directly will be conducted for early diagnosis and treatment.

- Each FRU/CHC needs to be supported with contractual staff (1 Doctor, 1 Nurse, 1 Technician, 1 Counsellor and 1 Data Entry Operator).

District Hospital

- District hospital is to be strengthened/upgraded for management of Cancer, Diabete, Cardiovascular Disease and Stroke.

NCD Clinic: All districts under the programme shall establish regular IMCD clinic for screening, treatment/management of IMCDs.

A. These clinics shall also provide for counselling services and undertake awareness generation activities regarding NCDs and associated risk factors.
B. The NCD clinic shall conduct comprehensive examination of patients referred by lower health facility/health workers as well as of those reporting directly to the clinic.
C. The clinics will advise laboratory investigations of the patients to rule out complications or advanced stages of common NCDs.

Cardiac Care Unit: 6 to 10 bedded Cardiac Care Unit (CCU) can be established/strengthened at the district hospital (up to 25% of districts taken).

A. Special skill based training shall be provided to health professionals and nurses in handling the patients in CCU/ICU.

Support for Cancer: District hospitals need to be supported for diagnostic facilities for common cancers.

A. In case the facility is not available for diagnosis of common cancers in the district hospital, these investigations may be outsourced. District hospital can consider outsourcing certain laboratory investigations that are not available at the facility.
B. Support is also provided for chemotherapy drugs for cancer treatment (up to 25% of districts taken under the programme). All efforts should be made by State Government to provide follow-up chemotherapy at district level. Till such time, patients should be referred to designated Tertiary Cancer Centre (TCC) for treatment.

C. Laboratory services at district hospital are supported to provide necessary investigations for cancer, diabetes, hypertension and cardiovascular diseases.

D. District hospital can consider outsourcing certain laboratory investigations that are not available at the facility.

Manpower Development

- Health professionals and health workers at various levels of health care delivery shall be trained for health promotion, NCD prevention, early detection and management of Cancer.

Diabetes, CVDs and Stroke

- The training shall include components of programme management and specialized training for diagnosis, treatment of cancer, diabetes, CVDs and strokes.

Drugs and Consumables

- Financial support is provided to district and CHC/FRU/PHC for procurement of common essential drugs for treatment of Cancer, Diabetes, CVDs and Stroke.
- The procurement is to be decentralized and to be done at the State level as per relevant norms/procedures in a transparent manner.

Public Private Partnership

- NGOs, civil society organizations and private sector can be involved in health promotion activities, early diagnosis and treatment of common NCDs at District levels, Block levels and Village levels.

Surveillance

- The surveillance for common Non-Communicable Disease and their risk factors needs to be done on a regular basis guidance with ICMR or any leading institution for uniformity and synergies in accordance with National priorities and needs.

18. Public Health Progress in the Study Area

District Women Hospital and District Male Hospital are functional in the District Sultanpur. There is one (24 × 7) Primary Health Centre in Bhadainya Block of Sultanpur District. There are sub-centre in each

Village panchayat of Bhadainya Block. Anganwadi Centre and Auxiliary Nurse Midwife Centres are also functional as per norms and guidelines of the Indian Public Health Standards.

The facility visits including visits to Anganwadi Centre and Auxiliary Nurse Midwife Centres are also ensured. Discussion Meeting with District Authorities and Health care providers are organized regularly. Household interviews with community members, beneficiaries, interviews with ASHAs/Anganwadi workers, visits to schools and interaction with school children are organized regularly.

Infrastructure and physical facilities are adequate and performance of facilities at various levels are sub-optimal.

It has been noted that at sub-centre level the services are largely focused on Immunization in Sultanpur District sub-centres and also the delivery points.

Most of the delivery point sub-centres have two ANMs, clear division of work plans between 2 ANMs. However, in Bhadainya Block deliveries and limited lab services are being provided at 24 × 7 Primary Health Centres.

There is lack of significant increase in OPD/IPD over the past few years in Sultanpur. There is wide variation in performance in BPD Services in one OPD of more than 1,000/month/doctor whereas in other OPD of around 300/doctor/months.

Janani Shishu Suraksha Karyakram and Janani Suraksha Yojana benefits are in place and work on Maternal and Child Health Wing started at District hospital in Sultanpur District. Labour rooms are well maintained and standard protocols displayed at facilities. Sanitary napkins are being provided for post-delivery cases.

The Community is aware of free ambulance services — *102/108.* Average 5 cases/per day/vehicles.

There is lack of identification and line listing of high risk pregnancies as Hb estimation, Urine albumin, not conducted for most mothers. MCP cards are symbolic and 1st ANC conducted in fifth or sixth month at times. The community has limited knowledge about doses of key medicines such as Misoprostol. Maternal death reviews are not conducted as per guidelines. There is lack of Gynaecologist/obstetric specialist at the District Hospital and Designated First Referral Units, knowledge and competencies also need improvement.

The Sick New Born Care Units are functioning at District Women Hospital, catering largely to in-borns. New Born Care corners are functional at all delivery points. Home based New Born Care Trainings are in progress at the District Sultanpur and ORS and Zinc available at the facilities.

New Born Care practices are not standardized and special New Born Care Unit is not operationalized in Sultanpur District Hospital. Home Based New Care has not been initiated in Sultanpur and Nutrition Counselling is almost non-existent at the Village Health Nutrition Days missed opportunity.

Nutrition Rehabilitation Centres at District Hospital has not been operationalized.

Doorstep delivery of Contraceptive by ASHAs are functional and Medical Termination of Pregnancy Services available in Sultanpur District. The fixed day services for Family Planning are also available.

The Post Partum/Intra Urine Contraceptive Device Services required yet to gain momentum and inadequate training at the facility level.

The lack of spacing between two children affecting health of mothers and Child lack of focus on family planning, Minimal Family Planning Counselling no fixed day for *Intra Urine Contraceptive Devices Service,* IUCD insertions.

Emergency contraceptives and medicines for Reproductive Tract Infection/Sexual Transmission Infection Treatment not available at all levels of Health facilities. Medical Termination of Pregnancy services are not available as per the records.

The immunization programme are well functional in Sultanpur District. *Teeka Express* is in place and delivering vaccine to the immunization sites. Zero dose of Bacillus Calmette-Guerin (BCG) not given before discharge missed opportunity. The coverage is poor, and there is lack of follow-up dropout cases.

Rashtriya Bal Swasthya Karyakram Teams are in position in all Blocks of Sultanpur District and plans are prepared in advance. In Sultanpur District Referrals are in place. However, due to inadequate number of vehicles all cases cannot be taken to the referral facility. Referral follow-ups and compliance are the basic issues. There is inadequate skills and competencies of staff.

The Adolescent Health services are available with male and female counsellors are in place, almost non-existent below District Hospital Level. The Adolescent Health Programme is almost non-existent in Sultanpur and there is no activity at Community Level.

The drug procurement and inventory control system including essential drugs and medicines are available in Sultanpur District. On-line drug inventory management system has been initiated in Sultanpur

District. The current system of indents are poor. Out of pocket expenditure on drugs and diagnostics has been a significant issue and prescription audits are not in place. Facility-wise Emergency Drugs List are in place in Sultanpur.

District Level Quality Assurance Centre has been formed and regular meetings has not been initiated. Quality Assurance unit has not been created in Sultanpur.

Patient Privacy a priority in most facilities has been visited. Facilities level quality assurance trans has not been formed in Sultanpur District. Quality Assurance Committee has been formed at District Hospital and Community Health Centre levels to review complaints in Sultanpur District. The awareness on helpline number with Community and ASHAs has been poor. Bio-Medical Waste Management has been outsourced and made functional in Sultanpur District.

District level Vigilance and Monitoring Committee is not functional and very few documented supportive supervision visited by District Level Health offices has been ensured in Sultanpur District.

The vacancies for specialist positions, Multi-purpose workers and other Health officials are high. Competency based recruitment and objective performance appraisal system has been initiated. Differential Payments/incentive based on difficult/most difficult/hard to reach areas are not in place. Absence of a career progression plan for ASHAs has been recorded. There is need for policies for retention and motivation of staff. The Reproductive Maternal Neo-Natal and Child Health and Adolescent Family Planning Counsellor are not in place at many high case load facilities.

Training on all Reproductive Maternal Neo-Natal and Child Health and Adolescent intervention are required in Sultanpur District. Insufficient training on all Reproductive Maternal Neo-Natal Child Health and Adolescent and Post Partum Intra Uterine Contraceptive Device, even in high case load facilities is required. There is lack of training data base at District level and rationalization of human resources on the basis of data base. Post Training Supportive supervision/follows up a missing link has been observed in Sultanpur District.

Various community processes has been initiated in Sultanpur District. There is no ASHA Vishram Kaksha/"ASHA Ghar" at PHC/CHC in Sultanpur District. ASHA Data base is maintained at District Level with all requisite information about ASHA.

The involvement of Panchayati Raj Institutions has been noted in Sultanpur District but very weak at the Block and Village Panchayat level.

Village Health Nutrition Days are being conducted but providing only immunization to children and pregnant women in Sultanpur District but the growth monitoring is not being done.

The knowledge level of ASHAs is a concern at Sultanpur District because the ASHAs are not well educated, trained and motivated properly.

The payments of ASHAs are significantly delayed and complete drug kits are not provided to ASHAs. The ASHA drug kit replenishment is not done at Sub-Centre level in Sultanpur District.

ASHA Grievance Redressal System is not operational in Sultanpur District. There is no collaboration and synergy of inputs between the Sub-Centres.

The Public Health Services are mainly confined to immunization, Ante-Natal and Contraceptive Care but no linkage with the National Disease Control Programme.

There is no planning to recruit separate programme management staff at District Management Unit for Urban Health Programme Management Unit for Urban Health Mission while the existing staff under National Rural Health Mission is managing the Urban Health Mission Programme in Sultanpur District.

Population Mapping of vulnerable population and Gap analysis of Health Facilities have not been carried out. The Recruitment of the Programme Orientation and Training Materials and Convergence Plan of operationalization of the public health programme has not been ensured.

A Skill Behaviour Change Communication Strategy and Planning Guideline for National Rural Health Mission has been developed and citizens charter is visible in most of the First Referral Units but not at Additional Primary Health Centres and Sub-Centres with the timings and available services at the facility level.

Block level HEIOs have no clear job description and are doing random work less than 5 per cent of their work on Information.

Education Communication/Behaviour Change Communication

District reported challenges such as the rates assigned for Information. Education and Communication activities are being much below the market rate flexibility may be needed. Local traditional media seems to be used sparingly.

State is using Health Management Information System data in monitoring and review purposes and for State and District level plans.

Training is the need of the hour at Block level and facility level in Sultanpur District.

Uploading of Data is delayed, i.e. after 5th of every month, due to internal reporting procedures. Data is not being utilized by the end users, i.e. ANMs as feedback not being provided to ANMs/works plans not being shared with ANMs.

Financial Management Training is conducted in Sultanpur District. Books of Accounts are maintained aimed in Tally at District and Block Level. Basic Books of accounts are being maintained all facilities. Concurrent Auditors are appointed by State and District have been completed and reports are submitted in due course of time.

Positions of District Accounts Manager and other supporting staff are vacant.

E-Transfer has been implemented up to the Block Level, but below the Block funds are being transferred through cheques. Some of the cheques issued to Sub-Centre/Village Health Sanitation and Nutrition Committee last year is still lying as Uncleared in the Community Health Centre Books and remain in the Community Health Centres Bank Accounts. Differential findings has not been followed for High Priority Areas and Differential Allocation of Untied funds is not being done.

Some of the Sub-Centres have common Bank Accounts which are still in the process of opening at the facility level and block level. The statutory Audit is under process and the Concurrent Auditors appointed is not pending and the District Report was available in Sultanpur District and compliance on report of concurrent Audit was available at the State level.

The funds transfer below block are treated as expenditure. They are lying as advances with facilities and some remain unclear with banks.

There is no estimation of liabilities for the Janani Suraksha Yojana at Sultanpur District. It has been noted that approximately 50 per cent are the uncleared stale cheques. There is no reconciliation of balance at the District Health Society and Block of the District Sultanpur.

The specific guidelines/orders are awaited at District Level to initiate expenditure in the initial part of the year. Despite the funds available from previous year, there is time lag in transfer of funds and issue of guidelines for utilization of Sanctioned Financial budget at the facility level in the Sultanpur District.

Financially, it has been recommended accounts should be maintained and managed at District and Block level and District Health Society level in Sultanpur district.

Several non-operational bank accounts are lying at the Block level may be closed and differential funding should be followed for the High

Focus areas. Regular Monitoring Visits should be undertaken by the supervisory units to its lower units.

It has been financially recommended that the Reconciliation of Balance at the District and Sub-District Level should be done on a quarterly basis. It has been recommended to streamline Janani Suraksha Yojana payments and receiving date by beneficiary should be maintained. The estimation of outstanding cheque of Janani Suraksha Yojana every month by the concerned facility and stale cheques should be reversed.

20. Conclusion

Public Health delivery system has increased many folds which have affected the quality of services. It is necessary to increase and promote health delivery points, so that the quality public health delivery services are provided at the facility level especially in the unserved, underserved and remote areas to the needy interested people equally effectively and efficiently.

A comparative study of Adherence and Cure rates of Tuberculosis using Technology enabled Monitoring and Supervision has also been implemented at the facility levels.

Immunization, Integrated Disease Surveillance Programme and National Disease Control Programme, National Vector-Borne Disease including Acute Encephalitis Syndrome and Japanese Encephalitis Programme have also been implemented at the Health facilities level.

Various non-communicable diseases including Injuries and Trauma, National Mental Health Programme and National Programme for the Health Care of the Elderly and National Programme for Prevention and Control of Deafness and National Tobacco Programme, etc. under National Rural Health Mission are being implemented at the Health facility level. The planning processes has focused on addressing inequities in terms of "*Time to Care*".

District Sultanpur has been planned to increase the institutional deliveries. Home deliveries and Institutional deliveries has been planned. Approximately 85 per cent of the Rural deliveries are planned to be brought by Accredited Social Health Activists.

The previous rates of ₹ 1,500 has been too meagre, therefore, the rate for C-Section in Private Accredited Centre for BPL Women has been increased to ₹ 25,000 per case.

Janani Shishu Suraksha Karyakram has been rolled out in Sultanpur District and 100 per cent coverage of the pregnant women is being ensured through providing free treatment, free drugs and consumables, free diagnostics, free Diet and free drop back. Maternal Death Review and incentives for ASHA under maternal health and treatment of severe anaemia and incentive to ASHA for early registration and opening beneficiary's Bank Account as new activity has been initiated.

Orientation training of ANMs at Block level, procurement and printing plan and incentive for first referral unit operationalizations as old activity and incentive for past maternal health has been initiated under National Rural Health Mission at the facility level.

Reducing infant mortality is one of the key goals under National Rural Health Mission. The infant and under five Child mortality has shown a steady decline over last three years. However, the progress is not uniform across the state and even intrastate. Inter-district variations are quite evident from the recent surveys. Moreover, the decline in Neo-Natal mortality is slow and has not kept *pace with* the overall decline *in child* mortality.

Diarrhoea is one of the major causes of the child mortality in Uttar Pradesh. National Policy for the management of Diarrhoea among children less than 5 years, recommends the use of zinc tablets along with ORS in treatment of Diarrhoea.

Revised Diarrhoea Management Policy recommends administration of Zinc for every case of diarrhoea a dose of 20 mg/day for 14 days (even if diarrhoea has stopped) for children aged 6 months to 5 years and 10 mg/days for 2-6 months).

Uttar Pradesh has proposed to sale up these programmes in the entire state so as to increase the use of ORS and Zinc in the treatment of child diarrhoea to at least 50 per cent in 2014-15.

Bal Swasthya Poshan Mah and Biannual Bal Swasthya Poshan Mah Programme focuses on strengthening joint health and ICDS planning and review meetings, streamlining logistics and ensuring monitoring during the rounds.

The Infant Mortality Rate has been declining very slowly and state is committed to meet our goals, hence 2013-14 was celebrated as a year of Navjaat Shishu Suraksha Varsh. An emphasis was given to strengthen facilities, services and capacity building of health staffs.

Various activities have been initiated to reduce the Neo-Natal Deaths including Sick New Born Care Units, New Born Stabilization Units, Nutrition Rehabilitation Centres, New Born Care Corners and New Born Screening and a preventive child health care initiative has been started for 13,500 neonates who have been screened for three disorders with easy effective and cheap treatment. The disorders tested were congenital thysodism, biotinidase deficiency and glacetosemia.

The *Girl or Boy: Healthy Baby is the Joy programme* has been launched. The burden of raising a handicapped child is immense and affects the financial, social and psychological aspects of all the family members. The prevention is better and cheaper than cure.

The children who dies before their fifth birth day, almost one-third of them die of infectious causes nearly all of which are preventable.

Infant Young Child Feeding and breast feeding week celebration is being organized jointly with ICDS, and technical support is being sought from WHO, UNICEF and other partners working in the state.

Child death review is a strategy to understand the geographical variation in the causes of child deaths and thereby initiating specific child health interventions. Analysis of child deaths provide information about medical causes of deaths which helps to identify the gaps in health service delivery and social factors that contributes to child death.

The goal of social marketing scheme will be to create a market where zinc and ORS are available in adequate quantities, informal providers prescribe its use and through repeated use mothers begin to recognize and demand for their infants.

The Total Fertility Rate of Uttar Pradesh has declined from 4.1 to 3.8 per cent. However, compared to National Average of 2.7, the rates are still very high. To enhance the performance of family planning it is imperative to meet the desired unmet needs. The unmet need for spacing method has increased from 9 per cent in 1988-99 to 12 per cent in 2005-06 to 29.7 per cent in 2010-11.

Tuesday and Friday are fixed days under fixed day sterilization services (legation/abdominal tubectomy will be continued at all districts women hospital/PHCs/CHCs having either a surgeon or Gynaecologist.

The plan for facilities providing Non-Scalpel Vasectomy services on fixed days at Health Facilities and Female Sterilization Camps and Non-Scalpel Vasectomy Camps are organized. Door step delivery of contraceptive by ASHA and enhanced contribution of Panchayati Raj Institutions and Family Members have been ensured to improve outputs of programme activities in family planning.

Family Planning Counsellors are being deployed in view of the opportunity of large number of institutional delivery under the Janani Suraksha Yojana and they will have the opportunity to reach all the mothers and will counsel the women and address their concern for small family norms.

A sum of ₹ 150 may be paid to ASHAs for escorting the client to the health facility for facilitating the insertion. *Pehal Sakhi Sammelan* is organized as community event. Male Group Meetings and Merry Gold Health Network activities are organized in order to engage the large and unregulated private sector through network and the same time to standardize the prices of health services.

Rashtriya Kishor Swasthya Karyakram has been proposed with a target group of 10-19 years of age which will get with various components of Reproductive Maternal Neo-Natal Child Health Adolescent.

It has been proposed to organize Adolescent Health Day at Block level initially twice a year which may be expanded to quarterly as per experience/feedback in the next year. An estimated number of 250 participants (ASHA, PEs, Adolescent boys and girls from various villages, selected school teachers, Panchayat Members, NGOs, ANMs and AWWs) will attend the function.

Weekly Iron Folic supplementation and Menstrual Hygiene Scheme and Convergence within Health and with other Partner Departments has been initiated through organizing regular meetings and their sustained involvement.

Rashtriya Bal Swasthya Karyakram is being implemented in the State from the last year which has been established by IIIrd quarter of the year 2013-14. Every Block of the State is also supposed to have two Mobile Health Teams with four members in each team (2 Doctors, 1 Paramedical and one staff nurse/Auxiliary Nurse Midwife).

Sex Ratio is an important indicator to measure gender equity. The rapidly increasing sex ratio in the state is likely to create severe gender imbalance that can destroy the social fabric. It should also be viewed both as child right issues as girls are killed either through sex selective abortions or die prematurely due to violence and neglect.

State Preconceive, Pre-Natal Diagnostic Technical Act and Zonal PC and PNDT Act Cell and also at Divisional, District and Block level. PC and PNDT Cell is to be established and the mobility for monitoring and inspection work has been ensured.

World Health Organization has estimated that most of the people in developing as well as in the developed countries received the bulk of their health care from traditional or indigenous health system.

Ayurveda, Yoga and Naturopathy, Unani, Siddha and Homoeopathy (AYUSH) systems of medicines have proven promotive, preventive and curative strengths of the health system. The objective of mainstreaming of AYUSH health care facilities at the PHCs, CHCs and District Hospitals should be fulfilled. The development of Health care institutions scheme has been revised along with addition of some new components, in order to mainstreaming of AYUSH more effectively, and equally at the facility level.

Orientation training and skill upgradation of the facility level officials is being organized.

Various referral transport and Patient transport system especially "108" Emergency Medical Transport services and "102" National Ambulance Services and Advance Life Support Ambulance and Paediatric Ambulance for Sick New Born Care Units and Monitoring Cell for Ambulance Services is being ensured. The fleet of 1972 Ambulance under "102" National Ambulance Services and "988" Ambulance under Emergency Medical Transport Services is very large and covers all the Districts of Uttar Pradesh.

Bio-Medical Waste must be managed and disposed of to protect the environment. General public and workers especially health care and sanitation workers who are at risk of exposure to bio-medical waste as an occupational hazard.

A critical challenge facing Tuberculosis Control Programme is to ensure that patients adhere to full course of treatment. Non-adherence not only jeopardizes a patient's treatment outcome, but also leads to the emergence of drug resistant strains, which are increasing threat to global public health while Directly Observed Therapy short cause (DOTS) Health and Sanitation greatly boosted adherence rates in Uttar Pradesh. There remain many challenges to measure patient' adherence and ensuring that it satisfies the expectations of the patients.

The immunization programme is the cornerstone of public health and vaccination was practiced in India since early 1900s especially against small pox in the late 1940s. In 1962 Bacilus Calmatte-Guerin (BCG) inoculation included in the National Tuberculosis Control Programme. It gained momentum in 1985 under Universal Immunization Programme and it was merged in Child Survival and safe motherhood programme in 1991-92. Since, 1997 immunization activities are an important component of Reproductive and Child Health Programme.

Iodine deficiency disorders one of the major public health problems in India with around 200 million people estimated to be at risk. Iodine deficiency can be prevented by using salt that has been fortified with Iodine.

Integrated Disease Surveillance Programme started in 2004 with the support from World Bank to improve and Integrate Disease Surveillance in pursuance of recommendations by High Powered Committee of Secretaries on Environment and Sanitation.

Vector-Borne Diseases are prevalent in Sultanpur District and prioritized as high risk districts. Sultanpur has been categorized as priority district for AES/JE and Malaria, Kala-Azar and Dengue fever diseases.

Fortnightly fogging of Malathion by the fogging machine in the villages reporting Japanese Encephalitis cases for last 2-3 years during transmission period. District Sultanpur has been facilitated with vehicle mounted large thermal fogging machine to each Primary Health Centre.

National Leprosy Eradication Programme and various other National Disease Control Programmes have been initiated at the facility level.

Non-communicable diseases include the National Programme for Control of Blindness, National Mental Health Programme, National Programme for Control of Dengue, Cancer, Diabetes, Cardio Vascular Disease and stroke, etc. have been launched under National Rural Health Mission Programme at the facility level.

Cataract operation, School Eye Screening and Corneal Blindness Programme have been initiated under the National Programme for control of Blindness.

National Mental Health Programme has been launched in 1982 because 6-7 per cent of general population suffers from mental disorders. Scheme consists of support for staff, medicines, IEC activities training and contingency for running District Mental Health Programme. The scheme is being revised to control and include life skills Education and Counselling in school, colleges, work place stress management District Counselling Centres and Crisis helpline with an enhanced outlay.

District Women Hospital and District Male Hospital are functional in Sultanpur and there is 24 × 7 Primary Health Centre in Bhadainya Block of the District Sultanpur. Infrastructure and physical facilities are adequate and performance of facilities at various levels are sub-optimal.

Janani Suraksha Yojana and Janani Sishu Suraksha Karyakram are in place and work in Maternal and Child Health Wing started at District Hospital. There is lack of identification and line listing of high risk pregnancies. Hb estimation albumin, not conducted for most mothers, MCP Cards are symbolic and 1st ANC conducted in fifth or sixth month at times. The community has limited knowledge about doses of key medicines such as Misoprostol.

The adolescent health services are available with male and female counsellors are in the place, almost non-existent below District Hospital level. The adolescent health programme is almost non-existent in Sultanpur and there is no activity at Community Level.

The Public health services are mainly confined to immunization, Ante-Natal and Contraceptive Care but no linkage with the National Disease Control Programme.

State is using Health Management Information System data in monitoring and review purposes and also for state and district level plans. Training is the need of the hour at Block level and facility level in Sultanpur.

Uploading of Data is delayed, i.e. after 5th of every month due to internal reporting procedures. Data is not being utilized by the end users, i.e. ANMs as feedback not being provided to ANMs/work plans not being shared with ANMs and other end users at the facility level.

The funds transfer below the blocks are treated as expenditure. They are lying as advances with facilities and some remain uncleared with banks. Several non-operational bank accounts are lying at the Block level may be closed and the differential funding should be followed for the high focus areas. Regular Monitoring visits should be undertaken by the supervisory units to its lower units.

Thus, the vision, mission and action plan for the appropriate delivery of the public health services to needy, interested deprived, unserved and underserved people at the facility level from Auxiliary Nurse Midwife Centre, Anganwadi Centres, Sub-Centres, Primary Health Centres, Community Health Centres and District Hospitals with the sustained involvement of community, Rogi Kalyan Samiti and Panchayati Raj Institutions for appropriate delivery of public health services at grassroots level equally effectively and efficiently as per norms, standards and guidelines of the Indian Public Health Standards.

4

PUBLIC HEALTH MANAGEMENT

1. Introduction

The Public Health Management may be ensured through controlling and checking the water pollution, water contamination which causes growth of water-borne diseases. Water-borne diseases are caused by the pathogenic micro-organism. The water-borne diseases are commonly transmitted in the contaminated fresh water.

Trivially most of the infections might be transmitted by the microbes or parasites which are accidentally, possible as a result of exceptional circumstances and it had got into water, but the fact is that there might be an occasional freak infection and not mean that it is useful to categorize the resulting disease as "water-borne" nor is it a common practice to refer disease such as malaria as "water-borne" just because mosquitoes as have aquatic phases in their life-cycle or due to treating the water, the people inhibit the happiness to be an effective strategy to control mosquitoes which are the vectors.

According to the World Health Organization the water-borne disease account for an estimated 4.1 per cent of the total daily global burden of disease and cause about 1.8 per cent million human deaths per annum. The World Health Organization has estimated that 88 per cent of the global burden of diseases are attributable due to unsafe drinking water supply, sanitation and hygiene.

The pathogens associated with water-borne illness, outbreak agents including factorial, virus, parasitic and chemical agents causes various water-borne illnesses through ingestion or consuming water by dermal contact of water with skin or mucous membranes or by inhalation which is by bathing in a mist or aerosolized water particles.

The water-borne diseases are more prevalent due to the lower level of access to drinking water and sanitation along with poorer and overall health hygiene and poor nutritional status.

It has been noted that a child dies approximately every six second from diarrhoeal diseases and more than 50 per cent hospital beds are occupied by the patient suffering from water-borne diseases associated with lack of access to safe drinking water, poor hygiene and inadequate sanitation.

It has been estimated that most of the disease burden could be reduced through improved good quality water supply, sanitation, hygiene and proper management of the water resources. It has been observed that more than 90 per cent deaths are caused due to diarrhoeal disease especially among to the children belonging to 5 years age.

The water-borne illness is typically associated with drinking water of etiologic agent which causes Chemical Contamination of Water through poor sanitary conditions of the water system and water supply from cesspits, unsanitary place and the cesspits of the old houses had never been drained causing cholera and diarrhoea diseases.

World Health Organization has been providing technical guidance, coordination and enforces surveillance in the dracunculiasis free area and also advocates for eradication. The arsenic has been one of the WHO's 10 chemicals of major public health concern. WHO's work to reduce arsenic exposure include setting guidelines value, reviewing evidence and providing risk management.

Guidelines for drinking water quality has been published by the World Health Organization. The recent recommended limit of arsenic in drinking water is 10 μg/litre, although this guideline value is designated as provisional due to measurement difficulties and practical difficulties in removing arsenic from drinking water where it is difficult to achieve the guideline value.

Anticipating the discussions on post 2015 development goals, the World Health Organization (WHO) and United Nations Children's Fund (UNICEF) convened a first consultation with broad stakeholders representatives at Berlin in May 2011 to start a process and formulation proposal for post 2015 target and corresponding indicators for Water Sanitation and Hygiene (WASH). As an outcome to Berlin Consultation, four working groups are established —

I. Water Supply Sanitation, Hygiene and Equity,
II. Non-Discrimination, Consisting of WASH sector and human right experts,
III. Representatives from Academia, and
IV. International Monitoring Community.

These groups have been tasked with the development of targets and indicators for the specific sub-sector except for Equity and Non-Discrimination.

Thus, the water-borne diseases may have significant impact on the economic status of the common people at the local level as well as international level. Infected and affected people by the water-borne diseases are usually confronted with the related costs and not seldom with a huge financial burden.

The financial losses are caused by, e.g. cost for the medical treatment and medication costs for transport, special food and by the loss of manpower. It has also been observed that many families must even sell their land and property to pay for the treatment in a proper hospital. It has been observed that on average a family spends approximately 10 per cent of the monthly household income per infected person suffering from the water-borne diseases.

Important features of the rural health includes the Reproductive and Child Health, Immunization, Disease Control Programme, action on the social determinants, and convergence that were to be leveraged from other sectors.

The architectural correlations has been related to decentralization with greater role for Panchayats and horizontal integration of vertical programmes. Important mechanism envisaged has been the creation of State → District → Sub-Division → Block and Village Societies which provided the representation of the multi-stakeholders. It has also been mandated for Hospital Development Societies (Rogi Kalyan Samiti) and Village Health and Sanitation Committees and the elected Panchayat Members should have an important/prominent place with the exact role definition being left to the State Decentralization and Integration of the District Health Action Plan and the State Programme Implementation Plan has been the key institutional device.

Management improvements and technical assistance, called for a number of new organization structures and interaction of professional management and accounting skills at Block-District-State Levels.

National Rural Health Mission is not singular package or even a set of mechanism whose effectiveness can be subject to a standard model of impact evaluation. It is primarily a financing mechanism for strengthening the public health system. The design of the National Rural Health Mission recognizes that beyond this increased investment, improved government institutional report and innovations are essential.

The available reports, documents, does not capture whether National Rural Health Mission has been "*successful*" or "*failed*" but analyzes the changes in the health outcomes and health systems from the point of view of the constraints that were faced and learnt lessons.

In view of the above, a factual and conceptual base line for the coming years only on such a well grounded understanding at Village → Block → District level, where the problems are faced in reaching at the grassroots level, can be planned for the future public health system for the resourcesless, deprived poor patients surviving in the remote rural areas. An attempt has been made in this study to explain the various needful recommendations and management of rural health for requisite delivery of the public health services at the facility level and village level.

2. Management Imperatives to Control Water Contamination

Water pollution occurs when the pollutant are directly or indirectly discharged into the water bodies. The water contamination affects plants and organisms living in these water bodies. Its effect is damage not only to the individual species and population but also to the natural biological communities.

It has been estimated that 580 people in our country die due to water pollution/contamination related illness everyday. Nearly 500 million people suffer due to lack of access to safe drinking water.

The treatment of the drinking water as applied to public water supplies consist of a series of water supplies and the nature and vulnerability of the source of water.

Generally these systems comprise for coagulation and flocculation, filtration and oxidation, the most common oxidative disinfectant used is chlorine. It provides an effective and robust barrier to pathogens and provides an easily measured residual that can act as marker to show that disinfection has been carried out and as a preservative in the distribution system of the water.

There are national standards or the international guidelines to judge the safety of the drinking water. The guidelines of the World Health Organization are most important for ensuring the quality of the drinking water. These guidelines are revised on a regular basis and these standards are supported by a range of detailed documents through describing various aspects of the safety of the water.

The Water Safety Plans are based on the guidelines of the World Health Organization which encompasses a much more proactive approach to the safety of the drinking water from source to tap water.

The contaminants of the water may be analyzed through several broad categories of the methods — physical, chemical and biological. Various agencies and research organizations have documented, standardized, validated analytical test methods to facilitate, the comparability of results from the disparate testing events at the different levels.

Testing of water for physical or chemical can be done through several methods depending on the accuracy required and the characteristics of the contaminants of water. Most of the water contamination events are sharply restricted in time, in association with the events of rain. The "grab" samples are often inadequate for fully quantifying the levels of the water contamination. The auto-sampler devices are oftenly employed for gathering this type of information that the pump increments of water at either time of discharge intervals of the water.

The biological testing of the water samples involves the collection of plants or the animals from the surface water body. The organism may be identified for the bio-surveys and returned to the water body or these may be dissected for bio-assays to determine toxicity levels. The common physical tests of water temperature concentrations, e.g. total suspended solids and the turbidity.

The biological testing of water involves the use of plant, animals or microbial indicators to monitor the health of an aquatic ecosystem. These biological organizations can be monitored for the bio-chemical, physiological or behavioural changes which may indicate a problem within their ecosystem.

The policy decisions on the type of degree of the control and treatment of wastes and the disposal and the use of adequate treated waste water should be based on considering all the scientific and technical factors of each drainage system in order to prevent any further contamination or harm to the local environment or ecosystem.

Generally, the domestic sewage are typically treated through centralized sewage treatment plants, properly designed and operating system, i.e. secondary treatment or better can remote, 90 per cent or more of these pollutants. There are some plants which have additional system to remove nutrient. Plants are not specifically designed to treat toxic pollutants found in the water in the residential areas. The residential areas with sanitary sewer overflows or combined sewer overflows employ one or more engineering approaches to reduce the discharge of untreated sewage —

- To utilize agree infrastructure approach to improve storm water management capacity and reduce the hydraulic overloading of the sewage treatment plant.
- Repair and replacement of leaking and malfunctioning of the equipments.
- To increase the overall hydraulic capacity of the sewage collection system.

Some of the business or household not served by the municipal treatment plant may have an individual septic tank which treats the Waste water on site and discharges into the soil. The domestic water may be sent to a nearly privately owned treatment system, alternatively.

The ordinary domestic sewage, that can be treated by the municipal facilities which generate waste water with high concentration of the conventional pollutants, e.g. oil, grease, toxic pollutants, i.e. heavy metals, volatile organic compounds or other non-conventional pollutants such as ammonia, required specialized treatment. The facilities can install a pre-treatment system to remove the toxic compounds and then send the partially treated waste water to the municipal system.

The loose soil sediments washed off fields has been the largest source of the agricultural pollution. The farmers may utilize the erosion control to reduce run-off flows and retain soil on their fields. The common scientific techniques include contour ploughing, crop mulching, crop rotation, planting perennial crops and installing riparian buffers in their farm land as per their feasibility.

The nitrogen and phosphorus nutrients are typically applied to the farm land as commercial fertilizers, animals manure or spraying of municipal or industrial waste water/effluents or sludge. The nutrients may also enter run-off from crop residues nitrogen, water, wild life and the atmospheric deposition. Interested farmers can develop and implement nutrient management plants to reduce excess application of nutrients and reduce the potential for the nutrient pollutions. To minimize the impacts of the pesticides, the farmers may use Integrated Pest Management Techniques which can include biological pest control to maintain control over pests and reduce reliance on the chemical pesticides and protect the quality of water.

The cultivated land with large livestock and poultry operations are termed as concentrated animal feeding operations. The animal slurries are usually treated by contaminants in anaerobic lagoons before disposal by spray on trickle application to the grass land. The constructed wet lands are sometimes used to facilitate and treatment of animal waste.

The animal slurries are treated by mixing with straw and composed at high temperature to produce a bacteriological sterile and friable manure to increase the fertility status of the soil.

The sediments from the construction site can be managed as per following details:

- Erosion control such as launching and hydro seeding.
- Sediment control such as sediment basis and construction of the silt fences.

The discharge of the toxic chemicals such as motor fuels and concrete washout are prevented —

- Spill prevention and Control Plans.
- Specially designed containers, i.e. concrete wash out and structure such as overflow control.

An effective control of run-off involves reducing the velocity and flow of storm water as well as reducing pollutant discharges. Different measures should be adopted to reduce the effects of run-off. Best management techniques and practices should be applied to focus on the water quality control while others focus on improving the quality of water.

The pollution prevention practices include low impact development techniques and installation of green roofs and improved chemical handling, e.g. management of motor fuels and soil, fertilizers and pesticides. The run-off mitigation system include the infiltration basins, bio-retention systems, constructed wet lands retention basins and similar devices for prevention of the water pollution.

The thermal pollution run-off can be controlled by the storm water management facilities which absorb the run-off or direct it into the ground water such as bio-retention systems and infiltration basis. The retention basin tend to be less effective for reducing the temperature, as the water may be heated by the sun before being discharged to a receiving stream at the grassroots level.

❑ *By-products of Drinking Water Treatment*

The drinking water treatment is required to remove organisms. In the most of the cases increasingly, the chemical contaminants cause water contamination which adversely affects the health of the people. The process may in itself result in the formation of other contaminants such as the tri-halomethanes and halocaetic acids from the reaction of Chemical oxidants, with naturally occurring organic materials. It has been noted that it requires a balance to strict between the benefits of the chemical oxidants in destroying micro organisms and the potential risk from by-products of the water treatment of these by-products only tri-halomethanes tends to be routinely monitored in the drinking water treatment.

The water treatment should take chemicals including chlorine, Chloramines, Chlorine dioxide and Ozone. The each water treatment methodology has certain advantage and disadvantages, but all of them form by-products of some sort. The quantities and various types of products form depend on a number of factors of the water treatment.

The formation of by-products during Chlorination depends on the amount and contents of organic matters, bromine levels, temperature, *p*H value of the water. The updates of *trihalomethanes can occur* not only *through ingestion* but also *by inhalation and skin absorption during the activities such as swimming, showering and bathing*.

The ingestion is the main route for the uptake. These have been associated with the cancers of the bladder, colon, rectum and the adverse birth outcomes, such as spontaneous abortion, low birth weight still birth and congenital malformations. In the epidemiological studies overall such evidences are inconsistent, inconclusive for the by-products of the drinking water treatment.

❑ *Operational Management of Drinking Water*

It has been noted that more than 61 per cent safe drinking water requirement is met from the ground water source through tube-wells, wells, public and private hand pumps, while the balance of 39 per cent requirement of the drinking water is met from the river, through water bodies, water works tanks, ponds and other sources of the surface water. Operational management of drinking water may be ensured as per the following details:

- Bacteriological test of the drinking water should be carried out.
- The drinking water samples of the residential, individual and commercial areas and drinking water samples through pipes which are contaminated to the extent of 33.27 per cent, 43 per cent and 42 per cent respectively should be properly tested.
- Testing of the drinking water of the underground water pumped through tube-wells in the highly populated commercial and industrial areas should be tested.

- Uttar Pradesh Pollution Control Board which is responsible for inspecting the water treatment plants and to review the data related to the water purification should be carried out regularly.
- The dumping of garbage and the Municipal Waste which causes algal growth and covered with the aquatic grasses in the water bodies, and generated sewage should be properly disposed of after appropriate treating through different drains.
- Overflow of the septic tanks should be disposed of properly.
- Low-lying areas and water-logged areas which has been a dumping site for garbage and sewage waste and infested with the garbage and municipal waste should be properly treated.
- Water testing of the drinking water of the functional India Mark-II Hand Pump should be properly ensured and tested as per the guidelines of the Indian Standard for Drinking Water Specification.
- Physical and Chemical Parameters of the water should be properly tested based on the required desirable and permissible limit of the Indian Standard for Drinking Water Specification.

3. Management of Water-Borne Diseases

The water-borne diseases are reserved largely for infection that predominantly are transmitted through contact with the consumption of the infected water. The water-borne diseases are the major causes of morbidity and mortality. The water-borne diseases are caused by the pathogenic micro-organism that most commonly are transmitted in the contaminated fresh water. The infection commonly occurs during bathing, washing, drinking and in the preparation of food or the consumption of food thus infected.

World Health Organization recognizes that the access to adequate water supply is a fundamental human right. The water related diseases are a human tragedy, killing millions of people each year which accounts for 80 per cent of all deaths.

The improved water supply and sanitation may lead to reduce the incidence of morbidity and mortality, which may be up to 100 per cent for some diseases such as Typhoid and Dracunculiasis.

An approximately management strategy to check, control and prevent the water-borne diseases are as follows:

- Lack of proper sanitation including sewage treatment which is inadequate instead human waste disposal in the open areas should be properly treated.

- Agricultural chemical, insecticides and pesticides fertilization and industrial wastes should be properly uses and treated.

Various appropriate measures can be adopted for prevention of water-borne diseases —

- Washing vegetables in clean water.
- Do not enter in the infected waters.
- Eating well cooked meat.
- In the areas where guinea worm is endemic, people can use piece of cloth to filter the water.
- To build the water channel in the fast flowing streams to make it difficult for snails to survive.

Most important actions for the prevention and control among the affected communities for further exposure to arsenic has been through the provision of safe supply of drinking water, preparation of food and irrigation system of the food crops. The various options to reduce the levels of arsenic in the drinking water are as follows:

- The substitute high arsenic sources of water such as ground water with low arsenic, micro-biologically safe sources such as rain water and treated surface water and low arsenic water should be used for drinking, cooking, and irrigation purposes, whereas arsenic rich water can be used for other purposes such as bathing and washing of clothes, etc.
- Low arsenic and high arsenic sources of water should be discriminated for example test of water for arsenic levels and point tube-wells or Hand Pump in different colours. It can be effective and low cost means to rapidly reduce the exposure to arsenic, if accompanied through effective education and awareness to the people.
- To blend low arsenic water with higher arsenic water to achieve an acceptable arsenic concentration level.
- To install arsenic removal system either centralized or domestic and ensure the appropriate disposal of the removed arsenic.
- The technologies for the removal of arsenic include oxidation, coagulation, precipitation absorption, ion exchange and membrane techniques. An effective and low cost option for removing arsenic from small or household level supplies of drinking water.

- The long-term actions are also required to reduce occupation exposure from industrial processes.
- Appropriate education training and awareness to the people and community engagement are key factors for ensuring successful intervention.
- It is necessary for the community members to understand the risks of high arsenic exposure. The sources of arsenic exposure including the intake of arsenic of Crops, i.e. rice from irrigation water and the intake arsenic into food from cooking water.
- The high risk population should be monitored for the early signs of arsenic poisoning especially the problems of skins.

World Health Organization works to reduce arsenic exposure includes setting guidelines, values, reviewing evidence and providing recommendations for the risk management. World Health Organization published a guideline value for arsenic in its "*Guidelines for Drinking Water Quality*".

The guidelines are intended for the use as basis for regulation and standard setting at various levels. The recent recommended limit of arsenic in the drinking water is 10 μg/litre.

There is no vaccine to prevent guinea worm disease nor there is any medication to treat the disease. However, the prevention is possible through prevention strategies —

- Heightening surveillance to detect every case within 24 hours of the emergency of worms.
- To prevent transmission from each worm by treatment, cleaning, bandaging regularly the affected skin area until the worm is completely expelled from the body.
- To prevent the contamination of drinking water through advising the patient to avoid wading into water.
- To ensure wider access to safe drinking water supplied to prevent infection.
- To filter the water from the open water bodies before drinking the water.
- To promote health education and awareness and change of the behaviour of human body.

During 1981, the International Steering Committee for Cooperative Action for the International Drinking Water Supply and Sanitation (Decade 1981-1990) had been proposed as the elimination of dracunculiasis as indicator of success of the decade.

World Health Organization's decision making body the World Health Assembly adopted a resolution (WHA-34-25) recognizing that the International Drinking Water Supply and Sanitation Decades presented an opportunity to eliminate dracunculiasis.

❑ *Control and Prevention of Water-Borne Diseases*

The prevention and control of the various water-borne diseases can be checked through adopting various approaches with the objectives to interrupt the transmission of water-borne diseases and thereby reducing their morbidity and mortality. Prevention and control measure to check the water-borne diseases are as follows:

- Proper sanitary disposal of human waste.
- Protecting public water supplies from faecal contamination.
- Treatment of suspected water supplies, both rural and urban before consumption.
- Keeping fetched water at home safe during storage.
- Mass treatment during epidemic outbreaks, e.g. at school, in prison, etc.
- Treatment of water supplies, etc.
- Washing hands with soap and water before preparing or eating food and after using the latrine.
- To ensure proper health education and creating awareness regarding the effect and preventive measures of water-borne disease. The promotion of health education should not be limited to those visiting health institutions out in all situations for individual or groups of people in the communities. The following points should be addressed:
    - The causative agents.
    - The mode of transmission.
    - The preventive and control measure.
    - The importance of early treatment.

The key management of a patient who has a water-borne infection is identifying the specific organism and instituting specific therapy appropriate for the organization.

The supportive therapy includes:

- Monitoring the patients' response to theraphy.
- Ensuring hydration and fluid balance.
- Continuously observing for complications and providing information to both the patient and family.

❑ *Nursing Intervention*

The goals of nursing management are to provide supportive care and to monitor for complications —

- ★ Encourage high fluid intake.
- ★ During the period of anorexia, the patient should receive frequent small feedings, supplemented, if necessary, by IV infusion of glucose containing fluids.
- ★ Encourage the patient to express fears/worries.
- ★ Skin Care (perennial care).
- ★ Teach the patient about his or her specific disease and therapeutic regimens. She or he is instructed about personal hygiene and the maintenance of the home environment and how they seek additional health care.
- ★ Inform the family about the disease problems and how they can seek additional health care.
- ★ Patient and family need specific guidelines about diet, rest, and follow-up.
- ★ In case of typhoid fever, delirium is common in its severest form. The patient requires special support during this period. Patients' safety must be maintained with the use of side rails and other restraints.
- ★ Tepid water sponges are administered for temperature over 40 °C.
- ★ Observe for bladder distension.
- ★ Monitoring for complications; for example, in typhoid fever a dangerous complication is intestinal hemorrhage and proportion of the bowel with resultant perforation.
- ★ Additionally, Hepatitis-A will rarely progress to fulminate Hepatitis terminating in cirrhosis or death.

❑ *Public Health Approaches to Control Water-Borne Diseases*

The water-borne diseases are of the major public health threats especially in the developing countries, where unsafe water, sanitation problems and hygiene practices exit. The Public health approach to the prevention and control of water-borne diseases should consist of three basic components —

- Provision of safe and adequate water supply.
- Improved Sanitation.
- Hygiene Education.

❑ *Treatment of Water Supply*

The water for domestic purposes can be treated against contaminants either in small scale or large scale.

❑ *Small Scale Treatment of Water Supply*

The following treatment method can be considered as small scale treatment of water supplies for individuals and families.

Boiling of Water: It is difficult to practice boiling of water due to fuel and time shortage. Nevertheless boiling water is an important method to prevent water-borne diseases at the household level.

Filtration: Home made sand filters and *candle filters* are helpful at the household level.

Storage of Water: Storing the water at the household level for 24-72 hours will help to settle suspended impurities including pathogens. It creates an unfavourable environment for pathogenic micro-organisms, most pathogens do not survive long in water.

Disinfection: Disinfection of spring or well with Chlorine right after construction or when the need arises.

❑ *Large Scale Treatment of Water Supply*

Large scale water treatment involves the municipal treatment of water for domestic use. Treatment of surface water involves several stages that include sedimentation assisted with various chemical reagents and the passage of water through sand filters (slow sand filtration or rapid sand filtration process). Finally, the filtered water will be treated with chlorine doses to maintain a residual amount of the Chlorine, throughout the supply lines to avoid any incidental contamination during distribution ozone could also be used to treat water supply. However, this is expensive and does not have residual effect like that of chlorine. Whatever chemical is used administrating the right dose of the disinfectant is vital in the prevention and control of water-borne diseases.

❑ *Care During Transport and Storage*

When the water is transported from the source to the individual household, care should be given to the cleanliness of the containers. Rather than dipping with a cup or free hand from a storage container, controlled outlets such as faucets should be used.

❑ *Monitoring of Water Supply*

The environmental health technician should follow the safe supply of water through the following activities:

Sanitary Survey: A sanitary survey is an on-site inspection and evaluation of all conditions and practices of the water system to prevent any incident of water-borne illness. Sanitary survey should be made —

- when developing a new water source.
- when laboratory analysis of a sample taken from the water system indicates a health danger.
- when a water-borne disease outbreak occurs in or near the area served by the water supply.

Water Sample: Samples are taken from drinking water system to determine if the water supply system is safe or not. The actual number and frequency of sampling must take the local conditions into account. Indicator organisms are used to interpret the results of laboratory analysis.

❑ *Improved Sanitation*

The main water-borne diseases causing pathogens are shed in the faeces and therefore, the hygienic disposal of human waste is of the utmost importance. Each family must be access to latrine which all members use and clean. The latrine must be *acceptable* and *attractive to the users*.

Following attention should be given while constructing the latrines:

- Latrine should be located at a convenient distance from the water source and at a distance which encourage users to use it.
- The latrine should be sited at a lower elevation than the water supply.
- The latrine should be cleanable and have a cover with a handle or a vent pipe to discourage insect reproduction.
- Empowerment of individual families and communities through their active involvement in the construction of Latrines.
- It is advisable to have hand washing facilities nearby a latrine to help people to develop hygiene behaviour.
- In case of water carriage system there should be proper means of final disposal.

❑ *Hygiene Education*

Providing safe water supply and encouraging people to build latrines only will not necessarily ensure good health. For instance, evaluation of water and sanitation programme by the Ministry of Health in Botswana (CVNICEF) depicted in the following results:

- Water that was clean at the source was highly contaminated by the time it was consumed in the home.
- Household adopting Ventilated Improved Pit (VIP) latrines still had a high incidence of diarrhoea.
- Approximately, 75 per cent of the people with latrines in their compound did not use them.

It was then discovered that nearly 85 per cent of the households that had built Ventilated Improved Pit latrines had received health education either before, during or after their construction.

Therefore, health education is vital in raising people's awareness and ultimately being behavioural change towards hygiene.

Thus, the Environmental Health Technicians should focus on the following areas with respect to:

- The Causative Agents.
- The mode of transmission.
- The early diagnosis and control through the use of different teaching aids such as flip charts, posters, etc.

An integrated approach to the provision of safe and adequate water supplies, improved sanitation and hygiene education (like washing hands with soap and water) are the keys to successful prevention and control of water-borne diseases.

❑ *Laboratory Diagnosis of Water-Borne Diseases*

Appropriate collection and handling of specimen related to water-borne diseases for the laboratory diagnosis is necessary. Proper specimen collection is essential because the final laboratory results are dependent on the initial quality of the samples taken for the laboratory diagnosis.

Unless the appropriate specimen is properly collected, preserved and processed the detection of organism is very difficult.

Thus, the generation of the test results must begin with focusing on the collection process of the samples. The water-borne diseases may be detected in the laboratory through examining the specimen such as stool, urine, blood, using macroscopic and microscopic techniques to identify morphological criteria, culture and bio-chemical test and serological test for immunodiagnosis. Thus the proper collection techniques are very important to yield the required results of the diagnosis of the water-borne diseases.

The detection of parasite in stool depends on its proper collection of the Specimen Procedure for the collection of specimen.

The following procedure should be followed in the collection of stool specimen:

- Provide patients with specimen containers having a tight fit lids and appropriately cleaned.
- Collect sufficient quantities of stool. It should contain 4 ml of stool especially in diarrhoeal cases.
- Examine the stool as soon as possible. The liquid specimen should not wait more than 30 minutes.
- If specimen cannot be examined immediately as mentioned above they should be preserved with the appropriate preservative.
- Use the appropriate aseptic techniques in the collection for the bacterialogical analysis.

❑ *Collection of Blood Specimen*

The following care should be taken while collecting blood:

- Collect sufficient quantities of blood.
- If Plasma is required use the approximately anticoagulant.
- Process the specimen appropriately.

❑ *Safety Procedure*

Health Care Personnel, by virtue of their profession, can acquire certain illness beyond those acquired by all others, who live and work in our society. Health Professionals especially the Lab Personnel are at risk of acquiring infections from patients or their specimens which may be viral, bacterial, parasitic or fungal. However, this risk can be minimized if they follow universal work precautions.

Much of the contamination in the Laboratory occurs as a result of penetrating injuries caused by sharp objects and splashing of the specimen material.

❑ *Guidelines for Basic Practices and Procedures*

- Prevention of puncture wounds, cuts and abrasions as well as creating barriers to existing wounds.

- Application of simple protective measures designed to prevent contamination of the person and his/her clothing.
- Good basic hygiene practices, including regular hand washing with soap.
- Control of surface contamination by contaminants and disinfection procedure.
- Safe disposal of contaminated water.

❑ *Bio-Safety Regulation*

- Wear gloves when handling infectious materials or where there is a possibility of exposure to blood and other specimens.
- Discard gloves whenever they are thought to have become contaminated or perforated wash your hands as put on new gloves. Alternatively where there are economic constraints, wash gloved hands whenever collecting further samples.
- Do not touch your eyes, nose or other exposed skin parts with your gloved hands.
- Sterilize non-disposable items.
- Wherever autoclaving is not possible boiling must be for 30 minutes at least.

Thus, the water-borne diseases can be prevented through the following methods.

❑ *Safe Disposal of Human and Animal Waste*

- Construction of appropriate fly roof latrines.
- Sanitary Utilization of latrines.
- Health Education pertaining to behavioural change in improved personal hygiene such as washing hands with soap and water after defecation and before handling of food and safe disposal of faeces.

❑ *Provision of Safe Drinking Water*

- Protecting Public Sources of Water Supply such as springs, well, etc.
- Installing piped water from protected sources.
- Health education of the public relating to —
    - Boiling, filtering (sieving) drinking water.
    - Safe collection and storage of domestic water.

- Protecting source of water from contaminants by persons affected by guinea worm.

❑ *Early Detection and Treatment Cases*

- Participation in active case finding.
- Participation in notification of control of epidemic outbreaks of water-borne diseases.
- Participate in the eradication programme of water-borne diseases (such as polio, myelitis and guinea worms).

❑ *Immunization*

- Children have to vaccinated as soon as they are born and then at 6 weeks, 10 weeks, 14 weeks and at 9 months of age according to immunization schedule.

❑ *Home Management to Control Water-Borne Diseases*

The water-borne diseases are the diseases which are caused as a result of contamination of water used for household consumption.

- ◆ At the source such as wells, springs, ponds, rivers, by human or animal wastes of latrines are not commonly used.
- ◆ During the processes of —
  - Fetching water from protected source when unclear containers are used.
  - Storing and utilizing water at home when the container is not well protected or covered.
  - Hands not clean during the food preparation or eating.

❑ *Home Management of Diarrhoea*

Diarrhoea is the most common and dangerous manifestation of water-borne diseases especially among children under five years of age.

- ◆ *A mother who has a child with diarrhoea should give more fluid to child.*
  - Give her/him Water Oral Dehydration Salts (ORS) solution, or locally available drinks or liquids such as soups, rice water or fruit juice.
  - Give her/him about 1/4 to 1/2 a cup of 50-100 ml of fluid to drink after each stool.

◆ *Continue feeding including breast-feeding:*

- If an infant is breast-feeding, breast feed him normally.
- If the child is 6 months or older and is no longer being breast fed feed him/her normally when he/she wants.
- Even after diarrhoea as stopped, give him/her an extra feed a day for one week.

◆ *Watch the signs to Dehydration and take the child to nearest Health Institution:*

If the child is losing too much water by passing watery stools too many times or if she/he is getting more and more risk, this is dangerous. Take him/her to the health control or hospital immediately.

◆ *Signs of Dehydration:*

- Thirst.
- Sunken, fearless eyes.
- Little or no urine.
- The child getting light and lean very fast
  Dropping in of the "Soft Spot" (Font angel), the soft part in the centre of the top of an infant's head.
- The skin not stretching when pulled.
- Death, if not treat in time.

◆ *Prevention of Water-Borne Diseases:*

Water-borne diseases can be prevented by —

- Construction and appropriate use of the latrines.
- Avoiding open field disposal of wastes.
- Using protected source of water for household consumption, using clean containers with appropriate coverings for fetching and storing water.
- Boiling water especially consumed by children.
- Hand-washing ,with soap before eating food, before preparation of food and after visiting latrine.

Thus, the control, prevention and management of the different water-borne diseases can be checked at the household level through the home management, because the water-borne diseases are caused as a result of contaminated water used for the household consumption.

4. Health Policy Management

During the 1983, National Health Policy was formulated with the view to provide health services for all needy people equally, effectively and efficiently. Initiatives outlined in the National Health Policy have yielded fruitful results, while in the several areas its outcome has not been achieved as per expected objectives.

In the existing circumstances various required recommendations at the grassroots level are as follows:

- Time-bound programme for comprehensive primary health services linked with extension and health education that designed in the context of the ground reality that the elementary health problems can be resolved by the people themselves.
- Intermediation through "Health Volunteers" having appropriate knowledge, simple skills and requisite technologies.
- Establishment of a well worked out referral system to ensure that the patients load at the higher level at the hierarchy is not needlessly burdened by those who can be treated at the decentralized facility level.
- An integrated network of evenly spread speciality and super speciality services. Encouragement of such health facilities through private investments for patient who can pay, so that the draw on the government facilities are limited those entitled to for the free use.
- To maximize the broad based availability of the health services to the common people of the country on the basis of the realistic consideration of the capacity of the infrastructural resources of the health services.
- To decentralize public health services through need based injection of the substantial resources into the health sector from allocated budget, as per the ground realities in regard to the availability of the financial resources at the grassroots facility level.
- To ensure an access to and the benefits from the public health system which has been very uneven between the better endowed and the more vulnerable sections of the society, particularly women, children and socially disadvantaged sections of the society.
- To ensure appropriate delivery of National Public Health Programme.
- To strengthen the existing public health infrastructure which is far from the satisfactory as per the needs of the people and funding has also been insufficient.

- To deploy the medical personnel in such underserved remote areas, which has usually been a loosing battle.
- To involve and strengthen the role of Local Self-Government institutions especially Panchayati Raj Institutions.
- To strengthen education of Health care professional and revised and updated need based undergraduate medical syllabus which is outdated and unrelated to the contemporary needs of the community.
- To promote the use of generic drugs and medicines.
- Information, Education and Communication Activities should be widely promoted, propagated for improving awareness and bringing behavioural change among the common people in the remote areas.
- To promote health research in the field of new molecules and vaccines and need based applied and operational research.
- To strengthen the role of civil society in the public health delivery system.
- National Disease Surveillance Network should be strengthened from the decentralized public health facilities to the State/Central Government Health Administration.
- To ensure the enforcement of quality for food and drugs.
- Alternative system of Medicine, i.e. Ayurveda, Yoga, Naturopathy, Unani, Siddha and Homoeopathy (AYUSH) should be promoted which have substantial role due to inherent advantages such as delivery modest cost low level of technological input and growing popularity of natural plant based products in the underserved and remote area.
- To increase access to the decentralized public health system by deficient areas and by upgrading the infrastructure in the existing health institutions. Overriding importance would be given to encourage a more equitable access to health services across the social and geographical expanse of the country.
- To increase the aggregate public health investment through a substantially increased contribution by Central Government.
- To strengthen capacity of public health administration to render the effective health services.
- Contribution of the private sector in providing health services should be enhanced particularly the people who can afford to pay for services.
- Primacy should be given to the preventive and first five curative initiatives at the Primary Health Centres level through increased sectoral share of the allocation.
- To rationalize the use of drugs within the allopathic system.

5. Public Health Status

The Public health care requirements and public health care delivery system should be managed as per the requirements of the deprived, downtrodden sections of the society at the Primary, Secondary and Tertiary level of the health system. The important health requirements are as follows:

- To provide optimal expert care to the people.
- To achieve and maintain an standard of quality of health care.
- To ensure that the services at the CHC are commensurate with universal best practices and responsive and sensitive to the need of patients.
- Janani Suraksha Yojana and Janani Shishu Suraksha Karyakram should be implemented as per guidelines of the Indian Public Health Standards.
- New Born Care and Child Health Care and full immunization of infant and children against vaccine preventable diseases and Vitamin-A and management of malnutrition cases should be implemented and managed as per the guidelines of the Government of India.
- Requirements for the National Tuberculosis Programme included diagnosis services and manpower, equipments and laboratory consumables and treatment services at the Community Health Centres level should be made available as per norms of the Indian Public Health Standards.
- Family Planning Programme, National Health Programme including communicable disease such as Tuberculosis, National Vector-Borne Disease Control Programme, National Leprosy Eradication Programme, National Programme for Control of Blindness, Integrated Disease Surveillance Project, National Programme for Control of Deafness, National Mental Health Programme and National Programme for Prevention and Control of Cancer and Diabetes, Cardio Vascular Disease and Stroke, National Iodine Deficiency Disorder Control Programme, National Programme for Prevention and Control of Fluorosis, National Tobacoo Control Programme, National Programme for Health Care of Elderly, and other services delivery of health should be implemented at the Community Health Centres level as per the requirements of the interested, needy, downtrodden, deprived sections of the society.

- Manpower including public health unit, general duty officers, Nurses and Paramedical, administrative and Group-D staff, equipments, drugs, infrastructure should be made available at the facility level as per the guidelines of the Indian Public Health Standards.
- The minimum common health facilities required for the Community Health Centres include the New Born Care facilities, National Aid Control Programme, National Vector-Borne Disease Control Programme, Integrated Disease Surveillance Project, National Programme for Control of Blindness, requisite equipments, drugs, Blood storage, Charter statutory compliance and check-list for Operation Theatres should be appropriately made available as per the guidelines of Indian Public Health Standards.
- Standard Surgical Set-I (Instruments) at First Referral Units (essential), Standard Surgical Set-II (essential) and Standard Surgical Set-III (essential), Normal Delivery Kit (essential), Standard Surgical Set-IV (essential), Standard Surgical Set-V (essential) and Standard Surgical Set-VI (essential), miscellaneous Equipments for the Anesthesia (essential), Equipment for Neo-Natal Resuscitation (essential), and Material Kit for Transfusion (essential), and equipments for the Operation Theatre and Equipments for Radiology and spare ice pack box, immunization equipments and equipments required for the Non-communicable Diseases and Communicable disease should be made available at the Community Health Centres level as per the guidelines of the Indian Public Health Standards.
- Required Drugs in the Community Health Centres which include Emergency obstetric care drug kits, Drug kits for Sick New born and Child Care at First Referral Units/ Community Health Centres and other essential drugs, and Ayurvedic Medicines, Unani Medicines, Siddha Medicines, Homoeopathy Medicines and Blood storage facilities and equipments for laboratory tests, Diagnostic Services, laboratory equipments and model citizens charter, and Statutory Compliances and surgical safety and check-list for monitoring at the Community Health Centres level should be made available systematically as per the norms and standard of the Government of India.
- Implementation of various rural health activities should be properly ensured and monitoring, supervision of the health delivery system under National Rural Health Mission should meet the people's

health needs in rural areas as per the norms of the Ministry of Health and Family Welfare, Government of India.

- Various priorities, constraints and actions to overcome the constraints in achieving the targets and the priorities of the National Rural Health Mission should be ensured for appropriate delivery of the Public health requirement to the needy, interested deprived sections of the society serving in the remote rural areas.

6. Public Health Planning

Public Health Planning should be managed through need based planning from bottom to top, i.e. from Hamlet villages → Revenue villages → Village Panchayats → Nyaya Panchayats → Block Panchayat → District Level → State level up to National level, i.e. at the facility level and also from Auxiliary Nurse Midwife Centres/Anganwadi Centres → Sub Health Centres → Primary Health Centres → Community Health Centres → District Hospital → State Level Hospital or medical colleges.

The various public health activities and possible processes and illustrative norms as per guidelines of the Indian Public Health Standards for appropriate public health planning management at the facility level are as follows:

★ To organize visioning workshops at the facility level for promoting, preventing, curative and the promotive health care for government health functionaries, contractual personnel with new skills as per the need orientation on the details of the plan of action which is critical for the public health system owning the challenges of health planning and implementation.

★ To ensure effective institutionalization of the Community ownership, constitution and orientation of all community leaders at the Sub-Centre/Primary Health Centres and Community Health Centres, committees, representatives on functionality of facilities including physical and financial management at the facility level.

★ To allocate Untied grants to village health and sanitation committees for household surveys, health camps, sanitation drives, revolving fund, etc.

★ To ensure selection of training, monthly orientation, drug kit, support materials, travel expenses, etc. of the Community Health Workers Multi-purpose workers including Accredited Social Health Activists, Anganwadi workers, etc.

- To provide performance related incentives at sub-health centre level for disbursement to ASHAs/Anganwadi Workers through allocation of ₹ 5,000 as permanent advance to every village panchayat.
- To ensure selection and training of non-government health providers of health cares for promoting common treatment protocols and also promoting current practices and priorities.
- To recapsulate the physical infrastructure for village level health activities, i.e. ASHA to Work from the Anganwadi Centre because the Anganwadi Workers, have the responsibility for under 6 years children, pregnant women and adolescent girls.
- To ensure selection, provide remuneration and training of ANMs through filling up Auxiliary Nurse Midwife vacancies, identification of selection teams, training packages and the remuneration, etc. and improvement of mobility of ANMs with a provision for interest free loans for two wheelers could be explored.
- To fulfil the need to strengthen the monitoring and supervision role of the Lady Health Visitors, who may be called the Public Health Nurse who should be equipped to improve skills of ANMs, supervise their work and assign specific tasks to them, etc.
- To ensure selection, training and remuneration of the Staff Nurses and other paramedics including AYUSH stream at Primary Health Centres/Community Health Centres level.
- To organize multi-skilled and special programmes or their orientation has to be developed in state specific contexts through selection training and remuneration of Medical Officers at Primary Health Centres including the AYUSH streams, etc.
- To resolve the problems to get the services of specialists at Community Health Centres level through selection, training and remuneration of specialist at Community Health Centres level.
- To ensure construction, renovation maintenance of physical infrastructure of Sub-Health Centres through Village Panchayats Sub-Health Centres Committee and Village Panchayats must be mandated to undertake construction and maintenance of the facilities.
- To ensure Primary Health Centres level Panchayat Committee/ Rogi Kalyan Samiti will have the mandate to undertake and supervise improvement and maintenance of physical infrastructure.
- To form Rogi Kalyan Samiti at Community Health Centres level and Block Panchayat level to undertake constructional and

maintenance of Community Health Centres to ensure quality services through functional physical infrastructure.

- ★ To manage procurement and distribution of quality equipments and drugs in the public health system.
- ★ To ensure needful support to Below Poverty Line families for institutional deliveries with system for timely availability of financial resources under the Janani Suraksha Yojana at the facility level.
- ★ To arrange and allocation united grants to get ₹ 10,000 at Sub-Health Centres level and to get ₹ 50,000 as united grants for local health Action Planning at Community Health Centres level.
- ★ To support provision of Mobile Medical Units/Health Camps to ensure better health care to the doorsteps of the public in the rural area.

States are required to involve District Health Society/Rogi Kalyan Samiti/Non-governmental organizations in deciding the appropriate modality of operationalization of the Mobile Medical Units.

- ◆ To support for school health programme/adolescent health programme for screening of school children for detection of refractive errors and provide free spectacles to poor children including oral health awareness programme and screening programme for oral/dental problems for early identification and prevention.
- ◆ To organize Nutrition and Health Education programmes for the women groups.
- ◆ To allocate appropriate resources for surveys, camps and public hearings as per the local needs and as articulated in the Block, District and State level Annual and Perspective Health Action Planning.
- ◆ An appropriate Grants-in-Aid should be allocated to the Non-governmental organizations at the District, State and National levels.
- ◆ For local action that emerge as priorities in the Block/District Health Action Plans, Government should appraise need for innovation and suggest costs as per need and existing norms of the State Government.
- ◆ To provide appropriate financial assistance for the monitoring and evaluation costs for the ongoing implementation of public health programme at the facilities.
- ◆ To allocate financial support for the resources for contractual engagement of personnel with new skills, travel costs and management costs/contingencies at the facility level.

- To establish State Level Health Resource Centre for operatonalizing new ideas and also strengthening health delivery services at facility level.
- To support District and Block Level Health Resource Groups for ensuring development of capacities and for field based supervision of delivery of health services at facility level.
- To support research studies and planning activities and need based capacity building at the facility levels.
- To allocate appropriate financial support for the cost of core, basic and secondary public health care at the facility level.
- To manage resources for risk pooling and strengthening of nursing schools including improvement of physical infrastructure of Auxiliary Nurse Midwife training centres and other nursing institutions.
- To improve physical infrastructure of Sub-Health Centres/Primary Health Centres/Community Health Centres/District Hospital, etc.
- To form Rogi Kalyan Samiti/Hospital Management Committee to ensure degree of permanency and sustainability and management structures should be evolved at facility level.
- To ensure need based preparation of District/Block/Village Panchayat level Health Action Plans.
- To ensure preparation of Village panchayats → Block panchayat level → District and State level Public Report on Health Delivery System annually through independent agencies.
- To ensure universal coverage of all pregnant women with package of quality ANC services as per National guidelines.
- To increase in deliveries with Skilled Birth Attendants including institutional deliveries.
- To increase prevalence of exclusive Breast feeding.
- To ensure appropriate mechanism of monitoring and evaluation.
- To mainstream the AYUSH Health System at the health delivery facility level.

7. Management of Imperative of Public Health System

State Government of the Uttar Pradesh has formulated State Programme Implementation Plan and framed Management Imperatives for the appropriate implementation of the Public Health System at the facility level. The details of the management imperatives of the public health system has been illustrated in Table 4.1.

Table 4.1: Public Health Management

Sl. No.	*Strategic Areas*	*Issues Planning and Strategies*
1	*2*	*3*
		Public Health Planning Strategies
		◆ District Action Plans have been prepared for all District based on the Block Plans. Thus, addressing the area specific issues of poor health indicators. it is being ensured that there is a 10 per cent annual increase in the State Health Budget. Programme Implementation Plan is being compiled including detailed activities for RCH Programmes so as to provide comprehensive maternal, child, Adolescent Health and Family Planning services. Convergence is being ensured for the activities of interrelated programmes such as NPCB with SHP, RTI/STI clinics with AFHS clinics and UPSACS Blood Banks with FRU operationalization NIDDCP with BSPM, etc.
		◆ Also a detailed plan to ensure quality has been implemented in the District by formulating quality assurance committees at every facility level and developing a system of Monitoring from Stated Division → District → Block.
2.	Management Strengthening	◆ Mission Director of NRHM in the State as well as full time Finance Controller of Finance Department at SPMU.
		◆ All the state level activities proposed in State PIP have been included with full consultation with State Programme officers posted at Medical and Health and Family Welfare Department. For mainstreaming of AYUSH Directorate is being posed at SPMU on deputation so as to ensure linkage at every level to provide appropriate services of Indian system of Medicine.
3.	Developing a strong public health focus	◆ All the key cadre staff is being trained on the Public Health issues to deal with various problems related to public health.
		◆ Separate Public Health Cadre is under consideration at the level of State Government of Uttar Pradesh.
4.	Human Resources policies for doctors, nurses, paramedical staff and programme management staff	◆ For the vacancies of the regular posts of Doctors, recruitment is being done after proper advertisement, but even after selection not many doctors are joining the services as new recruits are expected to serve in the rural areas, for which the congenial atmosphere and appropriate facilities are not available. The Specialists and Lady Doctors have very good opportunity of getting good emoluments and better facilities in the urban private sectors, which is leading to higher attrition rate. For the contractual staff under NRHM, HR policy is being formulated by IIM, Lucknow.
5.	Human Resource Accountability	◆ Once the HR policy is finalized and implemented the various issues of HR will be streamlined. Performance Appraisal

(*Contd.*)

Table 4.1 (*Contd.*)

1	*2*	*3*
		against benchmarks will be the basis for renewal of contracts/promotions as well as incentives. HR policy will also include special incentives for HR posted in the difficult/ high focused areas and also on the basis of performance. ◆ Regular facility based monitoring is being done to ensure availability of Quality services for the purpose of delivery, new born care, immunization and FP services.
6.	Medical, Nursing and Paramedical Education (new institutions and upgradation of existing ones)	◆ The capacity for training of Medical students, Nurses, ANMs and Para medical staff is to be increased in various institutions conducting the courses. The capacity of ANM/ Nursing/Para Medical Staff has been increased tremendously in the private sector during last 4-5 years. Private Medical Colleges have also come up in the State during this period. Efforts are being made to increase the seats of students in Government Medical Colleges and at ANMTCs. ◆ All the State and Central Medical colleges functional in the State are being utilized as resource centres for various training programmes under CCSP, SNCU, NRC, Quality maternity services, centre of excellence for NSV, State Resource Centre for RNTCP, NPCB, etc.
7.	Training and Capacity Building	◆ The strengthening of ANM training centers at District level, RFPTCs at Division level and SIHFW at State level is being done to provide good quality of training to the participants. Comprehensive training plan has been prepared by the State Institute, training cell at DGFW and GM training at SPMU. This body is also monitoring the post-training outcomes for various training programmes. PPIUCD training is being imparted with the help of HLFPPT.
		Strengthening Services
8.	Policies on drugs procurement system and logistics management	◆ The State has formulated its policy to provide free drugs to all the patients attending the OPD of Government facilities for five days. All the indoor patients are being provided free quality medicines in the hospitals. Free Medicines are available right from the districts hospitals up to sub-centre level. Under JSSK, all the medicines and consumables are being provided free of cost to the patients of normal as well as caesarean deliveries to minimize out of pocket expenditure. EDL has been formulated by DG-MH and generic medicines are available on rate contract. The efforts are being made to setup a dedicated corporation for drug procurement through UPHSSP. Essential drug list is available at the DG-MH. website:www.uphealthup@nic.in
9.	Equipments	◆ A gap analysis has been carried out in all the districts to find out the deficiencies of equipments at various levels as

(*Contd.*)

Table 4.1 (*Contd.*)

1	*2*	*3*
		per norms and the same has been proposed by the districts in the DAPs. All the equipments are being procured with provision of AMC.
10.	Ambulance Services and Referral Transport	◆ Two types of ambulance services are available in the state. Emergency medical transport services (108) are functional in whole of the State with a total number of 988 ambulances to help referral transportation in case of an emergency. All the vehicles are GPS fitted and a control room is there for proper functionality. Another type of ambulance — UP Ambulance Seva has been provided at facility level for dropping back the mother and baby after delivery. Very soon 102 services are also to be started with a call centre in the State.
11.	New infrastructure and Maintenance of buildings; sanitation, water, electricity, laundry, kitchen, facilities for attendants	◆ MCH wings at DWH and selected CHCs being constructed since 2012-13 and completion will be ensured by the end of the year 2014. In the same facilities, a proposal of renovations of doctors and staff residences has been included. Also proposal for trauma wings in selected 10 districts has been incorporated. ◆ In 500 sub-centers, where delivery load is high, proposal for one additional labour room has been included. ◆ Facility of ASHA ghar in 100 hospitals, where load is high. ◆ Proposal for maternity wings in 80 CHCs (30 units with 50 bed and 50 units with 30 beds) has been included. ◆ Bio-Medical waste management up to block level facilities is being proposed. Also hospital cleaning and upkeep is being addressed this year. ◆ 325 new sub-centres are to be constructed, where SCs are still functional in rented building. 353 new sub-centres under comprehensive village development schemes are to be constructed.
12.	Diagnostics	◆ The state is already ensuring Review on access, efficacy and adequacy. Mechanism of local decision making and authorization, responsibility and accountability. ◆ Mechanism for assured access at affordable cost. Placing prescription audit system. ◆ Placing PPP mechanism in case of need and linkages with private providers. ◆ There is a provision of free diagnostics for pregnant women and sick neonates and children under JSSK.
		Community Involvement
13.	Patient's feedback and grievance redressal	◆ Two call centres (NRHM helpline) with toll free number are functional at state level — At SPMU 1800-180-1900 At DG-MH 1800-180-5145

(*Contd.*)

Table 4.1 (*Contd.*)

1	*2*	*3*
		◆ The calls received from the districts are addressed by the concerning Programme Officers at SPMU and Directorates. Corrective actions are taken by the concerning DG or MD within 7 days. ◆ Tahseel Divas is being conducted on first and third Tuesdays and Thana Divas on two fixed days of the month. ◆ At the level of Chief Minister of the State regular sessions of Jan Sunwai is being organized.
14.	Community Participation	◆ To sensitize and empower the VHSNC members a detailed proposal of orientation programme is being included. To strengthen and support ASHAs, a proposal of ASHA strengthening and monitoring is being included this year, which comprises of State and Regional ASHA Facilitators and Block Community Process Managers. In remaining 58 districts 1 Facilitator on 20 ASHAs is proposed this year (17 districts already have such Facilitators). Proposal for Community Monitoring is being included.
15.	IFC/BCC	◆ There is defined BCC strategy in the state, according to which various IEC/BCC activities are being undertaken and planed. ◆ Plan for effective coverage of vulnerable, underserved and high risk area population to bring about behaviour change to achieve good health indicators. ◆ Strong emphasis on local role models and access to IPC at community level.
		Convergence, Coordination and Regulation
16.	Inter-Sectoral Convergence	◆ Good convergence is being maintained with WCD, PRI, Education, SSA and RD Departments. ◆ With the help of ICDS functionaries, acutely malnourished children are being identified and are being treated at NRCs. Promotion of exclusive breast feeding and timely complimentary feeding is being done with the help of ICDS Health, NGOs and Community. ◆ Convergence is being ensured in programmes like — VHND, BSPM, VHNSC, RL BSGY and SABALA. ◆ For PIP formulation convergence being ensured with all partner departments and developmental partners.
17.	NGO/Civil Society	◆ Proposal for Community Monitoring is being included In this year PIP which will be done with support of PFI and UPHSSP.
18.	Private Public Partnership	◆ Accreditation of private hospitals to provide sterilization and IUCD services. ◆ Social franchise through voucher scheme and merry gold health networking is being proposed.

(*Contd.*)

Table 4.1 (*Contd.*)

1	*2*	*3*
		◆ 8 ambulance services in partnership with GVK-EMRI have been launched in the state. New proposed ALS and BLS will also be operationalized in PPP mode.
19.	Regulation of Services in the private sector	◆ PHSSP has been assigned to understand, review, revise and finalize the Clinical Establishment Act at the State level. ◆ To ensure quality of sendees, Quality Assurance Cell has been established at State and District level. Appropriate check-lists have been developed and detailed plan of monitoring from State, Division and District has been finalized. Field visits have already started from the State, Division and Districts.
		Monitoring and Supervision
20.	Strengthening data capturing, validity/ triangulation	◆ The state has formulated a strategy for birth and death registration under Civil Registration System. A detailed proposal is being included this year. ◆ Strengthening data capturing, validity/triangulation — With the introduction of Facility based reporting under HMIS, more and more emphasis will now be on improvement of data, quality of health indicators which includes indicators like registration of births and deaths under Civil Registration System (CRS); capturing of births in private institutions. Government of India has upgraded the skills of State data Managers by providing training on tools like — SAS VDD which has really helped in making usage of data available through various sources, *viz.* AHS, NFHS, DLHS, HMIS so as to establish reliability of health data prior to actual use in planning and decision making. Data triangulation mechanisms are proposed to be used in year 2013-14 to increase reliability on HMIS data, revealing unique findings and providing a clearer understanding of the problem.
21.	Supportive Supervision	◆ For supportive supervision, monitoring and evaluation in year 2012-13 system has been developed to monitor various schemes from different levels, i.e. State, Division, District and Block levels. For the purpose of monitoring check-lists have been developed in consensus with NHSRC. The detailed guidelines have been disseminated to the divisions and districts for monitoring purposes and check lists have been specifically prepared to be used by different levels of officers.
22.	Monitoring and Review	◆ Regular meetings of State/District Health Societies are being convened under the chairmanship of DM in which the progress of schemes is also being reviewed and instructions are given to the concerned officers to take

(*Contd.*)

Table 4.1 (*Contd.*)

1	*2*	*3*
		corrective actions whenever required so as to implement the scheme successfully with good outcomes. ◆ At the State Headquarter regular review meetings are being conducted by the Mission Director/Principal Secretary — M and H of concerned district officials, Divisional PM/DPM units as well as of the State level officers of the Directorates, SIHFW and SPMU. ◆ In the Executive Committee Meetings being conducted almost every month regular physical and financial review of the schemes is being done and instructions for corrective action issued. ◆ The HMIS data is being regularly reviewed by the State Programme Officers for improvement of the schemes and better data uploading wherever there is fault in the data.
23.	Quality Assurance	◆ State Quality Assurance Cell at State level has been formed. Establishment of Divisional and District QAC is under process.
24.	Surveillance	◆ Integrated Disease Surveillance programme is being implemented in the State for various communicable diseases. State level unit is being strengthened, so as to tracking of services and evaluation activities. ◆ Maternal death audit system is present and programme will be effectively implemented in next year.
25.	Leveraging Technology	◆ In the year 2013-14, ICT based tools are being introduced in many areas. It is felt that programmes can only be planned and monitored in better way if we use these tools to have real time data during the implementation phase of any programme. This year Resource Mapping Management System for Health facilities in Uttar Pradesh is being proposed which will use geo-database on Google Earth. This will help in quick decision making while planning for resources. All MMUs, ambulances are fitted with GPS devises to have real time data on movement of vehicles. This year CUG phones are being given to all ASHAs, ANMs and MOICs so as to have better communication among health functionaries in entire State. IVRS based interventions like mobile kunj, Makhi, etc. are being proposed to promote Inter-Personnel Communication/BCC among ASHAs, ANMs relating to ANC, HBNC, etc. In recently launched Swasthay Guarantee Yojana Scheme, IVRS based application is being proposed to take real time data using Mobile Phones.

Source: National Rural Health Mission, State Programme Implementation Plan, Uttar Pradesh (2013-14).

8. Management Structure of Public Health System

National Rural Health Mission Programme seeks to decentralize with adequate devolution of powers and delegation of responsibilities has to have an appropriate implementation mechanism that is accountable in order to facilitate this process and implement the District Action Plan under the National Rural Health Mission has proposed a structure right from the Village to Block-District-State-National levels with details in key functions and the functional powers.

The National Rural Health Mission framework for District Planning for Health, Ministry of Health and Family Welfare-2006 formulated flowchart for programme management from Village level → Block level → State level → National level. The management structure of Public Health System at various levels has been depicted in Figure 4.1.

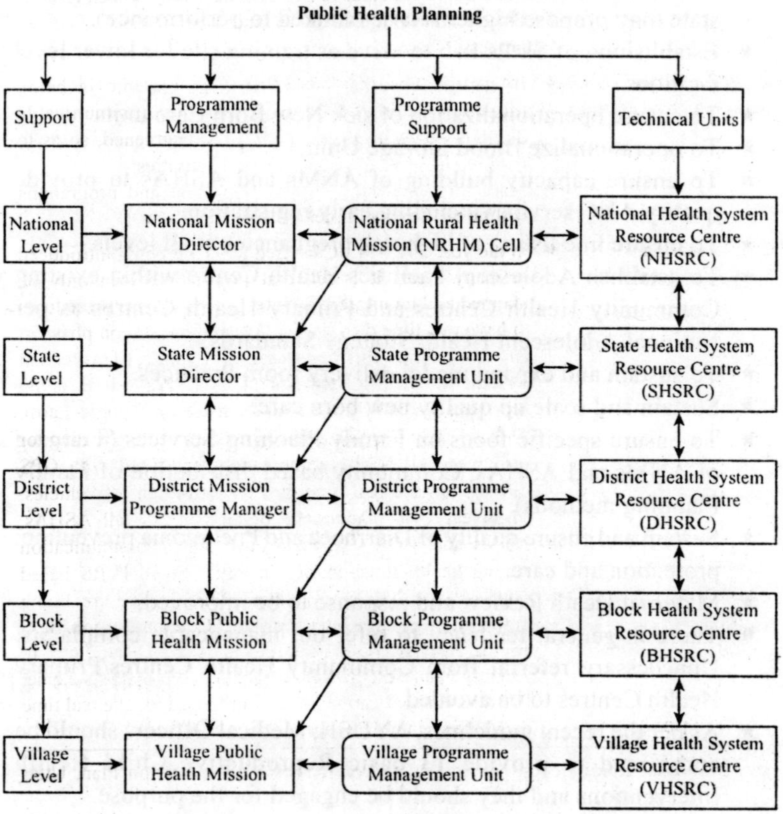

Figure 4.1: Management Structure of Public Health System.

9. Facilities Based Management of Health System

The facility based management of health system includes planning, recruitments and implementation of health delivery at various levels —

- ★ Strengthen the District Action Planning and Setting of priority based on need of the local people at the village level.
- ★ To support for additional human resource.
- ★ Ensuring functional human resources.
- ★ To strengthen the waste management system across all health facilities.
- ★ To strengthen district level vigilance and monitoring committees.
- ★ To increase the frequency of supportive supervision visits by district level government health officers.
- ★ To ensure recruitment of key staff obstetrician and Paediatricians state may propose higher salaries (linked to performance).
- ★ Establishing of Skills Lab to serve as training site for lower level facilities.
- ★ To ensure operationalization of sick New Born Care units.
- ★ To operationalize Blood Storage Unit.
- ★ To ensure capacity building of ANMs and ASHAs to provide quality ANC services including early registration.
- ★ To ensure line listing of high risk pregnancies at all levels.
- ★ To establish Adolescent Facilities Health Centre within existing Community Health Centres and Primary Health Centres as per National Adolescent Health Strategy Standards.
- ★ To sustain and expand model delivery room Practices.
- ★ Sustain and scale up quality new born care.
- ★ To ensure specific focus on Family Planning Services (Training of ANMs and ASHAs, Community based distribution of Family Planning methods).
- ★ Sustain and ensure quality of Diarrhoea and Pneumonia prevention, protection and care.
- ★ Maternal Death Review and response to be improved.
- ★ There is general tendency to refer out manageable complaints. Unnecessary referral from Community Health Centres/Primary Health Centres to be avoided.
- ★ As per the recent guidelines, AYUSH, Medical Officers should be authorized to provide 13 basic Reproductive Child Health Interventions and they should be engaged for the purpose.
- ★ Quality of services at private health sector to be ensured.

- ★ To strengthen Village Health Sanitation and Nutrition Days to include ANC, PNC Treatment of Childhood Illness and Nutrition Counselling.
- ★ To initiative and complete ASHA training in the module 6 and 7 and strengthen their skills in hygiene counselling.
- ★ Ensure intensive community based counselling on danger signs of pregnancy, postpartum and new born.
- ★ To strengthen community based nutrition counselling and support for infants and children.
- ★ General Neglect of Disease Control Programme to be addressed by constant review system.

10. Implementation Framework

Local Community should be sufficiently empowered to take leadership in strengthening the public health system. The Panchayati Raj Institutions right from the Village Panchayat to the District level would have to be given ownership of public health delivery system in their respective jurisdiction.

National Rural Health Mission seeks to empower the Panchayati Raj Institutions at each level, i.e. Village Panchayat – Block Panchayat – Zila Panchayat level to take leadership to control and manage Public Health Delivery System and Infrastructure at the District and Sub-District and also at the facility level —

- Village Health and Sanitation Committee should be formed in each village within the overall framework of Gram Panchayat/ Gram Sabha in which proportionate representation from all the hamlets should be ensured. An adequate representation to the disadvantaged categories like women, Scheduled Caste/Scheduled Tribes/Other Backward Castes and Minority Communities would also be given due priority at the village level.
- The Sub-Health Centres at village level will be responsible and accountable to the village panchayat as it should have a local committee for its management with adequate representation of the Village Health and Sanitation Committee.
- The Primary Health Centres at village panchayat level or cluster of the village panchayat level will be responsible to the elected representatives of the village panchayats, where it is located, the other village panchayats covered by the Primary Health Centres would be suitably represented in its management at facility level.

- Block level Primary Health Centres and Community Health Centres should have involvement of the Panchayati Raj Institutions elected leaders in the Management even through the Rogi Kalyan Samiti would also be formed for day-to-day management of the different affairs of the Hospital.
- Zila Panchayat at the District level should be directly responsible for the budgets of the health sector and for the planning for people's health requirements at the facility level.
- With the development of capacities and systems the entire public health management at the District level would devolve to the District Health Society which would be under the effective leadership and control of the Zila Panchayat with the participation of the Block Panchayat and Village Panchayat.

National Health Mission has sought amendments to Acts and Statutes in the State to institutionalize community led action for the health services and to fully empowered local bodies in the effective management of the Public Health Delivery System at grassroots level.

Therefore, the National Rural Health Mission would attempt to transfer funds, functions and functionaries to the Panchayati Raj Institutions. The concerted efforts with the involvement of the Non-governmental organizations and other resource institutions should be made to build capacity of the elected representatives and user group members for improved and effective management of the Public Health System at the village level.

To facilitate local level action the National Rural Health Mission should provide untied grants at different levels, *viz.* Village Level, Gram Panchayat Level, Block Panchayat Level and District Panchayat Level, Village Health and Sanitation Committee, Sub-Health Centres, Primary Health Centres and Community Health Centres and District Hospital.

The Monitoring Committee should be formed at the facility level with the Participation of the Panchayati Raj Institutions representatives, user groups, non-governmental organizations, representatives to facilitate their inputs in the monitoring and planning process and to enable the committee to be involved in broad based review and appropriate suggestions for the planning of the public health system.

A system of periodic "*Jan Sunwai*" or "*Jan Samvad*" at various levels would empower community members to engage in providing direct feedback and suggestions for improvement in the Public Health Delivery System at the facility level. Promotion of equity and partnership has been one of the main challenges, therefore, the empowerment of vulnerable and weaker section of the society through education and health education, providing priority to the area/hamlets/households inhabited by them running fully functional facilities, exemption for Below Poverty Line families from all charges ensuring access, risk pooling, human resource development capacity building, recruiting volunteers from amongst them are important management strategies which should be adopted at the facility level.

The success of decentralization experiment would depend on the strength of the pillars, supporting the pillars of the process of public health system. It is imperative to ensure that the management capacity should be built at each level. It should provide the management costs up to 6 per cent of the total annual plan approved for the District as has been introduced under the Reproductive and Child Health-II Programmes. Apart from the Medical and Para Medical Staff such services would include skills for financial management, improved community processes, procedures, procurement logistics, improved collection and maintenance of the data, the use of information technologies, management information system and improved monitoring and evaluation system.

Public Health System should also establish strong managerial capacity at the Block Level, as the Block would be the link between the village and the Districts. At the District Level Health Mission should support and insist on developing health management capacities and introducing policies in systematic manner so that over time all the District Programme Officers and their leadership are professionally qualified public health managers. The management stress at all levels should be accountable to the Panchayati Raj Institutions.

The available financial resources under the management cost could also be used for improving the work environment as such improvement directly leads to better outcomes at the village level. The management structures hold the key to the success of any programme and effective delivery of the public health system with detailing will be a priority. The task clarity, funds flow, powers, functions, account keeping, audit should be ensured at every level for successful delivery of the health services at facility level.

In view of the expected outcomes in the National Health Mission, the existing staff of the Sub-Health Centres/Primary Health Centres/ Community Health Centres/District Hospital are being carefully assessed to see how structure can be reoriented to health delivery more efficiently and effectively. The local authorities will constantly undertake review of management structure and devolution of powers and functions to carry out any mid-course correction at the facility level.

Block level policy will be of priority activity under the Public Health System. In view of the time line needed efforts to make all facilities fully functional, specialists working in the Primary Health Centres would be relocated at the Community Health Centres to facilitate their early conversion to First Referral Units. The outreach programmes are being organized with "*Block Pooled*" Community Health Centres as well as nodal point.

Public Health System would attempt to set-up Block level management capacities as per the local requirement. The behaviour of the Block Chief Medical Officer's Office to support the supervision of Public health activities in the Block would be the priority. The support of the Block Level Community Health Centres would also aim at improving the mobility and connectivity of the health functionaries with the support for Ambulance, Telephone, Computers, Electricity connection to provide needful infrastructural support at the facility level.

Monitoring and accountability framework should be managed through community based monitoring, external surveys and stringent internal monitoring. Rogi Kalyan Samiti and community, etc. should be expected to monitor the physical and financial performance of the public health facilities at the grassroots level.

The Health Monitoring and Planning Committees should be formed at the Primary Health Centres, Block, District and State Levels to ensure community based monitoring of the health delivery system along with facilitating relevant inputs for planning at the facility level.

Management of Public Health System should be attempted through transfer of funds, functions and functionaries to the Panchayati Raj Institutions. A system of periodic "Jan Sunwai" or "Jan Samvad" should be organized at various levels to empower the Community members to engage in providing direct feedback and needful suggestions for improvement in the Public Health Delivery System.

11. Strengthening Public Health System

The Public health delivery system aims at inclusive health and improved access to quality health care for those residing in the remote rural areas particularly women, children, and the poor by promoting intergradation decentralization and encouraging community participation in the health programme.

The "Disability Adjusted Life Years" (DALYs) in effect meant a focus on the Reproductive and Child Health and vertical Health Programme related to Tuberculosis, HIV/AIDS, Vector-Borne Diseases and Blindness Control Programme.

An important recommendation for the appropriate management of the public health delivery system has been illustrated as under:

- Through strengthening Public Health Delivery System and Health facilities as per norms and standard guidelines of Indian Public Health Standards.
- Mainstreaming the AYUSH health system at the facility level.
- Strengthening Community Health Care through Community level activities which has been designed with the ASHA Programme.
- To ensure Public Private Partnership in the Public Health System.
- To ensure Panchayati Raj Institutions and the Community Action.
- Through exploring New Health Financing Mechanism.
- To ensure District Health Action Plan, Block Health Action Plan and Village Level Health Action Plan.
- Through strengthening Medical Education.
- Public Health Delivery System should be ensured through the improved provision of Reproductive and Child Health services which broadly refers to the establishment of First Referral Units and 24 × 7 health care facilities at the village level.
- Improving quality of care in public health system through adoption of Indian Public Health Standards, ensuring skill gaps and standards treatment protocols, Hospital Management Societies, Rogi Kalyan Samiti, Untied funds, and quality improvement programmes.
- Access to safe delivery system should be ensured through Janani Suraksha Yojana, Emergency response and Patient Treatment's transport system and increasing access and utilization of outreach services disease control programme especially vector-borne diseases control programmes, i.e. Malaria, Japanese Encephalitis, Dengue and Chikungunya, Swine Flu, Kala-Azar, Lymphatic Filariatis, etc. and appointment of appropriate Human Resource for strengthening public health system and expansion, improvement in the Medical Nursing and Technical Education.
- To resolve the problems of retention overlaps through initiating innovative strategies for attracting and retaining the skilled professionals especially through incentives, workers management, educational strategies and ensuring regulatory system at the facility levels.

◆ To ensure management of community process, i.e. Accredited Social Health Activists, through training, support structure and payments to ASHAs in time.

12. Quality Assurance in Public Health System

Health care delivery system at Primary, Secondary and Tertiary level should be strengthened through quality care assurance as per guidelines of the Indian Public Health Standards which mainly included provision of optimal expert care to the community and making health care services more responsive and sensitive to the needs and aspirations of the community.

Quality assurance in the public health care system can be assured through the health services —

- Care to routine and emergency cases in surgery.
- Care of routine and emergency case in medicines.
- * Specific mention has been made for handling of all emergencies.
- 24-hour delivery services including normal and assisted deliveries.
- Essential and Emergency obstetric care — including surgical intervention like caesarean section and other medical interventions.
- Full range of family planning services including laparoscopic services.
- Safe abortion services.
- New Born Care.
- Routine and Emergency Care of sick children.
- Other management including nasal packing tracheostomy, foreign body removal, etc.
- All National Health Programmes should be delivered at the Community Health Centres and integration with the existing programmes.

The quality assurance should be managed as per norms of the Indian Public Health Standards —

- Specialist care in the Community Health Centres of acceptable standards.
- "Assured Service" provided at Community Health Centres.
- Apart from the existing 4 specialists in surgery, medicines, obstetrics and Gynaecology and Paediatrics, the services of Anesthetist and Public Health Manager on contractual basis should be appointed to ensure optimal utilization and good quality services.

- Necessary supporting staff should be made available as it already exists including Public Health Nurse, Auxiliary Nurse Midwife and the ASHA.
- Equipments and infrastructure already exists will have to be utilized as best as possible with re-modelling or rearrangement if necessary. New construction will follow the specifications spelt out in details as per guidelines of Indian Public Health Standards.
- Essential drug lists at the Community Health Centres level should be updated to ensure proper treatment.
- Laboratory facilities and other support services will be strengthened — laundry, diet, Referral Transport and waste management should be proposed to be outsourced after appropriate training.
- Capacity building should be ensured at the facility level through periodic training of all cadres.
- It is mandatory to every Community Health Centre to have Rogi Kalyan Samiti to ensure accountability.
- Every Community Health Centre shall have the "*Charter of Patient Rights*" displayed prominently at the entrance.
- Every Community Health Centre shall have standard Treatment. Protocols for Common ailments through Consumer Forum and Rogi Kalyan Samiti should be arranged and managed.

Minimum requirements of the delivery of health services should be ensured through clinical manpower and support manpower and appointment of the Public Health Manager and appropriate availability of the equipments, drugs, investigative facilities, and physical infrastructure should be made available as per norms of the Indian Public Health Standards.

Quality assurance for the Vector-Borne Diseases especially Malaria, Filariasis, Japanese Encephalitis, Kala-Azar, Dengue and Chikungunya Swine Flu should be ensured at the facility level through appropriate provision of Drugs, Equipments, and other physical and infrastructure should be made available at Health Delivery Centres as per norms of the Indian Public Health Standards.

Adoption of Model Citizen's Charter should be ensured with the view to provide a framework which enables citizens to know —

- What Services are available?
- Quality of Services they are entitled?
- The means through which complaints regarding denial or poor qualities of health services will be addressed.

Hospital Waste Management based on Bio-Medical Waste (Management and Handling) Rules, 1998 has been notified under the Environment Protection Act, 1986 (29 of 1986) by Ministry of Environment and Forest, Government of India. Various categories of Bio-Waste Management, its storage and collection, transportation and treatment of the Hospital Waste and safety measures, training, administrative management and coordination between Hospital and outside agencies should be properly coordinated, and managed as per standard norms.

Appropriate framework of Governance should be ensured through institutional framework, at the State level — State Health Mission, State Health Society and State Programme Management Unit and at the District level — District Health Society and District Programme Management Unit and Block level — Block Programme Management Unit and the village level — Village Programme Management Unit and Rogi Kalyan Samiti (Hospital Development Society) and Village Health Sanitation and Nutrition Committees should be formed to ensure proper management of the delivery of the public health services at the grassroots level, i.e. health facility level.

Public Health Management skills should be ensured through encouraging qualifications in public health or public health management among Medical Staff and supporting staff and management processes for the decentralized planning and developing Health Management Information System and building Institutions for technical assistance and knowledge management to ensure quality assurance in the appropriate need based delivery of public health services at the facility level for deprived, resourceless unserved and underserved downtrodden below poverty line women, children and weaker sections of the society surviving in the remote villages.

13. Public Health Programme Management

The management imperatives for the various Public Health Programmes include mainly Reproductive and Child Health Flexible Pool, Mission Flexible Pool, Routine Immunization and National Disease Control Programmes are being implemented under the National Rural Health Mission Programme at the facility level. The management of various public health programmes should be implemented at the facility level as per norms and guidelines of the Indian Public Health Standards.

A. *Management of Maternal Health*

Key Maternal Health Indicators and Janani Suraksha Yojana, Janani Shishu Suraksha Karyakram, operationalization of comprehensive Abortion Care services workshop/meetings, human resource arrangement, training and Information, Education, Communication and Behaviour change communication and procurement of equipments and drugs and other requisite infrastructure should be managed as per norms of the Indian Public Health Standards.

B. *Management of Child Health*

Priorities to reduce Neo-Natal Deaths through the facility based interventions and priorities Sick New Born Care Units, New Born Stabilization Units, New Born Care Corners and Nutrition Rehabilitation Centres and human resources, training for Navjat Shishu Suraksha Karyakram, Essential New Born Care Equipment Training and Integrated New Management of Neo-Natal and Childhood Illness training and Home based New Care and Infant Young Child Feeding Management of Diarrhoea, Bal Swasthya Poshan Mah — Information, Education, Communication and Procurement of Equipments and Drugs, etc. should be arranged and managed as per norms of the Government of India.

C. *Management of Family Planning*

The population policy looks at the issues related to population stabilization and improvement of the health status of people particularly women and children in a holistic manner. The family planning activities including the plan for facilities providing female sterilization services on fixed days and compensation for sterilization for male and female and plan for Post Partum Sterilization including spacing method and performance based reward to institutions and providers and incentives for ASHA, social marketing of contraceptives, other strategies, human resource, training and information, education and communication, 'World Population Day' celebration, procurement of drugs and materials and Public Private Partnership should be ensured for appropriate management of family welfare programme at the facility level.

D. *Adolescent Reproductive and Sexual Health*

Adolescent Reproductive and Sexual Health through establishing appropriate infrastructure, training and Menstrual Hygiene Training to adolescent and launch of SABLA Programme for addressing the issues of anemia in adolescent and procurement of Deworming Tablets under Menstrual Hygiene and implementation of Rashtriya Bal Swasthya Karyakram, proper arrangement of human resources, training and Information, Education and Communication Programme, should be organized to ensure appropriate implementation of Adolescent Reproductive and Sexual Health Programme at facilities level.

F. *Pre-Conception, Pre-Natal Diagnostic Techniques and Sex Ratio*

Sex Ratio is an important indicator to measure gender equity. Rapidly decreasing sex ratio is likely to create severe gender imbalance that can destroy the social fabric. It should also be viewed both as child right issue (girls are killed either through sex selective abortions or die prematurely due to violence and neglect). State and District level Pre-conception, Pre-Natal Diagnostic Techniques Cell should be made functional through proper inspection and monitoring and senitization and orientation workshops, training and capacity building programme should be organized to address discrimination against girl child and creating awareness regarding the provision of PCPNDT Act and its enforcement at the grassroots level.

G. *Infrastructure and Human Resources*

Appropriate deployment of human resources for Maternal Health, Child Health, Family Planning, Adolescent Reproductive Sexual Health, Routine Immunization, Dental Doctors and other routine programmes at the facility level should be ensured.

Proper training programme should also be organized for life saving anesthesia, skill training, Emergency, obstetrics care training skill Birth Attendant, obstetrics care training, Skill Birth Attendant Training, RTI/STI, MTP and Adolescent Reproductive Sexual Health Training, skill upgradation training for logistic management and sub-centre management training and ASHA training should be organized for appropriate management of various programmes at the grassroots level. Strengthening of existing training institutions should also be organized as per norms of the Government of India.

H. *Programme Management*

For effective management of activities under National Rural Health Mission, the State Programme Management Unit has been established in which Government Doctors, designated as General Manager, Technical Consultant and Programme Coordinators, etc. Most of the staff have been hired on contract, some have been posted on deputation from relevant government departments and some staff is on loan basis from SIFPSA. Programme Management Unit have been established at Division, District, Block Level Programme Management Unit.

Therefore, strengthening of State Programme Management Support Unit, and strengthening of Divisional Programme Management Unit of SIFPSA, and strengthening of District Programme Management Unit and strengthening of others including supportive supervision/mobility support/field visits should be promoted efficiently, effectively and curative health care delivery system at the facility level.

State, Divisional, District, Block and Village panchayat level evaluation, monitoring and review of the delivery of public health system should be implemented.

I. *Accredited Social Health Activists*

Various programmes especially training for Accredited Social Health Activists, drug kits, Annual ASHA Sammelan/Diwas, Uniform for ASHA, Payment Vouchers and Register for ASHA, News Letter and ASHA Award, Scheme, ASHA Mentoring Groups, Village Health Index Register, Area Specific Innovations under ASHA Programme. ASHA support system, untied funds and Annual Maintenance Grant for ASHA should be provided as per norms of the Government. Appropriate support should also be made available to Rogi Kalyan Samiti and Village Health Sanitation and Nutrition Committee to ensure quality and timely delivery of the health care services at the facility level.

J. *Hospital Strengthening*

Hospital strengthening should be ensured through provision of trauma wings, construction of Additional Buildings in District Hospitals, Spill-over — Maternity Wings in District Women Hospitals having 100 Bedded facilities and construction of 30 Bedded and 50 Bedded facilities at Community Health Centres and spillover — Primary Health Centres, Repair/Rennovation of State Drug Warehouse, Spillover District Drug Warehouse, Patient Relation Shed/ASHA Grah, and third party evaluation of the construction of works and sub-centre rent the contingencies should be ensured and managed at the facility level to provide needful delivery of Public health services.

K. *New Construction Rennovation of Setting-up*

New Construction of Maternity Wings in the Community Health Centres (30 and 50 Bedded) and Construction of Sub-Centre and setting up of Engineering Wing and setting up of Emergency Care learning centre should be made available at the facility level to fulfil the ever-increasing demand of the growing population.

L. *Health Action Plan*

Programme Implementation Plan should be formulated through sustained participation at Village, Block and District Level with active participation of Panchayati Raj Institutions, ICDS Rural Development and other important stakeholders.

Sustained participation of Rogi Kalyan Samiti and District Health Societies should be ensured in the Programme Implementation Plan formulation orientation workshop, training and capacity building of Panchayati Raj Institutions at State/District Health Society, Community Health Centres/Primary Health Centres, and Village Health Sanitation and Nutrition Committee should be organized at various levels.

M. *Mainstreaming of AYUSH*

Ayurveda, Yoga, Naturopathy, Unani, Siddha and Homoeopathy (AYUSH) systems of Medicines have proven promotive, preventive and curative health care with mainstream health care services, as per modified centrally sponsored Scheme for Development of AYUSH under National Rural Health Mission with innovations, human resources, drugs and consumables, etc. activities have been proposed with the view to strengthen the quality health delivery services. Strengthening of Information, Education, Communication, Implementation, Capacity for maternal health campaign "*Chhar Gaanth*", "*Chance Kyon Lena Hai*" and Child Health Family Planning "*Khushi Ka Mantra*" and routine immunization. Essential medical transport services, preconception, pre-natal diagnostic techniques, Medical Mobile Unit and Referral Transport/ Patient Transport System including "108" — EMTS Sewa, UP Ambulance Sewa and "102" Ambulance Sewa, etc. should be properly implemented and managed as per needs of the suffering patients.

N. *Innovations*

Various innovations such as inter-sectoral Convergence for Blood storage at the First Referral Units, Free Transport Facility through UPSRTC to the living with HIV/AIDS for their treatment related travel, Blood Mobile Van and District Specific Innovation and innovations related to immunization and to scale up of "*My Home My Village*" for tracking of immunization and Management of Information System, and the Innovations of Mobile Kunji, State Nutrition Mission, Mini Skills Lab and Mobile Nurse Training innovative programme should be implemented to ensure appropriate need based delivery of public health services.

O. *Planning Implementation and Monitoring*

Quality enhancement in health care has been recognized as an essential cornerstone for promoting equity and maximizing health gain. To address the issue of enhancing the quality of health care services rendered through establishment of Quality Assurance Network at all facility levels.

In continuation of our Quest for delivery high quality health services, Quality Assurance Cell and State Quality Assurance Working Groups have been formed to ensue appropriate planning and monitoring of the delivery of the public health system.

Procurement of equipments, Drugs and Consumables, Construction of the Drug Warehouse at state, Divisional and District level Drug Warehouse should be ensured qualitatively. Health Insurance Scheme for all ASHAs by LIC of India and Jan Shree Bima Yojana should be implemented as per norms of the Government of India.

State Health Resource Centre should be established. Research studies/ analysis and Programme evaluation should be used as a valuable tool for strengthening the quality of programme and improve the outcomes of the public health delivery system.

State Public Health Resource Institute should be established and support services for the Japanese Encephalitis/Acute Encephalitis Syndrome and Malaria under National Vector-Borne Disease Control Programme and additionally for Revised National Tuberculosis Control and additionally for National Leprosy Eradication Programme and additionally for National Programme for Control of Blindness and Multipurpose workers contractual and other expenditure including power back up and convergence support should be made available at the facility level to ensure proper delivery of public health services as per norms and guidelines of the Indian Public Health Standards.

P. *Routine Immunization*

Immunization Programme is the cornerstone of public health system. Strengthening of Routine Immunization, review meeting, and Routine

Immunization in slum and underserved areas, mobilization of beneficiaries, through ASHA and alternate vaccine delivery, consumables for computers including internet and Bio-Medical Waste Management, Training of frontline workers, incentives to ASHA, TEEKA Express and innovations under Routine Immunization including "*My Village My Home*" Programme should be ensured for successful immunization services as per the guidelines of the Government of India.

Q. *National Disease Control Programme*

Various National Disease Control Programmes have been launched which include National Iodine Deficiency Disorders Control Programme, Integrated Disease Surveillance Project, National Leprosy Eradication Programme, National Programme for Control of Blindness, Revised National Tuberculosis Programme, National Tobacco Control Programme, National Programme for Prevention and Control of Deafness and National Vector-Borne Disease Control Programme including Malaria, Dengue, Chikungunya, Filaria, Kala-Azar, Acute Encephalitis Syndrome/Japanese Encephalitis and Swine Flue Programme should be equally, effectively and efficiency implemented at the facility level as per the norms and guidelines of the Indian Public Health Standards to meet the increasing demand of the growing patients.

14. Management of Public Health Delivery System

An important Public Health Programme under National Rural Health Mission includes Maternal Mortality, Child Health, Family Planning, Routine Immunization and National Disease Control programmes are being implemented at the facility level.

It is being recommended to ensure need based planning for operationalizing additional delivery points. In the last 7 years after Janani Suraksha Yojana implementation, case of load at delivery points has increased many folds which have affected quality of services. Therefore, in the next three years it is necessary to increase number of delivery points so that we can provide quality delivery services to the women.

- To increase institutional deliveries under Janani Suraksha Yojana.
- To provide free drugs and consumables, diagnostics, free diet and free drop back facilities under Janani Shishu Suraksha Karyakram.
- To increase institutional deliveries under Janani Suraksha Yojana.

- To provide incentives for ASHAs for reporting suspected maternal death, treatment of severe anaemia, and incentives to ASHA for early registration should be timely paid to ASHAs as per norms.
- Maternal Health review and orientation workshops should be organized regularly.
- Incentives for ANMs for Maternal Health should be paid regularly.
- Supply of zinc and ORS should be timely made available in the required volumes.
- Bal Swasthya Poshan Mah and Biannual Bal Swasthya Poshan Mah should be organized and facility based interventions for sick New Born Care Units, New Born Stabilization Units, New Born Care Corners and Nutrition Rehabilitation Centres should be made functional at the facility level.
- New Born Screening, a preventive child health care initiative should be made available to the interested patients.
- First Passport to life (Child Health Cards) 0-5 years of age "Zindagi Ki Udaan" should properly be implemented to reduce the Infant Mortality Rate.
- "Bal Swasthya Kunji" scheme should be implemented to ensure developmental milestone of the child.
- Infant Young Child Feeding including breast feeding should be ensured as per guidelines.
- Increased cost of Medicine and investigation of ₹ 350 and Daily Wages Compensation for Mother and Food for Mother during stay ₹ 150 should be paid and provision of food to the mother (Breakfast, Lunch, Evening Snack, and Dinners) should be made available at the facility level. Transportation cost of ₹ 200 for bringing the child to Nutrition Rehabilitation Centre during admission, ₹ 100 for bringing child back home after discharge and an addition of ₹ 200 per visit is proposed for four follow-up visits of discharged children should be paid as per norms of the government.
- Incentive to ASHAs for follow-up visits: additional ₹ 100 for follow-up visits within two months incentives should be paid to ASHAs for motivating and bringing the mother and children to Nutrition Rehabilitation Centres.
- Golden Hour New Born Tracking and the first minutes, the Golden Minutes and hour as golden hour after delivery and service components of Post Partum care should be reinforced to reduce Maternal Mortality Rate and Infant Mortality Rate.
- To improve the quality of life with unambiguous and explicit emphasis on sustainable measure and action, population

stabilization, improvement of health status of people particularly women and children in holistic, open and transparent manner should be implemented through adopting family planning methods, i.e. Vasectomy, Tubectomy, Total limiting, IUCD, MTP, C.C. users, O.P. users and total spacing methods of family planning at the facility level.

- Deployment of Family Welfare Counsellor and Performance incentive to ASHAs under family planning of ₹ 150 should be paid to ASHAs for escorting the clients to the health facility for facilitating the insertion.
- *Pehel Sakhi Sammelan:* Happy user of Family Planning service interface with non-user and male group meetings and Merry Gold Health Network should be implemented under the guidance of USAID and State Innovations in the Family Planning Service Agency (SIFPSA).
- *Referral Transport/Patient Transport System:* "108" Emergency Medical Transport Services, "102" National Ambulance Service, Advance Life Support Ambulance and Pediatric Ambulances for Sick New Born Care Units should properly be implemented to reduce the Infant Mortality Rate.
- A comparative study to adherence and cure rates of Tuberculosis using Technology enabled, monitoring and supervision should be ensured.
- Immunization Programme which is the cornerstone of public health and Universal Immunization Programme which was merged in Child Survival and Safe Motherhood Programme should be properly implemented as per Mid Term Strategic Plan.
- National Iodine Deficiency Disorders Programme should be properly implemented to check and control damages during early pregnancy as it retards foetal brain development resulting in a range of intellectual, motor and hearing deficits.
- Adolescent Health/Rashtriya Kishore Swasthya Karyakrama should be properly implemented as per norms of the government.
- Biannual Adolescent Health Days should be organized at Block Level.
- Weekly Iron Folic Acid Supplementation Programme and Menstrual Hygiene Scheme and regional orientation meeting should be organized regularly.
- Rashtriya Bal Swasthya Karyakram should be implemented as per guidelines of the government.

- Pre-conception, Pre-Natal Diagnostic Techniques Act should be appropriately enforced to reduce rapidly decreasing sex-ratio because the girls are killed either through sex selective abortions or die prematurely due to violence and neglect. State-District-Divisional-Block level PC PNDT Cell should be established.
- Mainstreaming of AYUSH system at all levels in Health Care Delivery System should be promoted to ensure preventive and curative strengths at the facility level. Skill upgradation and orientation training of AYUSH Doctors including Ksharsutra, Panchkarma/Ilaz-ul-tadveer and skill Birth Training Programme should be implemented as per norms.
- Appropriate implementation of Integrated Disease Surveillance Project should be implemented with the view to provide greater emphasis on building the links between the collection and analysis of information and ground interventions by public or private sectors.
- To ensure appropriate implementation of National Vector-Borne Disease Control Programme including Malaria, Dengue, Chikungunya, Filaria, Kala-Azar, Acute Encephalitis Syndrome/ Japanese Encephalitis, Swine Flu and other Vector-Borne Disease Programme in the endemic/priority high risk area.
- National Leprosy Eradication, National Programme for Control of Blindness, National Mental Health Programme, National Programme for Prevention and Control of Deafness, National Tobacco Control Programme, National Iodine Deficiency Disorder Programme, Integrated Disease Surveillance Project, Revised National Tuberculosis Programme, National Vector-Borne Disease Control Programme and other diseased control programmes should be properly implemented at the facility level through community process, Rogi Kalyan Samiti, Health Societies and sustained involvement of Panchayati Raj Institutions to fulfil the increasing demand of the growing patients belonging to underserved/un-served area especially women, children, below poverty line people, deprived, resourceless multitudes surviving in the remote villages.

15. Conclusion

The Public Health system may be strengthened through preventing water pollution and water contamination which causes water-borne diseases. The water-borne diseases are caused by the pathogenic micro-organism. The water-borne diseases are commonly transmitted in the contaminated fresh water.

Trivially most of the infections might be transmitted by the microbes or parasites which are accidentally, possible as a result of exceptional circumstances and it had got into water, but the fact that there might be an occasional freak infection need not mean that it is useful to categorize the resulting disease as "water-borne" nor it is a common practice to refer disease such as Malaria as "water-borne" just because mosquitoes have aquatic phases in their life-cycle or due to treating by water; people inhibit the happiness to be an effective strategy to control mosquitoes which are the vectors.

According to the World Health Organization the water-borne diseases account for an estimated 4.1 per cent of the total Daily Global burden of disease and causes about 1.8 million human deaths per annum. World Health Organization has estimated that 88 per cent of the Global burden of disease are attributable due to unsafe drinking water supply, sanitation and hygiene. Water-borne diseases are more prevalent due to the lower level of access to drinking water and sanitation along with proper and overall health hygiene and poor nutritional status.

Water-borne illness typically associated with drinking water by etiologic agent causes chemical contamination of water through poor sanitary conditions of the water system and water supplies from cess-pits, unsanitary place and the cess-pits of the old houses has never been drained causing Cholera and diarrhoea disease.

Water-borne diseases may have a significant impact on the economic status of the common people at the local level. Infected and affected people by the water-borne diseases are usually confronted with the related costs and not seldom with a high financial burden.

The available reports, documents does not capture whether National Rural Health Mission has been "successful" or "failed" but analyzes the changes in the health outcomes and health systems from the point of view of the constraints that were faced and learnt lessons.

Water Pollution occurs when the pollutant are directly or indirectly discharged into the water bodies. Water contamination affects the water bodies, plants and organisms living in these water areas. Its effect is damaged not only to the individual species and population but also to the national biological communities.

It has been estimated that 580 people in our country die due to water pollution/contamination related illness everyday. Nearly 500 million people suffer due to lack of access to safe drinking water.

The treatment of drinking water as applied to the public water supplies consists of a series of water supply and the nature and vulnerability of the source of water.

The water testing physically or chemically can be done through several methods depending on the accuracy required and the characteristics of water. The biological testing of the water samples involves the collection of the plants or the animals from the surface water body. Biological testing of water involves the use of plants, animals or microbial indicators to monitor the health of an aquatic ecosystem.

The cultivated land with large livestock and poultry operations are termed as concentrated animals feeding operations. Animals slurries are usually treated by contaminants in an aerobic lagoons before disposal by spray or trickle application to grass land. The constructed wet lands are sometimes used to facilitate the treatment of animal waste. The animal slurries are treated by mixing with straw and composed at high temperature to produce a bacteriological sterile and friable manure to increase the fertility status of the soil.

The improved water supply and sanitation may lead to reduce the incidence of morbidity and mortality, which may be up to 100 per cent for some diseases such as Typhoid and Dracunculiasis.

World Health Organization works to reduce arsenic exposure includes setting guidelines, values, reviewing evidence and providing recommendations for the risk management. World Health Organization published a guidelines value for arsenic in it, "Guidelines for Drinking Water Quality".

Prevention and control of various water-borne diseases can be checked through adopting various approaches with the objective to interrupt the transmission of water-borne diseases and thereby reducing their morbidity and mortality.

The water-borne diseases are one of the major public health threats especially in the developing countries where unsafe water, sanitation problems and hygiene practice exist. The public health approach to the prevention and control of water-borne diseases consists of provision of safe and adequate water supply and improved sanitation and hygiene education.

Treatment of water supply for individuals and families can be considered through boiling of water, filtration, storage of water, disinfection of spring or well with Chlorine right after construction or when the need arises and monitoring of the water supply should also be ensured regularly.

National Health Policy was formulated during 1983 with a view to provide the health service for all needy people equally, effectively and efficiently, through providing decentralized public health services and to ensure an access to and the benefits from public health system which has been very uneven between the better endowed and the more vulnerable section of the society, particularly women, children, and socially disadvantaged sections of the society.

The Public health requirements for maternal health, child health including Janani Suraksha Yojana, Janani Shishu Suraksha Karyakram, Rashtriya Kishore Swasthya Karyakram and Rashtriya Bal Swasthya Karyakram and routine immunization and National Disease Control Programme should be implemented as per the needs of the people.

The public health planning should be managed through need based planning from bottom to top, i.e. from Hamlet villages → Revenue Villages → Village Panchayats → Nyaya Panchayats → Block Panchayat → District Panchayats → State level up to National level and also from Auxiliary Nurse Midwife Centres/Anganwadi Centres → Sub-Health Centres → Primary Health Centres → Community Health Centres → District Hospital → State Level Hospital or Medical Colleges.

Management imperatives of public health for planning and financing, management, strengthening human resources, policies for doctors, nurses, para medical and programme management staff, their accountability, training and capacity building, policies on drugs procurement systems and logistic management, equipments, ambulance services and Referral Transport, new infrastructure and maintenance of buildings, sanitation and water, electricity, laundry, kitchen, facilities for attendants, diagnostic services, patients' feedback and grievance redressal, community participants, Information, Education, Communication, Inter-sectoral, convergence, private public partnership and regulations of services in the private sector and strengthening of data capturing, validity/ triangulation, supportive supervision, monitoring and review, quality assurance, surveillance and leveraging technology should be planned as per the requirement of the local needy people from Village panchayat level to Block level to District Panchayat level to State level as well.

Management structure of Public Health System should be ensured through Technical Units Programme support and, Programme Management and support systems at various levels. Facility based management of health system included planning, recruitment and implementation of health delivery at the facility levels.

Local community should be sufficiently empowered to take leadership in strengthening the public health system. Panchayati Raj Institutions right from village panchayat level to the District level should be given ownership of public health delivery system in their respective jurisdiction.

National Health Mission has sought an amendment to Acts and Statutes in the States to institutionalize Community led action for health services and to fully empowered local bodies in the effective management of the public health delivery system at the facility level.

Therefore, the National Health Mission attempts to transfer funds, functions, functionaries to the Panchayati Raj Institutions. The concerted efforts with the involvement of the Non-Governmental Organizations and other resource institutions should be made to build capacity of the elected representatives and user group members for improved and effective management of public health system at the facility level.

A system of periodic "*Jan Sunwai*" or "*Jan Samvad*" should be organized to empower community members to engage in providing direct feedback and suggestions for improvement in the public health delivery system at the facility level.

The success of decentralization experiments would depend on the strength of the pillars, supporting the pillars of strength of the process of pubic system.

It is imperative to ensure that the management capacities should be built at each level. It should provide the management cost up to 6 per cent of the total annual plan approved for District as it has been introduced under the Reproductive and Child Health-II programme.

Apart from the Medical and Paramedical staff such services would include skills for financial management, improved community processes, procedure, procurement and logistics, improved collection and maintenance of data the use of information technologies, Health Management Information System and improved monitoring and evaluation system at the facility level.

Monitoring and accountability framework should be managed through community based monitoring, external surveys and stringent internal monitoring. Rogi Kalyan Samiti and Community, etc. shall be expected to monitor the physical and financial performance of the public health facilities.

The public health delivery system aims at inclusive health and improved access to quality health care for those residing in the remote rural areas particularly women, children and the poor by promoting integration, decentralization and encouraging community participation in the public health system.

Health care delivery system at Primary, Secondary, Tertiary level should be strengthened through quality care assurance as per guidelines of the Indian Public Health Standards, which mainly includes provisions of optimal expert care to the community and making health care services more responsive and sensitive to the needs and aspiration of the community.

Minimum requirements of the public health delivery services should be ensured through clinical manpower and support manpower and appointment of the Public Health Management and appropriate availability of the equipments, drugs, investigative facilities and physical infrastructure should be made available as per norms of the Indian Public Health Standards.

Hospital Waste Management based on Bio-Medical Waste (Management and Handling) Rules, 1998 has been notified under the Environment Protection Act, 1986 (29 of 1986) by Ministry of Environment and Forests, Government of India.

Public Health Management skills should be ensured through encouraging qualifications in public health or public health management among Medical Staff and supporting staff and management processes for decentralized planning and developing health management information system and building institutions for technical assistance and knowledge management to ensure quality assurance in the appropriate need based delivery of public health service at the facility level.

The management of Maternal Health and Child Health and priorities to reduce maternal mortality rate, infant mortality rate and also to reduce Neo-Natal Deaths through the facility based interventions at the grassroots level should be ensured.

Nutrition Rehabilitation Centres, and Human Resource Training for Navjat Shishu Suraksha Karyakram and Integrated Management of Neo-Natal and Childhood Illness training and Home Based New Care and Infant/Young Child Feeding, Management of the Diarrhoea, Bal Swasthya Poshan Mah, Information, Education, Communication and Procurement of Equipments and Drugs, etc. should be properly implemented and managed as per the norms of the Indian Public Health Standards.

Appropriate Management of the Family Planning and Adolescent Reproductive and Sexual Health and launch of SABLA programme for addressing issues of anaemia in adolescent and procurement of Deworming Tablets under Menstrual Hygiene and implementation of Rashtriya Bal Swasthya Karyakram, Proper arrangement of human resources, training, and Information, Education, Communication should be organized at the facility level.

Pre-conception of Pre-Natal Diagnostic Techniques Act should be properly enforced and executed at the grassroots level.

Appropriate deployment of human resources for Maternal Health, Child Health, Family Planning, Adolescent Reproductive Sexual Health, routine immunization and disease control programme should be ensured at the facility level.

Effective management of public health delivery system and strengthening of State Programme Management Unit, Divisional Programme Management Unit, District Programme Management Unit, Block Programme Management Unit, Village Programme Management Unit should be promoted equally, effectively and efficiently.

Accredited Social Health Activists and strengthening of hospital, new constructions, renovation and setting up of new sub-centre should be strengthened as per need of the local people.

Mainstreaming of AYUSH at the Primary Health Centres level and formulation of need based health action plans and innovation like "*My Village My Home*" and "*Mobile Kunji*" scheme should be promoted, propagated and implemented at the facility level.

Formulation of Health Action Plans and implementation of the facility level review, evaluation and monitoring of the programme implementation should be ensured for enhancing the quality of the health care services rendered through the establishment of quality assurance Network at all facility level.

An important public health delivery system includes maternal health, child health, Adolescent, Reproductive, Sexual Health, Family Planning, Routine immunization, Janani Suraksha Yojana, Janani Shishu Suraksha Karyakram, Rashtriya Kishore Swasthya Karyakram and Rashtriya Bal Swasthay Karyakram, Bal Swasthay Kunji including Golden Minute and Golden Hour Karyakram and routine immunization, referral transport/ patient transport system — "108" Emergency Medical Transport Services, "102" National Ambulance Services, Advanced Life Support Ambulance and Paediatric Ambulance for sick New Born Care Units should be properly implemented as per guidelines of the government.

Appropriate implementation of National Disease Control Programme including — National Leprosy Eradication Programme, National Programme for Control of Blindness, National Mental Health Programme, National Programme for Prevention and Control of Blindness, National Programme for Control of Deafness, National Tobacco Control Programme, National Iodine Deficiency Disorders Programme, Integrated Disease Surveillance Project Revised National Tuberculosis Programme and National Vector-Borne Disease Control Programme especially Malaria, Dengue, Chikungunya, Filaria, Kala-Azar, Acute Encephalitis Syndromes/Japanese Encephalitis, Swine Flue and other vector-borrne diseases should be implemented as per guidelines and norms of the Government of India at the facility level.

Continued involvement and sustained participation of Rogi Kalyan Samiti, Health Societies and Panchayati Raj Institutions at various levels should be ensured in a positive manner to fulfil the ever-increasing demand of the growing patients belonging to underserved, unserved areas, particularly women, children, below poverty line people, deprived resourcesless multitudes surviving in the unserved and underserved backward remote villages.

5

CONCLUSION

There is a significant progress in improving the life expectancy at birth reducing the morality due to Malaria, as well as reducing infant and maternal mortality over the last few decades in India. In spite of the progress made, a high proportion of the population especially the remote villages continues to suffer and die from preventable diseases, pregnancy and child birth related complication as well as malnutrition.

In addition to the old unresolved problems the health systems in our country is facing emerging threats and challenges. The rural health care system in many areas is in an unsatisfactory state leading to pauperization of poor households due to excessive extensive private sector health care.

Our country is in the midst of an epidemiological and demographic transition with the attendant problems of increased chronic disease burden and a decline in the mortality and fertility rates leading to an ageing of the population.

Premature morbidity and mortality from chronic disease has been a major loss of economic and human resources. The large disparity across different places the burden of these conditions mostly on the poor and on women scheduled castes, backward castes, especially those who are living in the remote villages. The inequity has also been reflected in the skewed availability of public resources between the advanced and less developed villages.

Most of the Public Health determinants are correlated to high levels of poverty and to degradation of the environment of the villages. It has been noted that State of Uttar Pradesh has to deal with multiple health crises, rising costs of health care and mounting expectations of the people.

It has been visioned to ensure effective integration of health concerns through decentralized management of District, Block and Village Level with the determinants of health like sanitation, hygiene, nutrition, safe drinking water, gender and social concerns.

It has been viewed to provide universal access to equitable, affordable and quality health care which is accountable at the same time responsive to the requirements of the village people and reduction of child and maternal deaths as well as stabilization of population, gender and demographic balance.

It has been strategically viewed to develop a framework for promoting inter-sectoral convergence for ensuring promotive, preventive and curative public health care system at the facility level.

An important objective of the Public Health Programme has been to ensure reduction in Maternal and Child Mortality Rate, ensure universal immunization, family planning prevention and control of communicable and non-communicable diseases including locally endemic diseases and to mainstream AYUSH health system for promotion of healthy life-styles and implementation of various National Disease Control Programmes at the facility level.

It is being expected that outcomes from the public health systems will be helpful in reducing the Infant Mortality Rate to 30/1,000 live births by 2012 and Maternal Mortality Rate reduction to 100/1,00,000 live births of 2012 and reduction in the Total Fertility Rate to 2.1 by 2012 and Maternal Mortality Reduction Rate — 50 per cent up to 2010 additional 10 per cent by 2012. It has also been planned to reduce Kala-Azar Mortality Rate — 100 per cent by 2012 and substantial elimination until 2012 and Filaria/Micro-Filaria Reduction Rate — 70 per cent, by 2010 and 80 per cent by 2012 and elimination by 2015, Dengue Mortality Reduction Rate — 50 per cent by 2010 and sustaining at that level until 2012.

It has been planned to provide improved access to universal immunization through induction of Auto-Diabled Syringes, alternate vaccine delivery and improved mobilization services and to provide improved facilities for institutional deliveries through provision of referral transport escort and improved hospital care under Janani Suraksha Yojana and Janani Shishu Suraksha Karyakram.

The Core Strategy of public health system includes strengthening of the existing Primary Health Centres through better staffing and development of human resources, health policy, clear quality standards, better community support and untied funds to enable the local management committee to achieve the norms of Indian Public Health Standards.

The supplementary strategy of the Public Health System has been to mainstream the AYUSH system of Medicine through revitalizing the local health traditions at the facility level and to reorient the medical education to support Public Health issues including regulation to medical care and medical ethics.

An unique opportunity for carrying out necessary reforms in the health sector has been prioritized at the facility level. The reforms are necessary for restructuring to health delivery system as well as for delivery better health financing mechanisms. The strengthening and effectiveness of health institutions like — Sub Health Centres/Primary Health Centres/Community Health Centres/Taluka/District Hospitals have positive consequences for all health programmes, i.e. Tuberculosis, Malaria HIV/AIDS, Filaria, Family Planning and Welfare, Leprosy, Disease Surveillance Project, etc. as all programmes are based on the assumption that a functioning of Public Health System actually exists at the facility level.

The key features in order to achieve the goals of the Mission included making the Public Health delivery system fully functional and accountable to the Community, human resource management, decentralization, rigorous monitoring and evaluation against standards, convergence of health and related programme from village level upward innovations and flexible funding and interventions for improving the health indicators at the various levels.

Public Health System seeks to improve outreach activities in unserved and underserved areas especially inhabited by vulnerable sections of the society through provision of Mobile Medical units covering all Anganwadi Centres. It also seeks to ensure availability of requisite equipment and drugs of all Public Health care facilities. Procurement of equipments/ drugs should be progressively decentralized at the facility level.

In order to provide managerial support for tracking funds and monitoring activities, a provision has been made to setting up Programme Management Units at facility level, over 500 professionals have already been recruited.

In view of the given large army of Accredited Social Health Activists, Auxiliary Nurse Midwife, Nurses and Rural Medical Practitioners require continuous skill development. Strengthening nursing institutions, linking medical colleges for providing skill development support to rural health workers involving the voluntary sector in skill development are few key interventions to be taken up at the facility level.

To make the health facilities more accountable to the health sector control would be gradually shifted to the Panchayati Raj Institutions and civil society. The sub-centres are proposed to be placed exclusively under the control of Panchayat Samitis and Rogi Kalyan Samiti.

The District Health Plan would be the main instrument for planning, inter-sectoral convergence, implementation and monitoring of the activities under the Public Health System.

Provisions have been made for state specific proposal for main-streaming AYUSH including the appointment of AYUSH doctors/ paramedics on contractual basis, providing AYUSH Wings in the Primary Health Centres.

The process of community involvement of health institutions itself would enhance the accountability and the National Rural Health Mission would facilitate this process by wide dissemination of the results. For effective monitoring a strong Management Information System is being put in place.

The citizen charter would help the public to know their rights and entitlements at each facility. Efforts are being made to integrate HIV/ AIDS programmes with Reproductive and Child Health at the facility levels. Convergence of Disease Control Programme, integration of service, combined awareness generation, education and advocacy at community and facility levels, taking care of the preventive, promotive and curative health care are expected to bring down Infant Mortality Rate/Maternal Mortality Rate/Total Fertility Rate and reduce the burden of diseases.

Public Health Manual is intended to be a user friendly tool to assist range of stakeholders to be engaged in the District Health Action Planning at the facility level. The Community Health Centres constitute the secondary level of health care which has been designed to provide referral as well as specialist health care to the rural people. Indian Public Health Standards for Community Health Centres have been prescribed under National Rural Health Mission to provide optimal specialized care to the community and achieve and maintain an acceptable standard of quality health care.

To maintain quality of services, external monitoring at appropriate intervals have been advocated. Guidelines are being provided for management of routine and emergency cases under the National Health Programme so as to maintain uniformity in Management in tune with the National Health Policy.

The minimum requirements are being projected based on an average bed occupancy of 60 per cent. It would be a dynamic process in the sense that if the utilization goes up to the standards would be further upgraded. As regards to manpower, 2 specialists, namely Anesthetist and Public Health Programme Manager should be provided on contractual basis in addition to the available specialists, namely surgery, medicine, obstetrics and gynaecology and paediatrics. The support manpower will include a Public Health Nurse and Auxiliary Nurse Midwife in addition to the existing staff. An Ophthalmic Assistant will also be required to be provided in the centres where currently there is none.

It is mandatory for every Community Health Centre to have "*Rogi Kalyan Samiti*" to ensure accountability. Every Community Health Centre will have the charter of Patient's Rights displayed prominently at the entrance.

A grievance mechanism under the overall supervision of Rogi Kalyan Samiti should be set-up at the facility level. Each Community Health Centre should have the standard. Operating procedure and standard treatment protocols for common ailments social audit by involvement of the Community through Consumer Forum and Rogi Kalyan Samiti has been recommended and to maintain quality of services external monitoring through Panchayati Raj Institutions and internal monitoring at appropriate intervals are being advocated. Guidelines are being provided for management of routine and emergency cases under the National Health Programme so as to maintain uniformity in management in tune with the National Health Policy.

Strengthening of Public Health System including First Referral Units achieving 24 × 7 public health care facilities and improved quality of health care and access to safe delivery of the health services and Disease Control Programme and Medical Education strategies, regularly and Community Process, Training Programmes for staff for the skill upgradation to ensure need based appropriate health delivery services at facility level.

Bhadainya Block of the Sultanpur District has been selected for analyzing the delivery of the health system at the village panchayat level because most of the population of the area are suffering from the various communicable and non-communicable diseases.

The total fertility rate of Uttar Pradesh is 5.3 and the infant mortality rate is 61 and the maternal mortality rate is 259 which are higher than the National average.

Historical background of the study area has been extremely famous, honoured and appreciated Archaeologically, Historically, Culturally, Geographically and Industrially District Sultanpur has very important place. In spite of several continued changes, the identity of Sultanpur has been permanent.

There are four Tehsils and fourteen Blocks in Sultanpur District. There are 8 Nyaya Panchayats and 63 Village Panchayats and 149 Revenue Villages in Sultanpur District.

Physiographically Sultanpur District has been divided into two main physical divisions such as Northern Tract and Southern Tract. The plain is characterized by unrelieved monotony of alluvial deposits which completely should be the old land surface to a depth of several thousand metres. The solid geology of the plain is totally obscured underneath mantle.

There are no noteworthy features in the Physiognomy of the Sultanpur District. Geologically Sultanpur District has been divided into the ravine tract of Gomati River, Central tract and the Lake tract.

The Rivers which flow in the district Sultanpur are Gomati, Majharai, and Manger. Sultanpur District experiences a rhythm of seasons with several prevailing winds. The several are regularly felt twice during the year. The rainfall during the months is scanty and sporadic. The annual rainfall of the study area is 1005 mm but it is unevenly distributed every year.

The older alluvial, saline and alkaline soils are the main soils found in the study area. The soils of the District are transported from the sedimentary rocks of the Himalayas and the products of decomposition of the rocks have been deposited over the tract through the water erosion. On the basis of the texture of the soils of the District the soils have been sub-divided into Bangar, Loamy, Clayeye loam, Clayeye soil, Khadar soils, Saline soils, Saline and Alkaline soils.

District Sultanpur has an almost inhabited human occupancy for over three millennia and centuries of plough and pastoral culture has reduced the natural vegetation except in the Pocket of Tarai and some river banks with a moderate and healthy climate and fertile soils, the District's Flora presents no peculiarities.

The District Sultanpur has very important role in the ancient, historical periods. Important religious places of the District Sultanpur are Bijethua, Mahaviran, Pancho-Piran, Sultan Shah Sharmad Shah Baba, Dhopap, Sitakund, Loharamau, Pahalwan Bir Baba and Gadha.

In view of the above an attempt has been made in this study to explain the public health programme related to Maternal Health, Child Health, Family Planning, Routine Immunization and National Disease Control Programme at Sultanpur District. An effort has also been made to explain the progress of the public health system and also to analyze the management of the Public Health Programme related to Maternal

Health, Child Health, Family Planning, Routine immunization and implementation of various Disease Control programmes at the grassroots level and to progress of the public health system at the facility level and need based management of the public health system has been analyzed at the health facility level.

Public Health Programmes

Significant progress has been noticed in improving the expectancy at birth, reducing mortality due to malaria as well as reducing infant and maternal mortality. HIV/AIDs, non-communicable disease such as cardio-vascular, cancer, blindness, mental illness and tobacco related illness have imposed the chronic disease burden on the already overstretched health care system.

Premature morbidity and mortality from chronic disease can be a major economic and human loss. The public spending on the preventive health services has a low priority over curative health.

Main objectives of the rural health programme has been reduction in child and maternal mortality, universal access to public health services, prevention and control of the communicable and non-communicable diseases and promotion of healthy lifestyle.

Under the Reproductive Child Health Flexible Pool Maternal Health Programmes specially Janani Suraksha Yojana and Janani Shishu Suraksha Yojana and operationalization of comprehensive abortion care services has been planned and strengthened. Maternal Health review-old activities and new activities, training, information, education, communication activities and procurement of equipments, drugs and supplies for maternal health programmes are being implemented at the facility level.

Navjat Shishu Suraksha Varsh is being celebrated to strengthen facilities, services and capacity building of health staff working at the delivery points to prevent the neo-natal morbidity and subsequent reduction in the neo-natal deaths.

Facility based interventions, i.e. Sick New Born Care Units, New Born Stabilization Units, New Born Care Corners, Nutrition Rehabilitation Centres have been established to fulfil the need of emergency care of the Neo-nate and to reduce neo-natal pre-natal death.

Navjat Shishu Suraksha Karyakram, essential new born care equipments and Home Based New Born Care Community based intervention and drug kits and infant young child feeding and management of diarrhoea and Bal Swasthya Poshan Mah and Information, Education and Communication activities under Child Health Programme are being implemented at the facility level.

Population Policy looks at the issues related to population stabilization and improvement of the Health status of the people, particularly women and children in a holistic manner.

Family planning management activities and Terminal/Limiting Method (Providing sterilization services) Provision of fixed day for Non-scalpel Vasectomy (NSV) services at each District Male Hospital (Combined Hospital and First Referral Units should be continued. Accreditation of Private Centre/Non-Governmental Organization for sterilization services, plans for post part sterilization, spacing method and performance based reward to institutions and providers including incentives for ASHA and social marketing of contraceptives, training Information, Education and Communication, and Public Private Partnership activities under Family Planning activities have been strengthened and implemented at the facility level.

Adolescent Reproductive and Sexual Health (ARSH) training, Major Hygiene and Rashtriya Bal Swasthya Karyakram, Pre-Conception and Pre-Natal Diagnostic Techniques, Information, Education and Communicable Training at various levels have been strengthened and implemented at the grassroots level.

To ensure effective management of activities under National Rural Health Mission of State Programme Management Unit, Divisional Programme Management Unit, District Programme Management Unit, Block Programme Management and Village Health Sanitation and Nutrition Committees have been formed to ensure need based delivery of health services.

Descriptive role of District Programme Manager, District Community Mobilizer, District Accounts Manager, District Data-cum-Accounts Assistant, District Programme Coordinator, District Data Assistant and responsibilities of Block Programme Manager, Block Data-cum-Assistant, Block Coordinator, Data Assistants have been deployed, supportive supervision/mobility support/field visits, etc. have been ensured at the facility levels.

Rural Health Mission Flexible Pool includes Accredited Social Health Activists, untied funds, Annual Maintenance Grants, Hospital, strengthening, New construction, Renovation and setting up of new sub-centres, mainstreaming of AYUSH, Information, Education and Communication, and Behaviour change, Communication, Medical Mobile Units, Referral Transport/Patient Transport System, Innovation,

Planning, Implementation and Monitoring, Procurement, Drug, Drug warehouse, health insurance scheme, Research/studies/analysis, State Health Resource Centre/State Public Health Resource Institute, support services and other expenditures (power backup and convergence), etc.

Accredited Social Health Activists programme included the provision of ASHA Drug kits, incentives for ASHA and Annual ASHA Sammelan/ Diwas, ASHA Uniform, News letters for ASHA and ASHA award scheme and ASHA Mentoring Group and State Specific Innovation under ASHA Programme and ASHA support system has been strengthened and implemented at the facility level.

The untied funds especially maintenance grant, strengthening of hospital including. Trauma wings spillover in District Women Hospital, Construction of 30 and 50 bedded Community Health Centres, Drug warehouse and construction of maternity wings and setting up of Emergency Caring Centre and strengthening of infrastructure have been implemented, Rogi Kalyan Samiti and involvement of community services and Panchayati Raj Institutions have been ensured at the facility level.

Orientation workshop, training and capacity building of Panchayati Raj Institutions at State District Health Societies, Community Health Centres/Primary Health Centres and village health sanitation and nutrition committees have been organized.

Establishment of Sub-centres, platform for effective Maternity and Child Health service delivery through frontline workers has been ensured at the facility level.

Mainstreaming of AYUSH (Ayurveda, Yoga and Naturopathy, Unani, Siddha and Homoeopathy) system of medicines have proven, promotive, preventive and curative strengths. With a view to integrating AYUSH health care with mainstream health care services as per the modified centrally sponsored scheme for development of AYUSH Hospitals and Dispensaries, operational guidelines, Department of AYUSH, Ministry of Health and Family Welfare, Government of India have been ensured for its implementation at the facility level.

Strengthening of Information Education and Communication/ Behaviour Change Communication and implementation capacity at the facility level has been ensured.

Maternity Health Campaign "*Chaar Ganth*" and "*Chance Kyon Lena Hai*", "*Surakshit Matritva*" and "*Ab Aur Der Nahi*" Campaign have been launched at the grassroots level.

Mobile Medical Unit have been envisaged which will provide preventive, promotive and curative health care in inaccessible areas which are underserved. Mobile Medical Units are operative by the Name of National Mobile Medical Unit along with requisite logistics and technical staff and doctors.

Emergency Medical Transport Service "108" and U.P. Ambulance Sewa and '102 Sewa' Ambulance services are made available to provide transportation of pregnancy cases as well as neo-natal cases from home to the health facility.

Sexual Transmitted Infection and Reproductive Tract Infection services at the district level are provided through the Out Patient Department of skin gynaecology and obstetrics department of medical colleges or district hospital are provided.

National Aids Control Organization has branded its Sexual and Reproductive Health Services as "*Suraksha Clinic*".

Rapid Plasma Region Kits (RPR) and Venereal Disease Research Laboratory (VDRL) Testing Services have been made available at the Sub-District Health Facilities.

Proposal for free Transport facility through UPSRTC to people living with HIV/AIDS for their treatment related travel to Anti-Retroviral therapy centres has been proposed by the Government of Uttar Pradesh.

Sanitation Programme for Rural Child Health and Hygiene Awareness programme "*Sanrachha*" has been launched and innovation for strengthening routine immunization and concurrent monitoring for follow-up action plan activities and regional review meetings and orientation of District Immunization programme have been planned and implemented.

Scale up of "*My Village My Home*" programme have been launched for tracking of immunization beneficiaries.

My Village My Home is a mechanism not only for ensuring registration and tracking of all beneficiaries in a particular catchment area but also focuses on developing and strengthening channels of communication between community and service providers for improving routine immunization coverage.

"*Mobile Kunji*" is designed to be used by ASHAs during their home visits with families. The audio-visual jobs aid bring together an Interactive voice response based mobile service and a printed deck of cards on a ring.

Planning, Implementation and Monitoring have been ensured through quality assurance at the State-Division-Block-Village or facility level.

Procurement of equipments, drugs and consumables have been ensured and Health Insurance Scheme known as "Jan Shree Bima Yojana" has been devised and launched by the Life Insurance Corporation of India for the benefit of the people living below poverty line.

State Health Resource Centre and State Public Health Resources Centre's establishment have been mandated under National Rural Health Mission.

Strengthening of routine immunization programme has been initiated through review meetings, and mobilization of beneficiaries through ASHA and alternate vaccine delivery.

Training of frontline workers and incentives for ASHA and TEEKA Express programme and various innovation under Routine Immunization has been launched and My Village My Home activity has been planned in each District.

Various Disease Control Programme have been launched under the National Rural Health Mission programmes. The National Disease Control Programme includes — National Iodine Deficiency Disorder Control Programme, Integrated Disease Surveillance Project, National Vector-Borne Disease Control Programme, National Leprosy Eradication Programme, National Programme for Control of Blindness, Revised National Tuberculosis Control Programme, National Tobacco Control Programme and National Programme for Prevention and Control of Deafness in which the surveillance, training, information, education and communication, specific constraints, strategies and innovations have been proposed for appropriate implementation of the various disease control programmes at the facility level.

Thus, the various programmes under National Rural Health Mission especially Maternal and Child Health, Adolescent, Reproductive and Sexual Health Routine Immunization and Rural Health Mission flexible pool and National Disease Control Programme should be launched equally, effectively, efficiently at the grassroots level in the remote unserved rural areas and to provide promotive, curative and preventive health care to all at the facility level to save the human lives and reduce the economic loss and also to improve the socio-economic conditions of the resourceless, deprived rural poor multitudes surviving in the remote villages.

Public Health Progress

Public Health delivery system has increased many folds which have affected the quality of services. It is necessary to increase and promote health delivery points, so that the quality public health delivery services are provided at the facility level especially in the unserved, underserved and remote areas to the needy interested people equally, effectively and efficiently.

A comparative study of Adherence and Cure rates of Tuberculosis using Technology enabled Monitoring and Supervision have also been implemented at the facility levels.

Immunization, Integrated Disease Surveillance Programme and National Disease Control Programme, National Vector-Borne Disease including Acute Encephalitis Syndrome and Japanese Encephalitis Programme have also been implemented at the Health facilities level.

Various non-communicable diseases, including Injuries and Trauma, National Mental Health Programme and National Programme for the Health Care of the Elderly and National Programme for Prevention and Control of Deafness, National Tobacco Programme, etc. under National Rural Health Mission are being implemented at the Health facility level. The planning processes has been focused on addressing inequities in terms of "*Time to Care*".

District Sultanpur has been planned to increase the institutional deliveries. Home deliveries and Institutional deliveries has been planned. Approximately 85 per cent of the Rural deliveries are planned to be brought by Accredited Social Health Activists.

The previous rate of ₹ 1,500 has been too meagre, therefore, the rate for C-Section in Private Accredited Centre for BPL women has been increased to ₹ 25,000 per case.

Janani Shishu Suraksha Karyakram has been rolled out in Sultanpur District and 100 per cent coverage of the pregnant women is being ensured through providing free treatment, free drugs and consumables, free diagnostics, free diet and free drop back. Maternal Death Review and incentives for ASHA under maternal health and treatment of severe anaemia and incentive to ASHA for early registration and opening beneficiary's Bank Account as new activity has been initiated.

Orientation training of ANMs at Block level, procurement and printing plan and incentive for first referral unit operationalizations as old activity and incentive for post-maternal health has been initiated under National Rural Health Mission at the facility level.

Reducing infant mortality is one of the key goals under National Rural Health Mission. The infant and under five child mortality has shown a steady decline over last three years. However, the progress is not uniform across the state and even intrastate. Inter-district variations are quite evident from the recent surveys. Moreover, the decline in Neo-Natal mortality is slow and has not kept *pace with* the overall decline *in child* mortality.

Diarrhoea is one of the major causes of the child mortality in Uttar Pradesh. National Policy for the management of Diarrhoea among children less than 5 years, recommends the use of zinc tablets along with ORS in treatment of Diarrhoea.

Revised Diarrhoea Management Policy recommends administration of Zinc in every case of diarrhoea a dose of 20 mg/day for 14 days (even if diarrhoea has stopped) for children aged 6 months to 5 years and 10 mg/days for 2-6 months).

Uttar Pradesh has proposed to scale up these programmes in the entire state so as to increase the use of ORS and Zinc in the treatment of child diarrhoea to at least 50 per cent in 2014-15.

Bal Swasthya Poshan Mah and Biannual Bal Swasthya Poshan Mah Programme focus on strengthening joint health and ICDS planning and review meetings, streamlining logistics and ensuring monitoring during the rounds.

The Infant Mortality Rate has been declining very slowly and state is committed to meet our goals, hence 2013-14 was celebrated as a year of Navjat Shishu Suraksha Varsh. An emphasis was given to strengthen facilities, services and capacity building of health staffs.

Various activities have been initiated to reduce the Neo-Natal Deaths including Sick New Born Care Units, New Born Stabilization Units, Nutrition Rehabilitation Centres, New Born Care Corners and New Born Screening and a preventive child-health care initiative has been started for 13,500 neonates who have been screened for three disorders with easy effective and cheap treatment. The disorders tested were congenital thysodism, biotinidase deficiency and glacetosemia.

The *Girl or Boy: Healthy Baby is the Joy Programme* has been launched. The burden of raising a handicapped child is immense and affects the financial, social and psychological aspects of all the family members. The prevention is better and cheaper than cure.

The children who dies before their fifth birth day, almost one-third of them die of infectious causes nearly all of which are preventable.

Infant Young Child Feeding and breast feeding week celebration is being organized jointly with ICDS, and technical support is being sought from WHO, UNICEF and other partners working in the State.

Child death review is a strategy to understand the geographical variation in the causes of child deaths and thereby initiating specific child health interventions. Analysis of child deaths provide information about medical causes of deaths which helps to identify the gaps in health service delivery and social factors that contribute to child death.

The goal of social marketing scheme will be to create a market where zinc and ORS are available in adequate quantities, informal providers prescribe its use and through repeated use mothers begin to recognize and demand for their infants.

The Total Fertility Rate of Uttar Pradesh has declined from 4.1 to 3.8 per cent. However, compared to National Average of 2.7, the rates are still very high. To enhance the performance of family planning it is imperative to meet the desired unmet needs. The unmet need for spacing method has increased from 9 per cent in 1988-99 to 12 per cent in 2005-06 to 29.7 per cent in 2010-11.

Tuesday and Friday are fixed days for sterilization services (legation/ abdominal tubectomy) will be continued at all districts women hospital/ PHCs/CHCs having either a surgeon or Gynaecologist.

The plan for facilities providing Non-Scalpel Vasectomy services on fixed days at Health Facilities and Female Sterilization Camps and Non-Scalpel Vasectomy Camps are organized. Door step delivery of contraceptive by ASHA and enhanced contribution of Panchayati Raj Institutions and Family Members have been ensured to improve outputs of programme activities in family planning.

Family Planning Counsellors are being deployed in view of the opportunity of large number of institutional delivery under the Janani Suraksha Yojana and they will have the opportunity to reach all the mothers and will counsel the women and address their concern for small family norms.

A sum of ₹ 150 may be paid to ASHA's for escorting the client to the health facility for facilitating the insertion. *Pehal Sakhi Sammelan* is organized as community event Male Group Meetings and Merry Gold Health Network activities are organized in order to engage the large and unregulated private sector through network and the same time to standardize the prices of health services.

Rashtriya Kishor Swasthya Karyakram has been proposed with a target group of 10-19 years of age which will get with various components of Reproductive Maternal Neo-Natal Child Health Adolescent.

It has been proposed to organize Adolescent Health Day at Block level initially twice a year which may be expanded to quarterly as per experience/feedback in the next year. An estimated number of 250 participants (ASHA, PEs, Adolescent boys and girls from various villages, selected school teachers, Panchayat Members, NGOs, ANMs and AWWs) will attend the function.

Weekly Iron Folic supplementation and Menstrual Hygiene Scheme and Convergence within Health and with other Partner Departments has been initiated through organizing regular meetings and their sustained involvement.

Rashtriya Bal Swasthya Karyakram is being implemented in the State from the last year which has been established by IIIrd quarter of the year 2013-14. Every Block of the State is also supposed to have two Mobile Health Teams with four members in each team (2 Doctors, 1 Paramedical and one staff nurse/Auxiliary Nurse Midwife).

Sex Ratio is an important indicator to measure gender equity. The rapidly increasing sex ratio in the State is like to create severe gender imbalance that can destroy the social fabric. It should also be viewed both as child right issues as girls are killed either through sex selective abortions or die prematurely due to violence and neglect.

State Pre-conceive, Pre-Natal Diagnostic Technical Act and Zonal PC and PNDT Act Cell and also at Divisional, District and Block level. PC and PNDT Cell is to be established and the mobility for monitoring and inspection work has been ensured.

World Health Organization has estimated that most of the people in developing as well as in the developed countries receive the bulk of their health care from traditional or indigenous health system.

Ayurveda, Yoga and Naturopathy, Unani, Siddha and Homoeopathy (AYUSH) systems of medicines have proven promotive, preventive and curative strengths of the health system. The objective of mainstreaming of AYUSH health care facilities at the PHCs, CHCs and District Hospitals should be fulfilled. The development of Health care institutions scheme has been revised along with addition of some new components, in order to mainstreaming of AYUSH more effectively, and equally at the facility level.

Orientation training and skill upgradation of the facility level officials is being organized.

Various referral transport and Patient transport system especially "108" Emergency Medical Transport services and "102" National Ambulance Services and Advance Life Support Ambulance and Paediatric Ambulance for Sick New Born Care Units and Monitoring Cell for Ambulance Services is being ensured. The fleet of 1972 Ambulance under "102" National Ambulance Services and "108" Ambulance under Emergency Medical Transport Services is very large and covers all the Districts of Uttar Pradesh.

Bio-Medical Waste must be managed and disposed of to protect the environment. General public and workers especially health care and sanitations workers who are at risk of exposure to bio-medical waste as an occupational hazard.

A critical challenge facing Tuberculosis Control Programme is to ensure that patients adhere to full course of treatment. Non-adherence not only jeopardizes a patient's treatment outcome, but also leads to the emergence of drug resistant strains, which are increasing threat to global public health while Directly Observed Therapy short cause (DOTS) Health and Sanitation greatly boosted adherence rates in Uttar Pradesh. There remain many challenges to measuring patient adherence and ensuring that it satisfies the expectations of the patients.

The immunization programme is the cornerstone of public health and vaccination was practiced in India since early 1900s especially against small pox in the late 1940s. In 1962 Bacillus Calmatte-Guerin (BCG) inoculation included in the National Tuberculosis Control Programme. It gained momentum in 1985 under universal Immunization Programme and it was merged in Child Survival and safe motherhood programme in 1991-92. Since, 1997 immunization activities are an important component of Reproductive and Child Health Programme.

Iodine deficiency disorders one of the major public health problems in India with around 200 million people estimated to be at risk. Iodine deficiency can be prevented by using salt that has been fortified with Iodine.

Integrated Disease Surveillance Programme started in 2004 with the support from World Bank to improve and Integrate Disease Surveillance in pursuance of recommendations by High Powered Committee of Secretaries on Environment and Sanitation.

Vector-Borne Diseases are prevalent in Sultanpur District and prioritized as high risk districts. Sultanpur has been categorized as priority district for AES/JE and Malaria, Kala-Azar and Dengue fever diseases.

Fortnightly fogging of Malathion by the fogging machine in the villages reporting decrease in Japanese Encephalitis cases for last 2-3 years during transmission period. District Sultanpur has been facilitated with vehicle mounted large thermal fogging machine to each Primary Health Centre.

National Leprosy Eradication Programme and various other National Disease Control Programmes have been initiated at the facility level.

Non-communicable diseases include the National Programme for Control of Blindness, National Mental Health Programme, National Programme for Control of Dengue, Cancer, Diabetes, Cardio Vascular Disease and stroke, etc. have been launched under National Rural Health Mission Programme at the facility level.

Cataract operation, School Eye Screening and Corneal Blindness Programme have been initiated under the National Programme for control of Blindness.

National Mental Health Programme has been launched in 1982 because 6-7 per cent of general population suffers from mental disorders. Scheme consists of support for staff, medicines, IEC activities training and contingency for running District Mental Health Programme. The scheme is being revised to control and include life skills Education and Counselling in school, colleges, work place stress management District Counselling Centres and Crisis helpline with an enhanced outlay.

District Women Hospital and District Male Hospital are functional in Sultanpur and there is 24 × 7 Primary Health Centre in Bhadainya Block of District Sultanpur. Infrastructure and physical facilities are adequate and performance of facilities at various levels are suboptimal.

Janani Suraksha Yojana and Janani Sishu Suraksha Karyakram are in place and work in Maternal and Child Health Wing started at District Hospital. There is lack of identification and line listing of high risk pregnancies. Hb estimation albumin, not conducted for most mothers, MCP Cards are symbolic and 1st ANC conducted in fifth or sixth month at times. The community has limited knowledge about doses of key medicines such as Misoprostol.

The adolescent health services available with male and female counsellors are in the place, almost non-existent below District Hospital level. The adolescent health programme is almost non-existent in Sultanpur and there is no activity at Community Level.

The Public Health services are mainly confined to immunization, Ante-Natal and Contraceptive Care but no linkage with the National Disease Control Programme.

State is using Health Management Information System data in monitoring and review purposes and also for state and district level plans. Training is the need of the hour at Block level and facility level in Sultanpur.

Uploading of Data is delayed, i.e. after 5th of every month due to internal reporting procedures. Data is not being utilized by the end users, i.e. ANMs as feedback not being provided to ANMs/work plans not being shared with ANMs and other end users at the facility level.

The funds transfer below the blocks are treated as expenditure. They are lying as advances with facilities and some remain uncleared with banks. Several non-operational bank accounts are lying at the Block level may be closed and the differential funding should be followed for the high focus areas. Regular Monitoring visits should be undertaken by the supervisory units to its lower units.

Thus, the vision, mission and action plan for the appropriate delivery of the public health services to needy, interested deprived, unserved and underserved people at the facility level from Auxiliary Nurse Midwife Centre, Anganwadi Centres, Sub-Centres, Primary Health Centres, Community Health Centres and District Hospitals with the sustained involvement of community, Rogi Kalyan Samiti and Panchayati Raj Institutions for appropriate delivery of public health services at grassroots level equally, effectively and efficiently as per norms, standards and guidelines of the Indian Public Health Standards.

Public Health Management

The Public Health System may be strengthened through preventing water pollution and water contamination which causes water-borne diseases. The water-borne diseases are caused by the pathogenic micro-organism. The water-borne diseases are commonly transmitted in the contaminated fresh water.

Trivially most of the infections might be transmitted by the microbes or parasites which are accidentally, possible as a result of exceptional circumstances and it had got into water, but the fact that there might be an occasional freak infection need not mean that it is useful to categorize the resulting disease as. "water-borne" nor it is a common practice to refer disease such as Malaria as "water-borne" just because mosquitoes have aquatic phases in their life-cycles or due to treating by water; people inhibit the happiness to be an effective strategy to control mosquitoes which are the vectors.

According to the World Health Organization the water-borne diseases account for an estimated 4.1 per cent of the total Daily Global burden of disease and causes about 1.8 million human deaths per annum. World Health Organization has estimated that 88 per cent of the Global burden of disease are attributable due to unsafe drinking water supply sanitation and hygiene. Water-borne diseases are more prevalent due to the lower level of access to drinking water and sanitation along with proper and overall health hygiene and poor nutritional status.

Water-borne illness typically associated with drinking water by etiologic agent causes chemical contamination of water through poor sanitary conditions of the water system and water supplies from cess-pits, unsanitary place and the cess-pits of the old houses have never been drained causing Cholera and Diarrhoea disease.

Water-borne diseases may have a significant impact on the economic status of the common people at the local level. Infected and affected people by the water-borne diseases are usually confronted with the related costs and not seldom with a high financial burden.

The available reports, documents does not capture whether National Rural Health Mission has been "successful" or "failed" but analyzes the changes in the health outcomes and health systems from the point of view of the constraints that were faced and learnt lessons.

Water Pollution occurs when the pollutant are directly or indirectly discharged into the water bodies. Water contamination affects the water bodies, plants and organisms living in these water areas. Its effect is damaged not only to the individual species and population but also to the national biological communities.

It has been estimated that 580 people in our country die due to water pollution/contamination related illness everyday. Nearly 500 million people suffer due to lack of access to safe drinking water.

The treatment of drinking water as applied to the public water supplies consists of a series of water supply and the nature and vulnerability of the source of water.

The water testing physically or chemically can be done through several methods depending on the accuracy required and the characteristics of water. The biological testing of the water samples involves the collection of the plants or the animals from the surface water body. Biological testing of water involves the use of plants, animals or microbial indicators to monitor the health of an aquatic ecosystem.

The cultivated land with large livestock and poultry operations are termed as concentrated animals feeding operations. Animals slurries are usually treated by contaminants in an aerobic lagoons before disposal by spray or trickle application to grass land. The constructed wet lands are sometimes used to facilitate the treatment of animal waste. The animal slurries are treated by mixing with straw and composed at high temperature to produce a bacteriological sterile and friable manure to increase the fertility status of the soil.

The improved water supply and sanitation may lead to reduce the incidence of morbidity and mortality, which may be up to 100 per cent for some disease such as Typhoid and Dracunculiasis.

World Health Organization works to reduce arsenic exposure includes setting guidelines values, reviewing evidence and providing recommen-dations for the risk management. World Health Organization published a guidelines value for arsenic in it, "Guidelines for Drinking Water Quality".

Prevention and control of various water-borne diseases can be checked through adopting various approaches with the objective to interrupt the transmission of water-borne diseases and thereby reducing their morbidity and mortality.

The water-borne diseases are one of the major public health threats especially in the developing countries where unsafe water, sanitation problems and hygiene practice exist. The public health approach to the prevention and control of water-borne diseases consists of provision of safe and adequate water supply and improved sanitation and hygiene education.

Treatment of water supply for individuals and families can be considered through boiling of water, filtration, storage of water, disinfection of spring or well with Chlorine right after construction or when the need arises and monitoring of the water supply should also be ensured regularly.

National Health Policy was formulated during 1983 with a view to provide the health service for all needy people equally, effectively and efficiently, through providing decentralized public health services and to ensure an access to and the benefits from public health system which has been very uneven between the better endowed and the more vulnerable section of the society, particularly women, children, and socially disadvantaged sections of the society.

The public health requirements for maternal health, Child Health including Janani Suraksha Yojana, Janani Shishu Suraksha Karyakram, Rashtriya Kishore Swasthya Karyakram and Rashtriya Bal Swasthya Karyakram and routine immunization and National Disease Control programme should be implemented as per the needs of the people.

The public health planning should be managed through need based planning from bottom to top, i.e. from Hamlet villages → Revenue Villages → Village Panchayats → Nyaya Panchayats → Block Panchayat → District Panchayats → State level up to National level and also from Auxiliary Nurse Midwife Centres/Anganwadi Centres → Sub-Health Centres → Primary Health Centres → Community Health Centres → District Hospital → Sate Level Hospital or Medical Colleges.

Management imperatives of public health for planning and financing, management, strengthening human resource policies for Doctors, nurses, paramedical and programme management staff, their accountability training and capacity building, policies on drugs procurement systems and logistic management, equipments, ambulance services and Referral Transport, new infrastructure and maintenance of buildings, sanitation and water, electricity, laundry, kitchen, facilities for attendants, diagnostic services, patient's feedback and grievance redressal, community participants, Information, Education, Communication, Inter-sectoral, convergence, private public partnership and regulations of services in the private sector and strengthening of data capturing, validity/ triangulation, supportive supervision, monitoring and review, quality assurance, surveillance and leveraging technology should be planned as per the requirement of the local needy people from village panchayat level to block level to District Panchayat level to State level as well.

Management structure of Public Health System should be ensured through Technical Units Programme support and Programme Management and support systems at the various levels. Facility based management of health system included planning, recruitment and implementation of health delivery at the facility levels.

Local community should be sufficiently empowered to take leadership in strengthening the public health system. Panchayati Raj Institutions right from village panchayat level to the District level should be given ownership of public health delivery system in their respective jurisdiction.

National Health Mission has sought an amendment to Acts and Statutes in the States to institutionalize Community-led action for health services and to fully empowered local bodies in the effective management of the public health delivery system at the facility level.

Therefore, the National Health Mission attempts to transfer, funds, functions, functionaries to the Panchayati Raj Institutions. The concerted efforts with the involvement of the Non-Governmental Organizations and other resource institutions should be made to build capacity of the elected representatives and users group members for improved and effective management of public health system at the facility level.

A system of periodic "Jan Sunwai" or "Jan Samvad" should be organized to empower community members to engage in providing direct feedback and suggestions for improvement in the public health delivery system at the facility level.

The success of decentralization experiments would depend on the strength of the pillars, supporting the pillars of strength of the process of pubic system.

It is imperative to ensure that the management capacities should be built at each level. It should provide the management cost up to 6 per cent of the total annual plan approved for District as it has been introduced under the Reproductive and Child Health-II programme.

Apart from the Medical and Paramedical staff such services would include skills for financial management, improved community, processes, procedure, procurement and logistics, improved collection and maintenance of data the use of information technologies, Health Management Information System and improved monitoring and evaluation system at the facility level.

Monitoring and accountability framework should be managed through community based monitoring, external surveys and stringent internal monitoring. Rogi Kalyan Samiti and Community, etc. shall be expected to monitor the physical and financial performance of the public health facilities.

The public health delivery system aims at inclusive health and improved access to quality health care for those residing in the remote rural areas particularly women, children and the poor by promoting integration, decentralization and encouraging community participation in the public health system.

Health care delivery system at Primary, Secondary, Tertiary level should be strengthened through quality care assurance as per guidelines of the Indian Public Health Standards, which mainly includes provisions of optimal expert care to the community and making health care services more responsive and sensitive to the needs and aspiration of the community.

Minimum requirements of the public health delivery services should be ensured through clinical manpower and support manpower and appointment of the Public Health Management and appropriate availability of the equipments, drugs, investigative facilities and physical infrastructure should be made available as per norms of the Indian Public Health Standards.

Hospital Waste Management based on Bio-Medical Waste (Management and Handling) Rules 1998 has been notified under the Environment Protection Act, 1986 (29 of 1986) by Ministry of Environment and Forests, Government of India.

Public Health Management skills should be ensured through encouraging qualifications in public health or public health management among Medical Staff and supporting staff and management processes for decentralized planning and developing health management information system and building institutions for technical assistance and knowledge management to ensure quality assurance in the appropriate need based delivery of public health service at the facility level.

The management of Maternal Health and Child Health and priorities to reduce maternal mortality rate, infant mortality rate and also to reduce Neo-Natal Deaths through the facility based interventions at the grassroots level should be ensured.

Nutrition Rehabilitation Centres, and Human Resource Training for Navjat Shishu Surakasha Karyakram and Integrated Management of Neo-Natal and Childhood Illness training and Home Based New Care and Infant Young Child Feeding, Management of the Diarrhoea, Bal Swasthya Poshan Mah, Information, Education, Communication and Procurement of Equipments and Drugs, etc. should be properly implemented and managed as per the norms of the Indian Public Health Standards.

Appropriate management of the Family Planning and Adolescent Reproductive and Sexual Health and launch of SABLA programme for addressing issues of anaemia in adolescent and procurement of Deworming Tablets under Menstrual Hygiene and implementation of Rashtriya Bal Swasthya Karyakram, Proper arrangement of human resources, training, and Information, Education, Communication should be organized at the facility level.

Pre-conception of Pre-Natal Diagnostic Techniques Act should be properly enforced and executed at the grassroots level.

Appropriate deployment of human resources for Maternal Health, Child Health, Family Planning, Adolescent Reproductive Sexual Health, routine immunization and disease control programme should be ensured at the facility level.

Effective management of public health delivery system and strengthening of State Programme Management Unit, Divisional Programme Management Unit, District Programme Management Unit, Block Programme Management Unit, Village Programme Management Unit should be promoted equally, effectively and efficiently.

Accredited Social Health Activists and strengthening of hospital, new constructions, renovation and setting up of new sub-centre should be strengthened as per need of the local people.

Mainstreaming of AYUSH at the Primary Health Centres level and formulation of need based health action plans and innovation like "*My Village My Home*" and "*Mobile Kunji*" scheme should be promoted, propagated and implemented at the facility level.

Formulation of Health Action Plans and implementation of the facility level review, evaluation and monitoring of the programme implementation should be ensured for enhancing the quality of the health care services rendered through the establishment of quality assurance Network at all facility levels.

An important public health delivery system includes maternal health, child health, Adolescent, Reproductive, Sexual Health, Family Planning, routine immunization, Janani Suraksha Yojana, Janani Shishu Suraksha Karyakram, Rashtriya Kishore Swasthya Karyakram and Rashtriya Bal Swasthya Karyakram, Bal Swasthya Kunji including Golden Minute and Golden Hour Karyakram and routine immunization, referral transport/ patient transport system — "108" Emergency Medical Transport Services, "102" National Ambulance Services, Advanced Life Support Ambulance and Pediatric Ambulance for sick New Born Care Units should be properly implemented as per guidelines of the government.

Appropriate implementation of National Disease Control Programme including — National Leprosy Eradication Programme, National Programme for Control of Blindness, National Mental Health Programme, National Programme for Prevention and Control of Blindness, National Programme for Control of Deafness, National Tobacco Control Programme, National Iodine Deficiency Disorders Programme, Integrated Disease Surveillance Project Revised National Tuberculosis Programme and National Vector-Borne Disease Control Programme especially Malaria, Dengue, Chikungunya, Filaria, Kala-Azar, Acute Encephalitis Syndromes/Japanese Encephalitis, Swine Flu and other vector-borne diseases should be implemented as per guidelines and norms of the Government of India at the facility level.

Continued involvement and sustained participation of Rogi Kalyan Samiti, Health Societies and Panchayati Raj Institutions at various levels should be ensured in a positive manner to fulfil the ever-increasing demand of the growing patients belonging to underserved, unserved areas, particularly women, children, below poverty line people, deprived resourcesless multitudes surviving in the unserved and underserved backward remote villages.

Thus, it has been noted that the Government of Uttar Pradesh has been focusing on the public health delivery system and it has been realized that the various public health programmes under the National Rural Health Mission especially maternal health, child health, immunization and National Disease Control Programme including National Vector-Borne Diseases, etc. has been given much emphasis due to an increasing trend of the patients at various levels. The infrastructural facilities especially clinical manpower, staff, medical facilities and hospitals as per the requirements of the growing population has been facilitated at various levels. The Progress of the Public Health System has not been up to the mark, the way it has been visualized as per the National Health Policy and the goals of the National Rural Health Mission. There is a lack of Doctors, staff, Medical Infrastructure including Hospitals, indoor and outdoor patient facilities and medicines as per an emergency requirements of the ever-increasing patients. The medical care to the needy patients has not been properly implemented. Due to which the people are forced to opt the private medical facility and are liable for excessive expenditure for medical treatment. In most of the cases it has been noted that the most of the families are bound to sell their land, ornaments and property to obtain proper medical treatment in the better hospital. The management of the public health system should be ensured through appropriate placing of the medical doctors, staff, hospitals, medicines and other facilities as per the growing requirements of the ever-increasing patients. Therefore, the Government should plan the health policy not from the top level, i.e. at the level of Government of India or at the State level but the health policy planning and implementation should be done at the village panchayat level with the involvement of Panchayati Raj Institutions and the village level health committees and Rogi Kalyan Samiti should be formed at the village panchayat level and also at the Sub-Health Centre, Primary Health Centre, Community Health Centre and District Hospitals level and ensure to provide appropriate need based Public Health Delivery system at the facility level for the downtrodden, deprived people, rural poor multitudes surviving in the remote villages.

BIBLIOGRAPHY

A — Books and Journals

A. Aseffa, "Viral Diseases in Ethiopia", *East African Medical Journal*, 1993: 70(10), pp. 624-26.

Abram S. Benensar, *Control of Communicable Disease Manual*, 16th edition, 1995.

Adel A.F. Mohammud, *Tropical and Geographical Medicine*, 2nd edition, 1993.

Bogale Worku, "Typhoid Fever in an Ethiopian Children's Hospital 1984-1995", *Ethiopia J. Health Dev.*, 2000: 14(3), pp. 311-15.

Braunwald, *et al.*, *Harrison's Principles of Internal Medicine*, 15th ed., pp. 1721-37.

Ethiopia Journal of Health Development, Vol. 10, No. 2, August 1996, p. 83.

G. Mitike, "Prevalence of Acute and Persistent Diarrhoea in North Gondar Zone, Ethiopia", *East African Medical Journal*, Vol. 78, No. 8, pp. 433-37, 2001.

Gabre-Emanuel Teka, *Water Supply in Ethiopia and Introduction to Environmental Health Practice.*

Helmut Kloos and Zein A. Zein, *The Ecology of Health and Diseases*, 1993, pp. 224-25.

Helmut Kloos and Zein A. Zein, *The Ecology of Health and Diseases*, 1993, pp. 225-27.

Helmut Kloos and Zein A. Zein, *The Ecology of Health and Disease in Ethiopia*, 1993, pp. 223-35.

K. Park, *Text Book of Prevention and Social Medicine*, 15th edition, 1997, pp. 152-57.

K. Park, *Text Book of Prevention and Social Medicine*, 15th edition, 1997, pp. 163-71.

K. Park, *Text Book of Prevention and Social Medicine*, 15th edition, 1997, pp. 184-85.

K. Park, *Text Book of Preventive and Social Medicine*, 15th edition 1997, pp. 157-58.

K. Park, *Text Book of Preventive and Social Medicine*, 15th edition, 1997, pp. 174-77.

Mekonenen Adimasu and Abera Geyid, "An Investigation of Diarrhoea Disease Outbreak at Bilate Military Training Center", *Ethiopia J. Health Dev.*, Vol. 6, No. 1, 1992, pp. 5-10.

MOH, *Guidelines for the Prevention and Control of Selected Epidemic Diseases in Ethiopia.*

Raminik Sood, *Medical Lab. Technology, Methods and Interpretation.*

WHO, *Fact Sheet: Childhood Diseases in Africa, Diarrhoeal Disease*, No. 109, March 1996, p. 1.

WHO, *Fact Sheet: Cholera in the Horn of Africa: "We can Prevent Mortality Even if we cannot Yet Eliminate the Disease*", Press Release WHO: 97, 23 December, 1997, pp. 1-2.

WHO, *Fact Sheet: Dracunculiasis Eradication*, No. 98, March 1998, pp. 1-2.

WHO, *Fact Sheet: Epidemic Dysentery*, No. 108, October 1996, pp. 1-2.

WHO, *Fact Sheet: Escherichia Coli*, No. 125, July 1996, pp. 1-3.

WHO, *Fact Sheet: Poliomyelitis*, No. 114, 1996.

WHO, *Fact Sheet: Poliomyelitis*, No. 52, 13 July, 1998.

WHO, *Fact Sheet: Typhoid Fever*, No. 149, March 1997, pp. 1-3.

Zeleke W/Tensay and Aschalew Mengistu, "Indigenous Weaning Foods: Hygiene and Diarrhoeal Diseases in Rural Ethiopian Setting, Jimma Zone", *Ethiopia Journal Health Development*, Vol. 11, No. 2, August 1997, pp. 149-56.

Government Documents

Broad Framework for Preparation of District Health Action Plan, August 2006, National Rural Health Mission, Ministry of Health and Family Welfare, Government of India, New Delhi.

Indian Public Health Standard (IPHS) Community Health Centre Level, Draft Guidelines, Director General of Health Service of Health and Family Welfare, Government of India, New Delhi.

National Rural Health Mission (NRHM) in the Eleventh Five Year Plan (2007-12) Strengthening Public Health System, National Health System Resource Centre, Ministry of Health and Family Welfare, Government of India, New Delhi.

National Rural Health Mission 2005-2012 — Reference Material (2005), Ministry of Health and Family Welfare, Government of India.

Bulletin on Rural Health Statistics in India (2005), Infrastructure Division, Department of Family Welfare, Ministry of Health and Family Welfare, Government of India.

Guidelines for Operationalising 24 × 7 PHC (2005) (unpublished), Maternal Health Division, Department of Family Welfare, Ministry of Health and Family Welfare, Government of India.

Guidelines for Ante-Natal Care and Skilled Attendance at Birth by ANMs and LHVs (2005), Maternal Health Division, Department of Family Welfare, Ministry of Health and Family Welfare, Government of India.

RCH Phase II: National Programme Implementation Plan (PIP) (2005), Ministry of Health and Family Welfare, Government of India.

Guidelines for Setting up of Rogi Kalyan Samiti/Hospital Management Committee (2005), Ministry of Health and Family Welfare, Government of India.

Indian Standard: Basic Requirements for Hospital Planning, Part-1 up to 30 Bedded Hospital, IS: 12433 (Part 1)-1988, Bureau of Indian Standards, New Delhi.

Indian Public Health Standards (IPHS) for Community Health Centre (April 2005), Directorate General of Health Services, Ministry of Health and Family Welfare, Government of India.

Indian Public Health Standards (IPHS), Guidelines for Community Health Centre, Revised 2016, Directorate General of Health Service, Ministry of Health and Family Welfare, Government of India, New Delhi.

National Rural Health Mission: Meeting Peoples Health Needs in Rural Areas Framework for Implementation (2005-12), Ministry of Health and Family Welfare, Government of India, New Delhi.

Other Documents

RCH Phase II — National Programme Implementation Plan (2005-2012), Ministry of Health and Family Welfare, Government of India (Document and CD available).

National Rural Health Mission (2005-2012), Guidelines for Operationalizing Support Mechanism for ASHA 2006, Training Division, Department of Family Welfare, Ministry of Health and Family Welfare, Government of India.

National Rural Health Mission (2005-2012), Mission Document, Ministry of Health and Family Welfare, Government of India.
http://www.mohfw.nic.in/NRHM%20Mission%20Document.pdf

Accredited Social Health Activist (ASHA) Guidelines, Ministry of Health and Family Welfare, Government of India.
http://www.mohfw.nic.in/eag/accredited_social_health_activist.htm

Reading Material for ASHA, Book No. 1, Ministry of Health and Family Welfare, Government of India.

Facilitators Guide for ASHA, Book No. 1, Ministry of Health and Family Welfare, Government of India.

National Rural Health Mission (2005-2012), Frequently Asked Questions, Ministry of Health and Family Welfare, Government of India. http://mohfw.nic.in/Frequently%20Asked%20Questions-March%2022,%202005.pdf

Indian Public Health Standards (IPHS) for CHC — Draft Guidelines, Directorate General of Health Services, Ministry of Health and Family Welfare, Government of India. http://www.mohfw.nic.in/draft%20chc%208marchjinal.pdf

Indian Public Health Standards (IPHS) for PHC — Guidelines, March 2006, Directorate General of Health Services, Ministry of Health and Family Welfare, Government of India. http://www.mohfw.nic.in/IPHS%20for%20PHC%20_04.April.2006_.pdf

Indian Public Health Standards (IPHS) for SUB-CENTRES — Guidelines, March 2006, Directorate General of Health Services, Ministry of Health and Family Welfare, Government of India. http://www.mohfw.nic.in/IPHS%20for%20SUB-CENTRES%20_07%20April%202006_.pdf

Janani Suraksha Yojana — Guidelines for Implementation. http://www.mohfw.nic.in/layout 09-06.pdf

Guidelines for Constitution of Rogi Kalyan Samiti/Hospital Management Society. http://www.mohfw.nic.in/Guidelines%20for%20Setting%20up%20Rogi%20Kalyan%20Samitis.htm

Implementation Guide on RCH II — Adolescent Reproductive Sexual Health Strategy for State and District Programme Manager, May 2006, Ministry of Health and Family Welfare, Government of India.

Efficient Management of Community Health Centre, Rajasthan. http://www.prod-india.com/searnum.asp7PNums140

Good Practices.

Letter of Mr. P.K. Hota, Secretary (FW), Government of India, Department of Family Welfare. Government of India regarding District Programme Management Units.

INDEX